Essential

Oils

and their
Relevance to the Bible

AROMATHERAPY BOOK WITH SPECIAL OIL BLENDS

FOR PRAYER, APPRECIATION, REMEDIES

AND ABUNDANCE

Esther Lehman

ISBN-13, 978-1724395368

ISBN-10, 172439536X

Published by HolyLand Oils

At CreateSpace

Second Edition

January 4th, 2021

Esther Lehman

HolyLand Oils

Maale Adumim, Israel

www.holylandoils.com

Printed in the United States of America

Table of Contents

Introduction

"When God created the first man, He took him and showed him all the trees of the Garden of Eden, and said to him, 'See My works, how beautiful and praiseworthy they are, and everything that I created, I created it for you. Be careful not to spoil or destroy My world for if you do, there will be nobody after you to repair it."
(Midrash Kohelet Rabbah 7:13)

Everything around us is a miracle and deserves our greatest respect and admiration. It says in the bible that God created the world in six days and on the seventh day he rested. Human beings were created on the sixth day of creation, only when the earth was completely ready for habitation. God planted the trees with many types of seeds, only allowing them to germinate once the garden of Eden was inhabited by Adam and Eve. The smallest seed can grow to be the largest tree, equally humankind starts out as fertilized eggs. As humans we must stand in awe and humility for trees, plants, and all vegetation, not only because of their beauty, but also for their stature and pride. God supplied us with all the elements created for our vital needs and comfort to survive and thrive. Even today, we are presented with so much abundance of food from trees and vegetation, as well as water from natural springs, rivers, and wells. Nature contributes even further by supplying us with materials such as large trees employing their wood for shelter, metals, oils and gasses for agriculture, industrial manufacturing and more.

Trees and plants grow from the same nutrients of the earth and rainwater as we do, desert plants have roots so deep and long that they can access water miles away from them. Most trees will outlive humans by hundreds of years, some even by thousands of years, they see civilizations come and go many times before they die. Trees learned the secrecy of survival, they possess vitality, strength, and energy, while flowers possess elegance, grace, and fragrance. Even though they don't talk with words, they communicate volumes to us with their presence, beauty, and stature. Trees and plants have families too, notice that many of the plants mentioned in the bible will refer to a plant of a certain family of plants which share the same Hebrew name. Each plant, flower and tree were appreciated and respected by the Israelites, they were very connected to nature, and it was a big part of their existence. They blended plants for harmonious prayer and service to God, employing their essence for fragrances and medications.

Imagine the hauntingly beautiful sight of a solitary Acacia tree standing in the middle of the desert, silently singing into the desert wind. Maybe we will hear its silent songs that may be revealing the secrets of our ancestors from all those hundreds of years ago. How many people over the years has it seen riding past it, either on a donkey, on horseback and now in cars and buses, do they notice it standing there in pride? Do they gaze at its beauty in awe? Trees and plants are very spiritual, they have a natural language that speaks with all of nature. It is a known fact for a long time now that trees have feelings and have been communicating with us since the beginning of existence. If we permit it, we may feel their relaxing presence to relieve our stress, they may help us focus and even heal. Trees have unique healing properties, the Israelites learned this in biblical days, they took advantage of their knowledge and passed it down the generations over the centuries for us.

Trees and plants are now mainly used for the purpose of making conventional medications, but in biblical times they were used for alternative healing only. We were created to be in sync with nature, trees inhale in our carbon dioxide and exhale oxygen, while we inhale their oxygen and exhale carbon dioxide to complete the cycle for our critical relationship for harmony with nature. Every person living today is a miracle unto himself, the intricate process of physical, mental, and spiritual development of a child in the womb is choreographed to perfection. The Hebrew prophet Isaiah, the son of Amoz, was a member of the royal family prophesied in middle of the eighth century BCE for around sixty-for years saying,

> "So said God the Lord, the Creator of the heavens and the One Who stretched them out, who spread out the earth and what springs forth from it, who gave a soul to the people upon it and a spirit to those who walk thereon." (Isaiah 42:5)

The land of Israel is known as the Land of Milk and Honey because the land is blessed with seven natural species that God created by seasons, so that the people of Israel would have what to eat throughout the year.

> "A land of wheat and barley, vines and figs and pomegranates, a land of oil producing olives and honey," (Deuteronomy 8:8)

> Wheat season is August to September

Barley Seasons are May to September, December to May
Grape's season is May to October
Fig's season is August to October
Pomegranate's season is September to February
Olive seasons is September to November
Honey's season is August to September

In Judaism we are raised to appreciate, and we have Four different blessings that we say when encountering and appreciating the aroma of trees and flowers. We say the blessings before perceiving the aroma, much like saying a prayer before starting to eat.

The first type of aroma is fragrant wood for which the blessing is,

"Blessed are you Lord our God, King of the Universe who created trees."

The second type of aroma are fragrant plants for which the blessing is,

"Blessed are you Lord our God, King of the Universe who created fragrant herbage."

The third aroma are fragrant fruits, for which the blessing is,

"Blessed are you Lord our God, King of the Universe who bestows good aroma in fruits."

The fourth aroma are miscellaneous fragrances which are none of the above, for which the blessing is,

"Blessed are you Lord our God, King of the Universe who creates species of fragrance."

Essential oils are gifts from God that allows us to expand and grow, it deepens our understanding of abundance and the joys of appreciation of our existence. Plants facilitates us to create more abundance in our lives, while accepting that once we respect nature, it becomes our right to receive abundance. We were created for this right and by simple mental adjustments of comprehension, we learn either the hard way or the easy way to live by God's rules of nature.

The path of abundance is evaluated by our choices, and it varies from person to person. By recognizing that every moment of our lives is the result of this brutal reality, everyone focuses on the importance of different things. Identifying what we need and how we go about it is a daily process of learning and growth. Our daily actions are choices that maneuver us towards our goals, every day is thinking and working, taking these baby steps to attain and earn our purpose.

Using Essential Oils Safely

Aromatherapy uses plant materials and aromatic plant oils, including essential oils, and other aromatic compounds to help improve psychological or physical well-being. It is as a complementary therapy used as a form of alternative treatment.

Complementary therapy should not be administered instead of conventional medicine, it should only be offered alongside standard conventional treatment.

A synergy is a blend of different essential oils that complement each other and used for protection, remedy, or meditation. We must understand and respect nature and understand that some synergies of plants are very powerful and affect our brain and may even cause hallucination or poisoning. Essential oils have no boundaries, their direct potency affect our nervous system and can enter our blood stream easily via our skin or sensory nerves and may overload our liver. Their potency must never be underestimated, so please be careful.

Any alternative holistic treatments should NEVER be offered instead of conventional medicine. Never take upon yourself the responsibility to replace a patient's conventional treatments. There are many ways to help people in harmony with convention.

Essential oils may be used for everyone between the ages of 0 to 100 and to work safely with oils, we must use a base oil to make our blends. Very few oils are safe to be used directly onto the skin, so it is always good practice to use a base oil to keep our self and our loved ones safe.

Recommended Dosages

Per tablespoon which is either 10mls or 10cc the recommended range of drops administered should be between 2-12.

⇒ Minimum Dosage   2-4 drops
⇒ Medium Dosage   6-8 drops
⇒ Maximum Dosage   10-12 drops

Do not administer oils to the following people without consulting with your doctor,

Patients taking steroids or cortisol
Pregnant women

People suffering from Diabetes or High Blood pressure
Patients suffering from Epilepsy
Patients taking Medications for Mental Illnesses or Depression

Dosage for Pregnant Women and Nursing Mothers is always less than for adults in general use 2-6 drops.

Never administer Lavender, Mint, Basil or Sage oils for pregnant women and nursing mothers. These oils can cause the uterus to start contractions and risk a miscarriage.

In nursing mothers Basil can change DNA causing mutations.

Dosage for Children between the ages of 5-10 years is also 2-6 drops.
Dosage for Children between the ages of 3-5 years is 1-3 drops.

Dosage for Babies between the ages of 0-3 years old is also 1-3 drops, however, never to be used on their skin. Either drop the oil onto their pillow or sheet very far from their face. You may rub the oil blend on the soles of their feet which are very sensitive.

Essential Oil Uses and Precautions

Always wash your hands after using oils
Make sure to not touch your face or eyes when you are mixing oils. This may be obvious to say but keep oils away from fire!

Do not blend oils that clash
Oils come in families. Some oils are relaxants and others are stimulants, it is never good to blend these two types together. For example, Lavender and Rosemary when they are not part of a synergetic formula should never be used together alone.

Pregnancy First Trimester
NEVER use any Essentials Oils in the first trimester of pregnancy!

Pregnancy Second and Third Trimester
Never use Lavender even though it is a relaxant it does induce labor. Rosemary is a stimulant and will cause contractions.

High Blood Pressure
Never administer Rosemary, Cinnamon, Camphor, Sage, or Thyme. However, they Should be administered for Low Blood Pressure.

Low Blood Pressure
Never administer Sweet Marjoram, Ylang Ylang, Melissa or Clary sage. However, they should be administered for High Blood Pressure.

People being treated with Chemotherapy
Never administer ANY essential oils, however they can use essential oils while being treated with radiation treatments.
USE HEMP OIL (Cannabis) this is an amazing Carrier Oil for Cancer Patients.

Connecting to the Oils
If the person you are administering treatment to does not like the scent of the oil – stop using it!

Never spread oil onto unclean skin

Please make sure that you have a shower before spreading an oil formula on yourself. Sweat or even body lotion on your skin will be absorbed into your skin along with the essential oils and distort their benefits and may contaminate your blood.

No essential oil should be spread directly onto your skin

Unless specifically specified.

Homeopathy does not blend with aromatherapy

If you are taking homeopathic medications wait until you have finished treatment before starting to use aromatherapy.

What are Essential Oils?

Essential oils are used for aromatherapy which is a form of alternative medicine in which the healing effects are attributed to the aromatic blends. Essential oils are the results of retrieving the essence from plants and reaping their aromatic scents, adopting their essence for remedies and healing oil blends. Their nutrients penetrate our cell membranes, employing their powerful capacity to help protect and combat threats. Essential oils cross the blood and brain barriers into our bodies inducing therapeutic substances for our minds and emotions.

Scent is only one of our sensors which instinctively identifies the type of scent we are exposed to. People who do not have a sense of smell still receive scents via their sensory nerves. Smell sensors are part of the involuntary nervous system that are triggered by the many various scents and aromas directly linking to its therapeutic effects on our physical, emotional, and spiritual being. Essential oils are plant or flower-based oils that are a concentrated hydrophobic liquid containing strong aroma extracted from their oil. They are used in perfumes, cosmetics, soaps, and other toiletry products. They may also be used as flavorings for food and drink, as well as for adding fragrance to incense and household cleaning products. In biblical times, essential oils were often mixed in a vegetable-based oil such as olive, flaxseed, walnut, sesame, or almond.

Their natural aromatic compounds are found in various parts of plants, either in the seeds, bark, stems, roots, or flowers. These oils are extracted by distillation mostly by using steam, other processes are expression, solvent extraction, absolute oil extraction, resin tapping, and cold pressing.

ESTERS

Have a low molecular weight and are most used for fragrances and essential oils. These are non-reactive oils that never attack the skin and are harvested from calm plants that are great for our skin, these are the oils we turn to when we suffer from skin infections.

Usually, esters are derived from an alcohol base using Glycerides, which are fatty acids. These are important esters in biology, because they are the main forms of lipids, making up the bulk of animal and vegetable fats.

TERPENE

This is an alcohol found in many flowers and spice plants. These have multiple commercial applications, the majority of which are based on its pleasant floral scent, with a touch of spiciness. Terpenes and terpenoids are the primary constituents of essential oils and of the many types of medicinal plants and flowers.

There are synthetic variations and byproducts of natural terpenes and terpenoids that also greatly expand the variety of aromas used in perfumery and flavors used in food additives. The complex structure of many terpenes often makes their chemical synthesis difficult, and the extraction from plants is also difficult, time-consuming and yields only small amounts of essential oils.

Terpenes have a very strong scent that are solvents and antiseptic and they affect mucus and saliva. Eucalyptus is a great example of an oil used as an antiseptic mixture to protect against catching a cold or a flu.

LINALOOL

Is used as the main scent in 60% to 80% of perfumed hygiene products and cleaning agents including soaps, detergents, shampoos, and lotions. It is also used as a chemical intermediate because the downstream product of linalool is vitamin E.

Linalool is used by pest professionals as a flea, fruit fly and cockroach insecticide and is a very effective method of pest control. These oils are great for sinuses because they are very active and enter the blood stream very easily and is best not to have direct contact with the skin. They know how to kill viruses, infections and heal lung problems. They cleanse out the respiratory system allowing our bodies to get rid of infections.

Please remember, that even though everybody may benefit from using essential oils. Extra precautions must be taken when administering to elderly adults, children, and babies. Please use essential oils responsibly.

Carrier Oils

Carrier oils are the base oils used in all formulas and are usually vegetable oils derived from the fatty portion of a plant, usually from the seeds, kernels, or the nuts. All base oils are nutritious, edible and may be used directly on the skin. Base oils are cold compressed and always vegan, animal-based oils are never used for aromatherapy.

Each base oil has their own personality allowing us to improve our formulas to be efficient, effective as well as personal. Combining the base oil with the essential oils, we must know what their unique qualities are and how they will work together. Carrier oils have healing properties of their own and it is important to blend them with oils that allow them to be part of the healing process. Carrier oils are enhanced by the specific essential oils we choose to accompany it, base oils also dilute the concentration of the essential oils assisting them to be absorbed into the blood stream more efficiently.

Cold Compressed
Are oils that are compressed with an unheated method, this ensures that the oils retain their beneficial properties.

Unrefined
These oils have undergone only a little refining making sure that the oils retain their richness and strength without additives.

Almond

Latin Name, Prunus Amygdalus

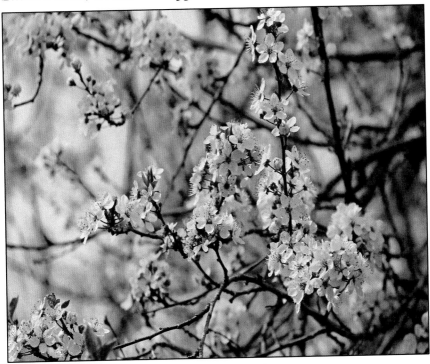

Almonds are native to the Mediterranean and Middle East and are classified as like peach trees. Almonds are eaten either fresh or roasted and are used for cooking and baking and are included in a large variety of sweets and desserts recipes. They are rich in B vitamins riboflavin and niacin, vitamin E, and in essential minerals calcium, iron, magnesium, manganese, phosphorus, and zinc. Almonds have two variations, sweet or bitter and since bitter almonds contains slight traces of cyanide, it is best to stick to using the sweet variation.

Almond makes a beautiful oil that has a very light nutty odor. Almond oil is an omega nine fatty acids, being a rich source of vitamin E. It is a light yellowish oil used a lot by massage therapists, because of its ability to blend amazingly well with most oils. Almond oil is very light and absorbs easily into our bodies.

BIBLICAL

"So, Israel, their father, said to them, "If so, then do this, take some of the choice products of the land in your vessels, and take down to the man as a gift, a little balm and a little honey, wax and lotus, pistachios and almonds." (Genesis 43:11)

"And on the following day Moses came to the Tent of Testimony, and behold, Aaron's staff for the house of Levi had blossomed! It gave forth blossoms, sprouted buds, and produced ripe almonds." (Numbers 17:23)

The words of Jeremiah, son of Hilkiah, of the priests who were in Anathoth in the land of Benjamin." (Jeremiah 1:1)

"And the word of the Lord came to me, saying, what do you see, Jeremiah? And I said, "I see a rod of an almond tree." (Jeremiah 1:11)

When Jeremiah is ordered by God to go and confront the people of Israel, he reassures Jeremiah that he has nothing to fear, the places where he needs to go and the words he needs to speak in those places, will not be his own. However, God warns him that his mission is going to be tough, and sometimes dangerous, but he will not be alone since he is an agent of God and a fortress like resilience will befall him and he will come to no harm.

"Let the son of the corrupt woman, whose deeds are proper."

Jeremiah who was the descended from Rachav the harlot, is the very man God chooses for this specifically important task. By this God demonstrates that he is giving Jeremiah a unique opportunity as the son of this righteous woman to reprove those whose deeds are corrupt. God identifies to him the Israelites who are corrupted and doing bad deeds, and who are thus corrupting future descendants from legitimate seed. Since the days of the first man God revealed to Adam who will be the prophet in each generation, maintaining the importance that each generation must have "a prophet from their midst." There will be those generations who will deny the bible, their prophets and their customs of their nation, the prophet will be expected to discipline those people by giving them to drink the cup of wormwood and hemlock poison as retribution.

An almond takes twenty-one days from its blossoming until it is completely ripe, which coincides with the same number of days between the seventeenth of Tammuz, when the city of Jerusalem was broken into, until the ninth of Av, when the Temple was burnt. This is the same exact time of year that the almond ripens, and in the bible, the almond is a symbol of watchfulness and promise due to its early flowering. The almond tree is mentioned in the bible ten times, beginning with the Book of Genesis, being described as "among the best of fruits." Almonds in the bible are compared to the development of a child, first he grows, then he is weaned and then he develops into, in this case, a Kohen.

The fruits of your planted trees become recognizable only after they are fully developed.

Aloe Vera

Latin Name, Aloe Vera

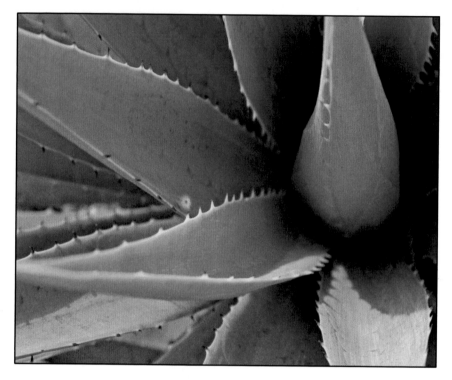

Aloe Vera is a succulent evergreen plant that grows in the Middle East and other tropical type countries. Aloe Vera is a very hardy and fast-growing plant that can reproduce itself at a very fast rate. It has long thick leaves that stems from a core and are filled with a clear gel-like meat. When peeled the gathered gel can be used in shakes, creams, and gel-based mixtures. Aloe Vera has very sharp teeth along the edges of which we need to be careful when handling them.

It has become a very popular plant and can be found in most gardens around the world, Aloe Vera needs to be kept away from direct sunlight and in contrast Aloe Vera is used to sooth sunburns, psoriasis, skin irritations, insect bites and genital herpes.

BIBLICAL

*"They extend like streams, like gardens by the river, like aloes
which the Lord planted, like cedars by the water."
(Numbers 24:6)*

*"I fanned my couch with myrrh, aloes, and cinnamon."
(Proverbs 7:17)*

*"Myrrh and aloes and cassia are all your garments; more than
ivory palaces, those that are Mine will cause you to rejoice."
(Psalms 4:9)*

Aloe Vera is one of the oldest medicinal plants known to man, and the Bible speaks of its health benefits quite a few times. It was used in fragrant blends as well as in poultices and creams to heal skin conditions. Aloes are like streams extended and drawn out for distances; the Midrash says that a wicked man's blessings can determined by how he intended to curse. It is when he decided to turn his face toward the desert. When the Omnipresent is reversed, his words may be a blessing corresponding to his curse. God planted Cedars in the Garden of Eden like the firmament which is stretched out along the rivers like a tent to shade the aloes.

From the wells, king will be anointed and from his sons shall be greatness, and his seed shall have abundant water. This is an expression denoting prosperity, like a seed which flourishes when planted close to water. The first king of Israel being Saul who will capture Agag, king of Amalek. From the blessing of Isaac to Jacob, the kingship of Jacob will become greater and greater, for following Saul, will come David and Solomon

Argan

Latin Name, Argania Spinosa

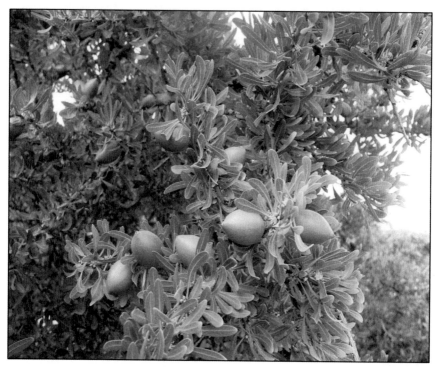

The Argan tree grows in the valleys of Southwestern Morocco and is a very thorny tree, with a gnarled trunk and a wide spreading crown that can live up to approximately two-hundred years. Goats love to eat their fruits, so they are kept away until after the trees are harvested, then the flesh of the fruits are fed to the animals.

The nuts are cracked open to take out their seeds which are used to make the oil. Argan oil is edible and is eaten by dipping bread in it or eaten with couscous and salads. Un-roasted Argan oil is used to treat skin diseases and used as a cosmetic oil for skin and hair. Argan oil contains Vitamin A and E making it great for skin, it is also an antioxidant and has UV protection qualities.

BIBLICAL

"That they may see, and know, and consider, and understand together, that the hand of the LORD has done this, and the holy one of Israel that has created it." (Isaiah 41:20)

"And that they should publish and proclaim in all their cities, and in Jerusalem, saying, go out to the mountain, and fetch olive branches and branches of Etz Shemen "Oil Tree" and myrtle branches, and palm branches, and branches of thick trees, to make booths, as it is written." (Nehemiah 8:15)

"And within the sanctuary he made two Cherubim of Etz Shemen, Oil Tree" (I Kings 6:23)

"And for the entering of the inner sanctuary he made doors of Etz Shemen, Oil Tree" (I Kings 6:31)

This is the Etz Shemen tree also called Oil Tree and is differentiated from the olive tree which is already been mentioned in the Bible in its own right. There is a specific referral to the branches of Oil Trees and Palm Trees, needing to come from thick trees to build the huts. When all the people gathered as one in the square in front of the Water Gate asking Ezra the scholar to bring out the Torah scroll, which is also known as the Law of Moses. Ezra who was at that time the priest, brought out the Torah before the congregation, where both men and women were congregated, and for everyone who could hear and understand, on the first day of the seventh month which is the day of Rosh Hashanah was declared as a holy day. "This day is holy to the Lord your God; neither mourn nor weep."

As Ezra the scholar read the Torah, he stood on a wooden tower that they had made for this purpose. When Ezra opened the scroll before the eyes of the entire people of Israel, all the people stood silently and in awe. Ezra blessed the greatness of God, and all the people answered, "Amen, Amen," with the uplifting of their hands to thank God and they then bent their heads and prostrated themselves before God with their faces to the ground. The Ezra said to them, "Go, eat fat foods and drink sweet drinks and send portions to whoever has nothing prepared, for the day is holy to our Lord, and do not be sad, for the joy of the Lord is your strength."

The five species mentioned by Nehemiah for their use to accompany the Lulav, to celebrate the Festival of Sukkot, specifically explaining which type of myrtle is suitable for the Lulav. Then again, we see another referral to this Oil Tree in I Kings for instructions when building the Holy Ark of Temple of Jerusalem, making the carved Cherubim and inner sanctuary doors.

Avocado

Latin Name, Persea Americana

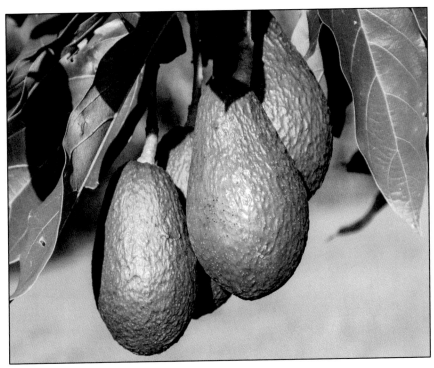

Avocados originated in South Central Mexico and come from a flowering plant and is sometimes called Alligator Pear, and they are best cultivated in tropical and Mediterranean climates such as Israel. Avocados are cold compressed containing Vitamins A, B, E and K, they help heal skin problems such as acne, scars after operations and stretch marks. It is used for all situations where the skin needs to recover, protect itself from sun damage or wrinkles.

Avocado is a great synergy on its own because of its natural constituents of Vitamin A which is Retinol, and Vitamin E. This combination shows its tremendous abilities where it can heal by breaking down damaged fibers and heal by regenerating new cells. This makes Avocado an amazing solo synergy oil and a must have at home oil.

BIBLICAL

"I will send an angel before you, and I will drive out the Canaanites, the Amorites, the Hittites, the Perizzites, the Hivites, and the Jebusites to a land flowing with milk and honey; because I will not go up in your midst since you are a stiff-necked people, lest I destroy you on the way." (Exodus 33:2-3)

"So, I said to you, you shall possess their land, and I shall give it to you to possess it a land flowing with milk and honey. I am the Lord your God, who has distinguished you from the peoples." (Leviticus 20:24)

"If the Lord desires us, He will bring us to this land and give it to us, a land flowing with milk and honey." (Numbers 14:8)

"When you cross, you shall write upon them all the words of this Torah, in order that you may come to the land which the Lord, your God, is giving you, a land flowing with milk and honey, as the Lord, God of your forefathers, has spoken to you." (Deuteronomy 2:3)

"When I bring them to the land which I have sworn to their forefathers to give them, a land flowing with milk and honey, they will eat and be satisfied, and live on the fat of the land. Then, they will turn to other deities and serve them, provoking Me and violating My covenant." (Deuteronomy 31:20)

Moses sent the twelve spies representing one from each of the twelve tribes of Israel, to scout out the Land of Canaan. There are six nations listed in the bible already living in the land, although there were seven nations mentioned previously in the bible. This is because the Gigacities got up and emigrated to escape the Israelites on their own accord. When they left to scout the land, God sent angels to accompany them, their task was to check out what kind of land Canaan is and see who lives in it. Are the people of Canaan weak or strong? How many people are there? Is it good or bad? What type of cities and fortresses are there? Is the land fat or lean? Are there trees or not? They were encouraged to be brave and bring back fruit of the land.

When they came back Moses and Aaron gathered up all the congregation of Israel from the desert of Paran, to Kadesh. They reported in front of the entire congregation and showed them the fruits of the land saying,

"We came to the land to which you sent us, and it is flowing with milk and honey, and this is its fruit."

God warned the people of Israel, meaning we will consume them like bread. Their shield and strength of their virtuous ones have died, and their protection of the Omnipresent has departed from them.

"You shall not rebel against the Lord, and you will not fear the people of that land for they are as our bread. Their protection is removed from them, and the Lord is with us; do not fear them."

While Avocado was not one of the original seven species of Israel, however, now in modern times, this fruit has definitely earned its status as a fruit of the land of Israel. Israel developed the European avocado market first using cultivars developed abroad, and recently also newer and better cultivars of avocado developed here in Israel.

Belladonna

Latin Name, Atropa belladonna

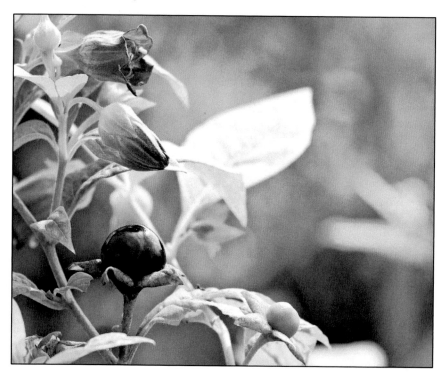

Belladonna is a native to Europe, North Africa, and Western Asia. This plant grows wild in fields its foliage and berries are extremely toxic when ingested, it contains tropane alkaloids. Its toxins include atropine, scopolamine and hyoscyamine, which cause delirium and hallucinations. Belladonna has been used in herbal medicine for centuries as a pain reliever, muscle relaxer, and anti-inflammatory, and to treat menstrual problems, peptic ulcer disease, histaminic reaction, and motion sickness.

Atropa belladonna and related plants, such as datura stramonium commonly known as jimson weed, have been used as recreational drugs. They cause vivid hallucinations and delirium which have been described as very unpleasant. This plant is considered extremely dangerous and toxic and has been the cause of many unintentional fatal overdoses. Belladonna is named after the beautiful women of Renaissance Italy, who took it to enlarge their pupils, which they found to make them more alluring.

Never use this plant for any formulas.

BIBLICAL

"And Reuben went in the days of the wheat harvest and found dudaim in the field". Reuben's stone was a ruby; the color of his flag was red and embroidered thereon were dudaim."
(Genesis 30:14)

And she said to her, "Is it a small matter that you have taken my husband, that you wish also to take my son's dudaim?" So, Rachel said, "Therefore, he shall sleep with you tonight as payment for your son's dudaim." (Genesis 30:15)

Belladonna is also known as dudaim in the Bible, which is known to enhance a woman's attractiveness. Reuben brought it home from the fields for his mother Leah because was desperate to help his mother be loved by Jacob. It was also the plant flowers that Rachel desired to help herself conceive; the sisters' argument ended in an agreement that Leah will have Jacob that night in exchange for the dudaim. God decided that Issachar. Leah's fifth son should be born from the union of that night.

When Jacob came from the field in the evening thinking he will spend the night with Rachel, but he sees Leah coming forth toward him, and she says, "you shall come to me, because I have hired you with my son's dudaim," and he slept with her on that night. Rachel's harsh punishment for her treatment of the cohabitation with such a righteous man lightly, was that she did not merit to be buried at his side.

Borage

Latin Name, Borago Officinalis

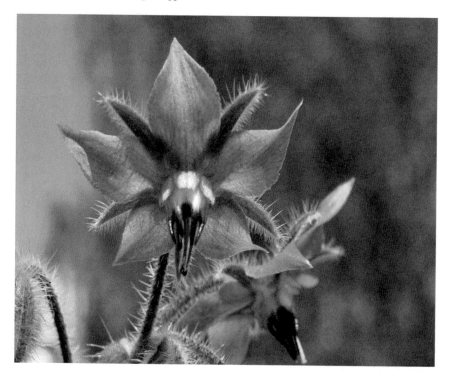

Borage, also known as star flower or tailwort, is a wild plant containing a large amount of GLA (Gamma Linolenic Acid) and is an anti-inflammatory oil. Borage is native to the Mediterranean, its flowers are usually blue, but can be sometimes pink and they make a perfect star shape. In the past Borage was used to dress salads and make soups, even though it does have a slightly bitter taste. The leaves and flowers were put into wine and were intoxicating, making people very happy and drove away their feelings of sadness, dullness, and melancholy. A syrup was made of these Borage flowers and was said to comfort the heart.

Borage helps hyperactive gastrointestinal, respiratory, and cardiovascular conditions. This plant protects cells and membranes, preventing thrombosis acting as blood thinners. It is also used to help teenagers for acne, skin infections, period problems and menopausal women with hot flushes, because of its photo estrogen and prostaglandin characteristics which regulate the metabolism and hormonal system.

Do not administer to people suffering from epilepsy, schizophrenia or those taking phenothiazine.

BIBLICAL

"The sons are gathering wood, the fathers are kindling fire, and the women are kneading dough to make starshaped cakes for the queen of the heaven and to pour libations to other gods, in order to provoke Me." (Jeremiah 7:18)

"And you said to yourself, 'To the heavens will I ascend, above God's stars will I raise my throne, and I will sit on the mount of the assembly, in the farthest end of the north." (Isaiah 14:13)

"They pluck salt-wort on shrubs, and the roots of juniper bushes were their fare." (Job 30:4)

When they were in the deserts, they would pluck for themselves saltwort that grew on the trees of the forests and eat. Saltwort is the name of an herb, and the Mishnah it says, "they brought up mallows on golden tables." On the mount where they all assembled Mount Zion in the forecourt, the chosen place was the north side, as the matter is stated, "On the side of the altar to the north."

Maimonides wrote a wealth of medical writings of his principles of health which he called "Regiment of Health." He was well learned of the connection between mental and physical health in relation to stress and anxiety. He knew Borage oil contains high quantities of the essential fatty acid gamma-linoleic acid, GLA. Borage oil works to help stabilize the adrenals and produce adrenaline, which helps the body to cope with stress. Maimonides wrote in a suggestion to make life changes,

"The physician should not think that medical knowledge alone can set aside emotional instabilities. Psychology and ethical philosophy are necessary."

Contemplation alone reduces bad thoughts, anxiety, and distress. Most thoughts that cause distress, sorrow, sadness, or grief, occur from one of two things,

Either one thinks of the past like the loss of money
or a beloved one

Or one thinks of something that may occur in the future like a
possible loss or injury and one fears their coming.

Yet it is known through rational observation that thinking about the past is of no benefit at all. Sorrow and grief over the past are activities of those who lack the influence of the intellect. There is no difference between a person who grieves over lost money and the like, and someone who grieves because he is human and not an angel, or a star, or similar thoughts which are impossibilities.

Similarly, any anxiety that results from thoughts about what may happen in the future are pointless because every possible thing lies in the realm of possibility, maybe it will happen and maybe it will not. Let a person replace anxiety with hope in God and with this hope it is possible that in fact the opposite of what one fears will actually happen, because both what one fears, and its opposite are equally in the realm of possibility.

"This anti-anxiety formula should be taken regularly, at all
times. Its effects are that sadness and anxieties disappear. This
is a remedy of which no equal can be found in gladdening,
strengthening, and invigorating the psyche. It should always be
found in your possession." (Maimonides, 12th century)

Calendula

Latin Name, Calendula Arvensis

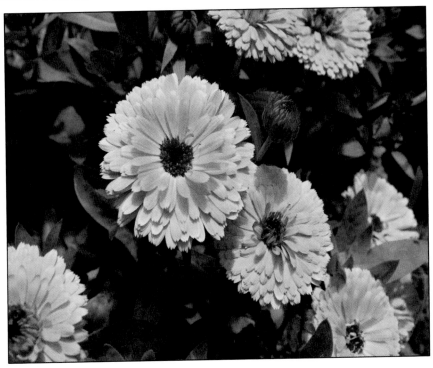

The leaves of this plants are edible, you can make tea with them or sprinkle them over a salad. The flowers are orange, this means it contains Beta Carotene and Omega 6, it also contains Vitamins C and E and Flavonoids. Calendula is the main base oil used for eczema. It is also used for burns, scrapes, diaper rash, skin irritations and rehabilitation. It helps internal skin problems such as Digestive Tract problems like Ulcers, Chron's and liver disease.

How to make your own,

⇒ 50G CALENDULA FLOWERS
⇒ 200MLS ALMOND OIL
⇒ PLACE CALENDULA FLOWERS AND ALMOND OIL INTO A BOWL.
⇒ PLACE BOWL CONTAINING THE MIXTURE INTO A POT OF HOT WATER.
⇒ COOK FOR ONE HOUR, DO NOT COVER.

⇒ LEAVE IN POT FOR 5 HOURS, THEN REPEAT THIS WHOLE PROCESS.

⇒ STRAIN USING A MUSLIN CLOTH AND STORE IN A BROWN BOTTLE.

Do not allow the oil temperature to exceed 180 degrees, we want to prevent the oil from oxidizing, oxidized oil is very unhealthy.

BIBLICAL

"For He knows our creation; He remembers that we are dust."
(Psalms 103:14)

"As for man-his days are like grass; like a flower of the field, so does he sprout." (Psalms 103:15)

"For a wind passes over him and he is no longer here; and his place no longer recognizes him." (Psalms 103:16)

"Everything has an appointed season, and there is a time for every matter under the heaven."
"A time to give birth and a time to die; a time to plant and a time to uproot that which is planted".
(Ecclesiastes 3:1-2)

Calendula is the Marigold plant which is a native of the Mediterranean areas. In the Bible they are known as one of the flowers of the field. In this case, it is referred to the passing time, how our lives are like a flower in the field, and how quickly life passes us by. The wisdom of the world that God put into the hearts of the creatures, God did not put it all into the heart of everyone. But God gave a little to this one and a little to that one, in order that man should not comprehend the entire plan. A man will never know the day of his death or how he will die, this is so that he will repent with his heart just in case he would die today or maybe tomorrow.

Another reason why the day of death is concealed, is if a man would know that the day of his death was near, he would neither build a house nor plant a vineyard, he'll just say why bother, God will make everything beautiful soon enough. The fact that there is a time for death is a beautiful thing, for a person to rely on and say, "perhaps the time of my death is far off," and he builds a house and plants a vineyard, and it is therefore important that it is concealed from people.

Man must make the most of his time on this earth, because soon enough he will die, he must rejoice in his deeds, by the toil of his hands he should rejoice and eat. He must not desire to covet riches, or to accumulate that which is not his, because after he dies, what he had his sons will have. They too will prosper with the riches that he gathered and left over for them, or maybe they will not prosper.

It is said a righteous man that can fall seven times and rise, but the wicked will always stumble upon evil. Never waste time being angry, place your anger in a fiery furnace and let the fire consume them. Interestingly this plant's name derives from the Latin word "calends" or "kalendae" the root of the word "calendar" known as the "little Calendar, or "Little Clock" which we now use in modern times, its original meaning was referred to the first day of every month. It was known as such because the flower blooms each month, which is why it its name was, 'calends.' Its blossoms open and close in synchronization with the rising and setting of the sun.

Castor Oil

Latin Name, Ricinus Communis

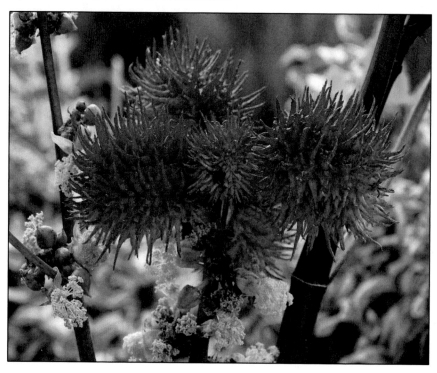

This is a castor bean plant that has firm stalks which enables it to grow up to four meters in height and have large abrasive leaves. It grows quickly and is short-lived, it is indigenous to the Mediterranean Basin and East Africa and is mainly grown as an ornamental plant which self-pollinates. The castor bean plant is notorious for its highly potent poison, as it is called Ricin which is the most powerful poison in nature and is very toxic. Its oil is pale yellow with a recognizable odor and taste and is used in the manufacturing of soaps, lubricants, hydraulics, and brake fluids. It is also a composite of paints, dyes, coatings, inks, cold resistant plastics, waxes and polishes, nylon, pharmaceuticals, and perfumes

In India, Pakistan and Nepal food grains are preserved by applying castor oil to rice, wheat, and pulses, stopping them from rotting. It was also used to induce labor because of its toxicity, it causes the body to reject it.

BIBLICAL

"Now the Lord God appointed a Kikayon, and it grew up over Jonah to be shade over his head, to save him from his discomfort, and Jonah was overjoyed with the Kikayon."

"Now God appointed a worm at the rise of dawn on the morrow, and the worm attacked the kikayon, and it withered."

"Now it came to pass when the sun shone, that God appointed a stilling east wind, and the sun beat on Jonah's head, and he fainted, and he begged to die, and he said, "My death is better than my life."

"And God said to Jonah; Are you very grieved about the kikayon? And he said, "I am very grieved even to death."

"And the Lord said, you took pity on the Kikayon, for which you did not toil, nor did you make it grow, which one night came into being and the next night perished." (Jonah 4:6-10)

When Jonah was deep in the belly of the whale, and his soul grew faint, he remembered his prayers at the Holy Temple. Jonah made a vow to God to make peace-offerings, thanksgiving offerings, "with a voice of thanks will I sacrifice to you." Then suddenly God ordered the fish, to spew up Jonah onto dry land. God told Jonah, "Arise, go to Nineveh the great city, and proclaim upon it the proclamation that I speak to you."

Jonah made his way into the city, which was about one day's walk, and he proclaimed and said, "In another forty days Nineveh shall be overturned!" Jonah did not say, "destroyed," as he was supposed to, he said "overturned." He said this because his prophesy saw the possibility of having two outcomes. If they do not repent, Nineveh will be destroyed, however, if they repent, then it just will be "overturned." Jonah didn't have any faith that the people of Nineveh will change from bad to good, and repent. As it happened, the people of Nineveh believed in God, and they proclaimed a fast and donned sack cloths, everyone from their greatest to their smallest repented. When he heard the prophesy, even the king of Nineveh, rose from his throne, took off his royal robe, covered himself with a sackcloth, and sat on ashes. The people of the town were saying, whoever will repent, perhaps God will relent from his burning wrath, and we will not perish. God saw their deeds, that they had sincerely repented of their evil ways, and God relented did not destroy the city.

Jonah was displeased with this outcome, he said to God, "now the nations will say that I am a false prophet, if they repent, you will not destroy them, and I will appear to them as a liar." Jonah left the city and stationed himself on a hill on the east of the city, and there he made himself a hut and sat under it in the shade until he would see what would happen in the city. God sent him the Kikayon tree under which he sat and was delighted with the shade that it provided. This plant translated from Hebrew is the Caster Bean plant, known as gourd which is a member of the cucurbit family. The commentaries explain that this is a plant that grows high with many branches, and it affords shade, its name being Kikayon. Suddenly God sent a worm to destroy the tree, the worm attacked the tree all through the night and the Kikayon withered and died. This devastated Jonah and he begged God to let him die, God asked Jonah, "really, are you very grieved about the kikayon?" to which he answered, "I am very grieved even to the point of death." God was very upset with Jonah, "you took pity on the kikayon, for which you did not toil, nor did you make it grow, for which one night came into being and the next night perished. However, you do not take pity on Nineveh, the great city, in which there are many more than one hundred twenty thousand people."

Coconut

Latin Name, Cocos Nucifera

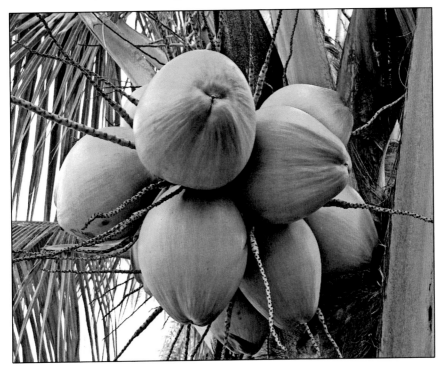

Coconuts are completely different from other fruits in existence because of their endosperm which is their large quantity of water found inside the fruit called coconut milk. It is an amazing superfood, and its oil is cold compressed which has a light delicate scent as well as tasting very good. This oil is known for its versatility ranging from foods to cosmetic products using the oil and the milk. It contains lactic acid and is excellent for skin revival. It has antioxidants, anti-inflammatory, and anti-biotics.

It is one of the most pragmatic trees in the world and is often called the "tree of life." It provides food, fuel, cosmetics, medicine and building materials, and many other uses. Coconuts have been used by humans for thousands of years, when taken internally it can prevent Alzheimer because coconut oil may feed the nerve cells which are starved of Glucose. It is said that the origin of coconuts as being from the region of

Southwest Asia and Melanesia. Coconut palm thrives on sandy soils and is highly tolerant of salinity, just like date palms they can produce sweet tasting fruits despite the soil being salty.

BIBLICAL

"They came to Elim, and there were twelve water fountains and seventy palms, and they encamped there by the water." (Exodus 15:27)

"And ye shall take you on the first day the fruit of goodly trees, branches of palm trees, and boughs of thick trees, and willows of the brook, and ye shall rejoice before the LORD your God seven days." (Leviticus 23:40)

"The righteous shall flourish like the palm tree, he shall grow like a cedar in Lebanon." (Psalm 92:12)

"In the visions of God, He brought me to the land of Israel, and He placed me on a very lofty mountain, and upon it was like the building of a city from the south." (Ezekiel 40:2)

"And the man spoke to me, "Son of man, see with your eyes and with your ears hear, and set your heart to all that I am showing you, because in order to show you, you have been brought here; tell all that you see to the House of Israel." (Ezekiel 40:4)

God showed Ezekiel the vision of the new temple of Jerusalem, a man appeared to him whose appearance was that of copper, he stood at the gate holding a linen cord and a measuring rod in his hands. The man sparkled like the color of burnished copper the man spoke to him and told him all he was about to show him about the building of the new temple.

He showed Ezekiel the structure of one building on the north side of the mountain and a wall on the outside going all around. It is delineated as such at the end of the book that the city is in the south and the House in the north. It was to be six cubits by a cubit and a handbreadth, this is a cubit of medium length which equals a cubit and a handbreadth using a cubit that equals five handbreadths. The height one rod measured the outside wall, which surrounds the Temple Mount, and it was low. All the walls were very high except for the eastern wall where the priest will burn the red cow. He will stand on the Mount of Olives will be able to look directly at the entrance of the Temple while sprinkling the blood.

When Moses was leading the Israelites away from the Red Sea into the desert of Shur where they could not find drinking water for many days. They finally arrived at the river Marah meaning "bitter,' and like its name the waters were bitter. After much complaining about not having water to drink, Moses cries to God. God instructed Moses to take a certain piece of wood, which he was to cast into the water, and the water became sweet. Soon after the Israelites arrived at Elim which were twelve water fountains corresponding to the twelve tribes, that were prepared for them. There were also seventy palm trees corresponding to the seventy elders.

Palm trees in the dessert always indicates that there is water in close proximity, making it an aspiration for survival. Palm trees are able to thrive in very harsh conditions, ranging from subzero temperatures to burning hot climates. The Bible mentions a few types of the palm trees that grew in the biblical regions, they were the Coconut, Date and Banana. The Lulav which is the closed frond of the date palm tree is used on the Jewish Holiday Sukkot.

Evening Primrose GLA

Latin Name, Oenothera Biennis

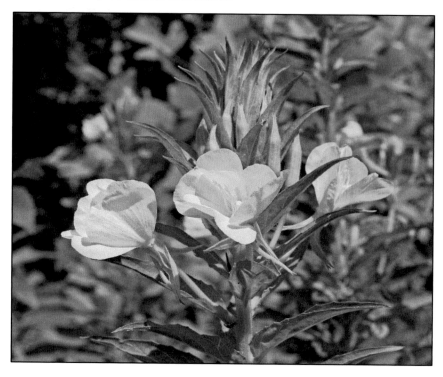

This plant has a beautiful yellow flower that flowers at night, which has Gamma Linolenic Acid and is rich in omega-6 essential fatty acids. It also has anti-carcinogenic and anti-inflammatory qualities. Because of its hormonal influence it balances estrogen, it soothes breast and period pains, it helps with menopausal symptoms. Evening Primrose also reduces acne and adds elasticity to your skin. Cherokee Indians heated the plant's root and applied it to hemorrhoids and made poultices to heal bruises.

Evening Primrose has a life span of two years, it grows into a tight rosette the first year, and spirally on a stem the second year. The flowers are hermaphrodite which are produced on a tall spike that only last until the next noon. They open noticeably fast every evening with a beautiful demonstration, earning their name "evening primrose." It is an edible plant, the root may be cooked and eaten like potatoes, the leaves may be eaten either raw or cooked. Native American tribes make tea from the leaves, using it as a dietary aid. Evening Primrose stabilizes the pancreas and can help lower cholesterol. It may also help recover from a hangover quicker.

During World War II, the seeds of the evening primrose were roasted and used as a coffee substitute. It was known to the world as the imperial medication for the Kings and Queens and was nicknamed "Kings Cure All."

BIBLICAL

"Moses cried out to the Lord, saying, "I beseech you, God, please heal her." (Numbers 12:13)

"Then the kohen shall order, and the person to be cleansed shall take two live, clean birds, a cedar stick, a strip of crimson wool, and hyssop." (Leviticus 14:4)

"Heal me, O Lord, then shall I be healed; help me, then I shall be helped, for You are my praise!" (Jeremiah 17:14)

"They come to war with the Chaldeans and to fill them with the corpses of the men whom I have smitten with My anger and with My wrath, and that which I have hidden My face from this city because of all their evil."
"Behold, I will bring it healing and cure, and I will cure them, and I will reveal to them a greeting of peace and truth."
(Jeremiah 33:5-6)

"It's marshes and its pools will not be healed; they will be set aside for salt mines."
"But by the stream, on its bank from either side, will grow every tree for food; its leaf will not wither, neither will its fruit end; month after month its fruits will ripen, for its waters will emanate from the Sanctuary, and its fruit shall be for food and its leaves for a cure."
(Ezekiel 47,11-12)

Moses prays to God to heal his sister Miriam of leprosy; he beseeches God to answer him as to whether he will heal Miriam or not. Eventually, God replied, "If her father were to spit in her face, would she not be humiliated for seven days? She shall be confined for seven days outside the camp, and afterwards she may enter." The people waited for her and did to travel until she returned, she earned this honor as a reward for the time she remained with Moses when he was cast into the river, as it says, "His sister stood by from afar to know what would be done to him"

This valley is full of pools with marshes all around it, there are also ditches in which water naturally gathers, these waters are very often salt mines that must be turned sweet. It is only then can the waters heal, Judaism is always a source of hope, one that derives from the structuring principles of the Torah. The principle of God is that he creates the cure before he creates the disease. God gives us everything we need through nature, we just need to find it, this plant is a cure than was well known as a "cure for all" and God promised he will reveal the cure. In biblical times Kings and Queens in Israel as well as in Eastern Europe and North America used Evening Primrose and this oil certainly knows how to heal. We should appreciate all plants, herbs, and trees in the world, not only for their healing properties but also for their beauty and aroma.

Fig

Latin Name, Ficus Carica

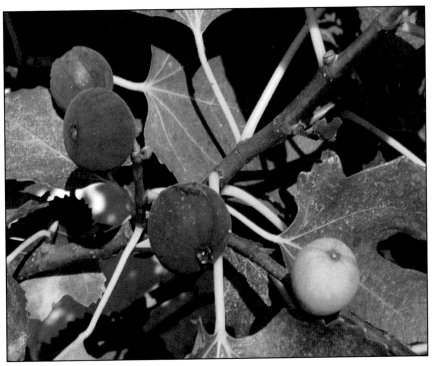

Figs belong to the mulberry family and are native to the Mediterranean, Western Asia, and the Middle East. It is a very sought-after tree and was soon growing all over the world, both for its fruit and as an ornamental plant. The fruit is a small cup like figure called a syconium, the Figs flowers grow inside their fruit which produces dozens of small seeds that give figs their unique, crunchy texture. Figs are sweet and juicy when eaten ripe, but mostly are bought dried. They contain essential minerals, including magnesium, manganese, calcium, copper, and potassium as well as vitamins, principally K and B6. They also contain high amounts of dietary fiber which helps your system regulate and figs are mixed as poultices to help cure tumors, warts, and wounds.

Early studies show that fig trees precede the domestication of wheat, barley, and legumes, the fig tree liquid or milky substance that comes from

51

the stem of the fruit, this connects the fig to the branch and its sap is an amazing cure for warts and verrucae.

BIBLICAL

"And the eyes of both of them were opened, and they knew that they were naked, and they sewed fig leaves and made themselves girdles." (Genesis 3:7)

"They came to the Valley of Eshkol, and they cut a branch with a cluster of grapes. They carried it on a pole between two people and they also took some pomegranates and figs." (Numbers 13:23)

"For the Lord your God is bringing you to a good land, a land with brooks of water, fountains and depths, that emerge in valleys and mountains," (Deuteronomy 8:7)

"A land of wheat and barley, vines and figs and pomegranates, a land of oil producing olives and honey," (Deuteronomy 8:8)

"And Isaiah said, "Take a cake of pressed figs." And they took one and placed it on the boil, and it was healed." (II Kings 20:7)

In the Bible Adam and Eve clothed themselves with fig leaves after eating the "forbidden fruit" from the Tree of Knowledge. Since then, because of this scenario, fig leaves depictions have long been used to cover the genitals of nude figures in paintings by famous artists and sculptors, as an example in Masaccio's The Expulsion from the Garden of Eden. The Midrash speculates that fig leaves are from the tree of which they had eaten and that which they had sinned, but that mistake has been rectified. Other trees in the garden of Eden prevented Adam and Eve from taking their leaves to cover themselves. God did not divulge the identity of the tree because he did not wish to grieve any creature, so that others should not put it to shame and say, "This is the tree because of which the world suffered.

Their sudden awareness of their nakedness exposed their guilt and shame, the Midrash says even a blind man knows when he is naked! What then is the meaning of "and they knew that they were naked." They had one commandment in their possession, and they became denuded of it. When they heard the voice of God in the garden towards the evening from the direction of the sun, Adam told Eve to quickly hide amongst the trees. God was calling, "where are you?"

Adam replies, "I heard Your voice in the garden, and I was afraid because I am naked; so, I hid."

God asks, "who told you that you are naked? Have you eaten from the tree of which I commanded you not to eat?"

Adam says, "The woman whom You gave to be with me she gave me of the tree; so, I ate."
(Genesis 3:10-12)

God wants to know; how do you know what shame there is in standing naked? Obviously, God knows the answers, and by asking Adam he wished to enter into conversation with him. God wanted honest answers from him, so he didn't want to scare him right away. However, instead of being sincere, Adam immediately shows his ingratitude and blames Eve for everything by claiming, "the woman that God gave to him for forcing him to eat from the forbidden fruit." This did not end well as we know, God said, "I shall place hatred between you and between the woman, because women are easily enticed, and they know how to entice their husbands."

Isaiah pressed fresh figs pressed into a round cake and placed it on Hezekiah's boil, and it was healed. This was a miracle within a miracle, for even healthy flesh when a cake of pressed figs is placed upon it, decays, yet God allows Isaiah to put an injurious substance upon vulnerable tissue and somehow it becomes healed. However, the bible makes it clear that Hezekiah owes his recovery to God alone who responded to Hezekiah's prayers and not to Isaiah's action and God promises Hezekiah fifteen more years of life. Miracle cures by prophets, such as Elijah and Elisha are always a combination of physical actions with the spiritual actions of prayer, and the ultimate healing to be done by God.

The fig is one of the Seven Species that the land of Israel is blessed with. These seven plants indigenous to the Middle East that together they provide food all year round. The list is organized by date of harvest, with the fig being fourth due to its main crop ripening during summer. The biblical quote "each man under his own vine and fig tree" has been used to denote peace and prosperity. We read in the Book of Kings, Judah and Israel shall dwell securely, each man under his own vine and fig tree, from

Dan to Beersheba." The bible compares the ease of their conquering of all fortresses, "it should be as easy to conquer all fortified cities and to ravage all that is in their midst, like the fig trees when they are with their first ripe fruits; when the tree is shaken, the first ripe fruits fall into the mouth of the eaters."

Grape

Latin Name, Vitis Vinifera

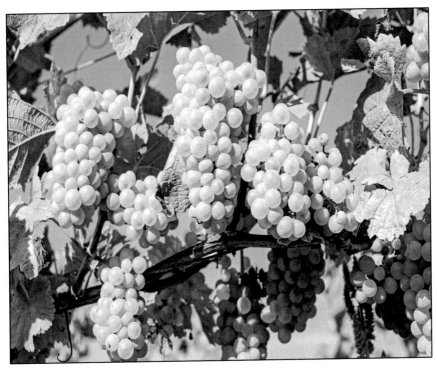

The grape is the third natural plant of the seven kinds with which the Land of Israel is blessed and is mentioned many times in the Bible. Harvested Grapes are used to make juice from crushing and blending them into a liquid which is fermented and made into wine, brandy, or vinegar. It is a well-known fact that the French tend to eat higher levels of animal fat and their incidences of heart disease remains one of the lowest in the world. This is known as the "French paradox", one of the reasons for this could be their regular consumption of red wine. Red wine is known to alter molecular mechanisms in blood vessels and reducing vascular damage.

Resveratrol which is a natural phenol is found in grapes mainly in their skins and seeds, they naturally produce this to protect themselves from injury or damage by pathogens, bacteria, or fungi.

Grapeseed oil is a good source of vitamin E which is a fat-soluble antioxidant. It protects the cells from damaging free radicals that have been associated with cancer, heart disease, and other chronic illnesses. Grapes also contains omega-6 linolenic acids, these fatty acids are necessary to protect your skin by moisturizing, healing acne, lightening, and tightening. Your skin absorbs grapeseed oil very quickly without being too oily. Just make sure to use Grapeseed oil that's cold-pressed or expeller-pressed and not chemical solvents or with high heat during processing.

BIBLICAL

"And Noah began to be a master of the soil, and he planted a vineyard." (Genesis 9:20)

"And he drank of the wine and became drunk, and he uncovered himself within his tent." (Genesis 9:21)

"And on the vine are three tendrils, and it seemed to be blossoming, and its buds came out; then its clusters ripened into grapes." (Genesis 40:10)

"And the Lord spoke to Aaron, saying," "Do not drink wine that will lead to intoxication, neither you nor your sons with you, when you go into the Tent of Meeting, so that you shall not die. This is an eternal statute for your generations," (Leviticus 10:8-9)

"And it grew and became a spreading vine of low stature, to turn its tendrils to him, and its roots were under him, and it became a vine and it sprouted branches and sent forth boughs." (Ezekiel 17:6)

Now there was one great eagle with great wings and many feathers, and behold, this vine gathered its roots upon him, and its tendrils it sent forth to him, to water it from the furrows of its planting. (Ezekiel 17:7)

"In a good field, beside abundant waters it is planted, to sprout branches and to bear fruit, to become a sturdy vine." (Ezekiel 17:8)

"Woe to the heroes to drink wine and valiant men to mix strong wine." (Isaiah 5:22)

"For behold the harvest when the blossom is past, and the buds turn into ripening grapes, and he shall cut off the tendrils with pruning-hooks, and the roots he removed, he cut them off. (Isiah 18:5)

"They shall be left together to the birds of the mountains and to the beasts of the earth, and the birds shall spend the summer upon them, and the beasts of the earth shall spend the winter upon them." (Isiah 18:6)

"Who drinks from basins of wine, and with the first oils they anoint themselves, and they feel no pain concerning the destruction of Joseph." (Amos 6:6)

Vines are described in the Midrash as large with overhanging length and gathering roots expression of hunger, as in plunder and famine. Then its tendrils sent a plea to the eagle to come to it and water it. The eagle is said to have made water ditches for the plant that provided it with constant water. When the vine's blossom is past and the grain is close to becoming ripe in its ears and before the buds of his vine become ripening grapes, ripened to the extent of being as big as a white bean. To stay healthy this plant, the tree must be pruned by cutting off its tendrils often.

Grapes are first mentioned in the bible from when Noah grew them on his farm, then prepared wine and got drunk. The bible says that Noah brought with him when he entered the ark, vine branches and shoots of fig trees; this confirms that he was already familiar with grapevine crops and what the grapes produce. Having a drink for celebrations is very much endorsed in the bible, however drinking too much, and mixing strong wines and getting drunk is frowned upon. Aaron is warned by God to not drink to intoxication, the Midrash explains what intoxication is,

"Wine in a manner that leads to intoxication, is the drinking of sufficient undiluted wine without interruption thus causing intoxication."

The bible says that a kohen is forbidden to enter the Temple after drinking wine and this prohibition applies also to approaching the altar.

The grapevine is often represented as the symbol of Israel and destiny, kings of the Hasmonean dynasty imprinted the grape symbol with a date onto their coins. A gold grapevine was hung at the entrance of the Holy Ark of Jerusalem, and there are forty terms in the bible related to grapes and their process, found in all the various ancient Jewish literatures. When the Israelites were expected to bring their first fruits to the Temple, those who lived far were told "to bring raisins." Grapes are awarded to a special prayer, "the Creator of Vine" and the blessing on the grape,

"Blessed are You, Lord our God, King of the universe, who creates the fruit of the vine."

The grape has "precedence" all over the other fruits of the seven kinds of Israel. The seven blessings are the central part of the ceremony of marriage, they draw divine blessings for the duration of the couple's married life, and they commence their lives together with a blessing over a cup of wine.

Hemp

Latin Name, Cannabis Sativa

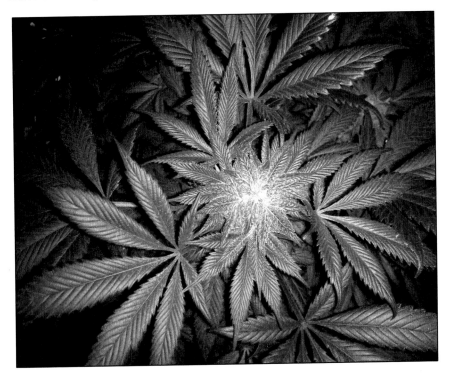

Also known as cannabis oil, in Aromatherapy it is used without the THC, initials for Tetrahydrocannabinol which is the principal psychoactive constituent of the cannabis plant. It is known to help cure many diseases such as Heart Disease, Cancer, Auto Immune Problems and Digestive Diseases. Hemp oil is cold compressed and must be stored in a dark bottle, we are always discovering more and more amazing qualities of this oil. It contains Amino Acids, Vitamins E and Beta Carotene, Albumin, Creatine, Iron, Minerals, Potassium and Magnesium. It is advisable to take one tbsp of this oil morning and evening every day.

BIBLICAL

"You shall offer up on it no alien incense, burnt offering, or meal offering, and you shall pour no libation upon it." (Exodus 30:9)

"Take thou also unto thee the chief spices, of flowing myrrh five hundred shekels, and of sweet cinnamon half so much, even two hundred and fifty, and of kaneh-bosem two hundred and fifty." (Exodus 30:23)

"And of cassia five hundred-shekel weights according to the holy shekel, and one hin of olive oil." (Exodus 30:24)

"You shall make this into an oil of holy anointment, a perfumed compound according to the art of a perfumer; it shall be an oil of holy anointment." (Exodus 30:25)

"Kaneh-Bosem" literally means "Cane of Spice" and it can be seen how the name "Cannabis" evolved. Its ingredients are very specific, and the Bible refers to it as a perfume, bosem, and not a spice. One of their methods to make the Kaneh-Bosem was to soak the spices in water so that they would not absorb the oil, they poured the oil over them until they were absorbed with the scent after which they rubbed the oil off the roots.

The Israelites were expected to mix the spices thoroughly into a powder, blending them well like beaten eggs with a spoon, then to blend them with water with his finger or with a spoon. This is their daily incense, which left on the inner altar in the Tent of Meeting, appointments to speak were set up to enter the holy of holies. This formula was made personally by each person according to his choice of ingredients which were to be used only for offerings to God and this recipe was not permitted to be used for personal fragrance!

On the golden altar any donated or alien incense which is neither burnt offerings nor meal offerings should not be offered. To clarify the difference, a burnt offering is one of an animal or fowl and a meal offering is one of bread. Burnt offerings were for atonement, usually sacrificing either a bull or a kid on Yom Kippur, in a ritual to atone for contamination and sins, these were not to be eaten they were for sanctifications only. Everybody over the age of twenty was expected to give donations to the Holy Temple, a coin of fire weighing half a shekel, the rich and the poor gave equally the same amount to atone for their souls. "Like this one they shall give."

Hypericum

Latin Name, Hypericum Perforatum

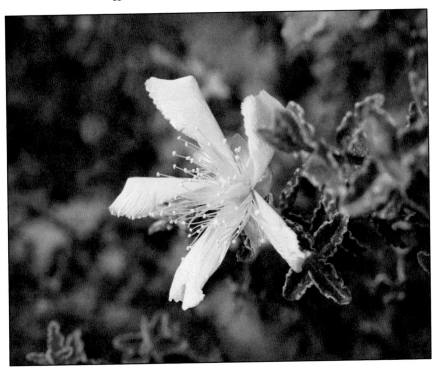

Its other name is St. John's Wort, this is a plant with star shaped yellow flowers and it mainly grows in Europe, North and South America, Australia, New Zealand, and Eastern Asia. The plant is known to help depression and strongly affects the nervous system, it is one of the main ingredients for psychotic medications such as Prozac because of its ability to stabilize the mood. There are two main compounds found in Hypericum are, hyperforin and hypericin, this psychiatric medication is usually taken in a pill form but may also be consumed as a tea. St. John's Wort is also known to helps bee stings, bites, and bruises, and in tea form it is great for relaxation, PMS, Anemia, and mouth sores.

BIBLICAL

"As the good oil on the head runs down upon the beard, the beard of Aaron, which runs down on the mouth of his garments." (Psalm 133:2)

"You shall take the anointing oil and pour it on his head and anoint him." (Exodus 29:7)

"You shall then take some of the blood that is upon the altar and some of the anointing oil, and sprinkle it upon Aaron and upon his garments, upon his sons and upon the garments of his sons with him; thus, he will become holy along with his garments, and his sons and their garments with him." (Exodus 29:21)

"To fail to take care of one's beard was a sign of insanity." (I Samuel 21:13)

"Any injury to or cutting of one's beard signified disgrace." (II Samuel 10:4)

"They went up to the temple, and Dibon to the high places to weep; for Nebo and for Medeba shall Moab lament; on all their heads is baldness; every beard is shaven." (Isaiah 15:2)

"For every head is bald and every beard clipped; on all hands are scratches, and on the loins sackcloth." (Jeremiah 48:37)

Aaron had such a long beard that it reached the hems of his garments. The Midrash talks about the ointment with which Moses anointed his brother Aaron the high priest, to establish the priestly lineage. The Hypericum species, as we know them today, goes by the common name of "St. John's Wort" named for John the Baptist. In the bible it is known as "Aaron's Beard," which is the more intended name for this plant. The oil extracted from the Hypericum was used in the anointing mixture, blended with other aromatic oils, the objective was to manufacture this ointment explicitly for sacred consecration only. The bible describes Aaron's very long beard filled with oil that was poured on with the precious ointment from his head, describing how it ran down his beard all the way down to the hems of his garment, indicating that Aaron's beard was as long as the hem of his priestly robes

"The oils from his head to his beard, to the mouth of his tunic, for the beard rests on the mouth of the tunic."

In those days being clean shaven was unheard of, because being clean shaven in those days was seen as a sign of grief. We see this when the people of the city of Dibon walked up to the temple to weep at its highest place, and they were all clean shaven. Shaved heads in biblical days were only to be performed on a deceased person, as the Midrash says, "baldness between your eyes, or anywhere else on the head, are for the dead." The high Priest, the Scripture says, are also prohibited from shaving their heads. Thus, the linking of the laws for the regular Israelite and the Kohen, strictly prohibits baldness unless it was a natural cause. The main reason being is for safety, so that people should not accidentally cut their flesh, and if someone does unwittingly make several cuts of five and above, he would be liable.

Only a person who has leprosy it permitted to shave off all his hair, this is to immerse himself in purified water to become cleansed, after which he then remains outside the community for seven days. After the seventh day, he must shave off all his hair, including his head, his beard, his eyebrows, and every place where hair grows, he will then once again immerse himself with his garments into the water and thus becoming finally clean.

Jojoba Butter

Latin Name, Simmondsia Chinensis

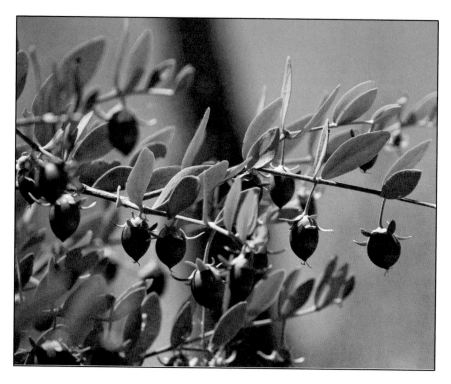

Jojoba is also known as wild hazel or a quinine nut and is a desert plant that grows in the South of Israel. It is very waxy, and this is its way of keeping its moisture inside. The plant is silver to reflect heat and prevent being cooked. Native Americans extracted the oil from jojoba seeds to treat sores, burns and wounds, it protects the skin from the sun because it does contain UV protection. Don't use this oil for babies in the sun, its UV protection is only about eight and will not give enough protection. Jojoba is now being used all over the world for facial skin too, especially dry skin.

It has a long shelf life and is now being used as a replacement for whale oil where it is proving to be a far more superior quality oil than sperm whale oil. It is in the process of being developed and grown in Israel by a company called "Jojoba Israel" established in 1988 by "Kibbutz Hatzerim" in Southern Israel and export their oils and creams to many countries.

BIBLICAL

"And the watchers saw a man leave the city. And they said to him, "Show us now the entrance to the city and we will deal kindly with you." (Judges 1:24)

"I went down to the nut garden to see the green plants of the valley, to see whether the vine had blossomed, the pomegranates were in bloom." (Song of Songs 6:11)

"Smooth were the buttery words of his mouth, but his heart was set on war; his words were softer than oil, but they are curses." (Psalms 55:22)

"For pressing milk will give out butter, and pressing the nose will give out blood, and pressing anger will give out strife." (Proverbs 30:33)

Jojoba was one of the most popular oils used as a base oil, or as a dilution for incense and balm blends. It was used together with olive oil in mixtures to heal leprosy or as a constituent to make perfume to obtain have a lighter fragrance. Jojoba's consistency makes a very thick oil mix which is closer to butter, creating a firm and smooth base oil, great for luxurious creams. We all know smooth talkers, with buttery words that fall easily from their mouths, but his heart was set on war. "His words may be softer than oil, but they are really cursing." The Midrash explains, just as butter is the result of pressed milk, so is blood the result of pressing the nose too much. Strife is the consequence of pressing the nostrils with anger, the Midrash says,

"If you have evil thoughts and quarrel in your heart, then place your hand over your mouth and stay silent. Whereas if you have been put to shame, your reactions are in your own control, and you will ultimately ascend in the matter."

If you felt a fool by asking a question and doubting your intelligence, you will ultimately be exalted; but if you placed a muzzle on your mouth and never ask questions, it will in the end be as though you are dumb anyway. If you don't ask you will never know anything about anything. God tells the Israelites, "My soul made me chariots for a princely people." However, the congregation of Israel complains that they did not know to beware of sin or retain their honor and greatness. They erred in the matter of groundless hatred and controversy, which intensified during the reign of the Hasmonean kings, Hyrcanus and Aristobulus. It was not until one of them brought the kingdom of Rome and received the kingship from their hands and became their vassal, and since then, God says, "my soul made me to be chariots, that the nobility of other nations rides upon me."

Moses had to order Aaron to approach the alter and perform sin offerings, because in truth, Aaron was bashful and afraid. So, Moses said to him, "Why are you ashamed? This is the function you have been chosen for!" Aaron then presented the burnt offerings to God according to their prescribed ingredients, causing them to go up in smoke on the altar. Then Aaron blesses the Israelites with the blessing of the high Priest,

"May the Lord bless you and watch over you."
"May the Lord cause his countenance to shine to you and favor you."

"May the Lord raise His countenance toward you and grant you peace."

"They shall bestow my name upon the children of Israel, so that I will bless them."
(Numbers 6:24-27)

Linseed/Flaxseed

Latin Name, Linum Usitatissimum

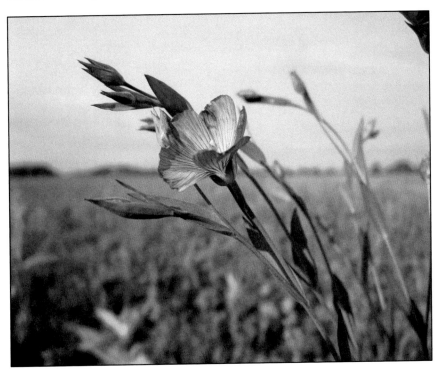

This plant is very strong, its fibers are used to make ropes and its wood is used for carpentry. In Rome and Egypt, it was used to spread on ships with oil paints. There is evidence that Flaxseed existed and was cultivated in Egypt over five-thousand years ago, ancient Egyptians cultivated their seeds and embalmed their mummies with them. The Phoenicians traded the seeds with Egypt for their linen, Flax fibers are reaped from the stem of the plant and are known to be twice as durable as cotton fibers. The seeds are often used as feed for swine and poultry because it is rich in protein.

Flaxseeds have high levels of Omega 3 and softens milk, eggs, or meat, generating a higher unsaturated fat content. It is also high in Vitamin E and this oil is great for the digestive tract, helping constipation and easing digestion in the small and large intestines. It also may be used to lower blood pressure, cholesterol, sugar levels, as well as skin rashes.

BIBLICAL

"Though the flax and the barley have been broken, for the barley is in the ear, and the flax is in the stalk." (Exodus 9:31)

"When Aaron enters into the holy place, he shall put on the holy coat of linen, and shall gird himself with the belt of linen, and he shall put on himself the miter of linen; these are the garments of holiness." (Leviticus 16,4)

"You shall observe My statutes, you shall not crossbreed your livestock with different species. You shall not sow your field with a mixture of seeds, and a garment which has a mixture of Sha'atnez shall not come upon you." (Leviticus 19:19)

"You shall not wear a mixture of wool and linen together." (Deuteronomy 22:11)

"And she had brought them up to the roof, and she hid them with the stalks of flax, that she had laid arranged upon the roof." (Joshua 2:6)

"The priests, Levites and sons of Zadok, when they enter at the gates of the inner court, they shall be clothed with garments of linen, and no wool shall come up upon them when they minister in the gates of the inner court and inward; miters of linen shall be upon their head, breeches of linen shall be upon their loins." (Ezekiel 44:17-18)

Cain brought of the fruit of the soil as an offering to God, and folklore claims that it was flaxseed. A flax worker will know if his flax is of high quality when he beats it, if it is not of high quality, it crushes and breaks too easily. When God did not accept his offering but accepted his brother Abel's offering, Cain allowed his jealousy to take control of him and he murdered his brother.

When the Israelites were waiting to enter their promised land, Caleb and Pinchas secretly entered Canaan as spies. They were sent by Joshua to report back in detail about the people of the land. When they arrived in Canaan, they came to the house of an innkeeper named Rahab, who was also unfortunately reputed to be a harlot, though the bible describes her as a righteous woman. They rented a room at her inn and the Midrash says that they disguised themselves as deaf-mutes so that the people of Canaan would not conceal their affairs from them. When the king of Jericho found out about two strangers arriving in town, he questioned Rahab about them. Since she had hidden them, she was not willing to disclose their whereabouts to the king. She hid them in a narrow place, and she told the king, "At darkness, the men went out, pursue after them quickly, for you will overtake them." She then brought them up to her roof, and she hid them within stalks of flax that she had laid arranged upon the roof. After the king's men had gone, she told Joshua and his men to go to the mountain and hide yourselves there three days until the pursuers will return, and you can on go your way.

In the bible the river Nile of Egypt is called Pishon because its waters are blessed, they rise and water the land, it is also called the Pishon because Flax grows along the riversides. The color of the Flax dims when they were quenched. The people of Israel are called upon to contribute thirteen materials, gold, silver and copper, blue, purple, and red-dyed wool, flax, goat hair, animal skins, wood, olive oil, spices, and gems. Out of which, God says to Moses, "They shall make for Me a Sanctuary, and I shall dwell amidst them."

"Their steeds are swifter than leopards, and they are fiercer than the wolves of the evening; and their riders shall increase, and their riders shall come from afar; they shall fly like an eagle that hastens to devour." (Habakkuk 1:8)

Jews are forbidden to wear garments that contain wool, and linen sewn together, this is called "Sha'atnez" which means mixture. The Torah prohibits Sha'atnez that applies only to materials combed, spun, and woven together. These are the type of rules decreed without any apparent rationale, and with which the evil inclination may ask "What is the sense of these prohibitions? Why are we forbidden to wear garments that are a mixture of wool and linen? The scriptures say that this is how God can distinguish his own people from other peoples. The laws given to the Israelites are supposed to be wholeheartedly and voluntary obeyed. It should not be said, "I find pork disgusting," or "It is impossible for me to wear a mixture of wool and linen." But rather, God wants his people to say, "I indeed wish to eat pork, but my Father in heaven has imposed this decree upon me, and I wish to comply completely," or to say, "because the Scripture says so." God says that by separating his people from transgression is their accepting upon themselves the yoke of the Kingdom of Heaven.

"And you shall be holy to Me, for I, the Lord, am holy, and I have distinguished you from the peoples, to be Mine." (Leviticus 20:26)

Macadamia

Latin Name, Macadamia Tetraphylla

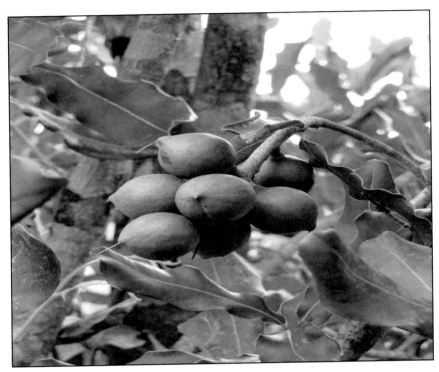

Macadamia is an evergreen tree indigenous of Australia and there are four species of this tree. It contains large quantities of Omegas 3, 6 and 9 and Macadamia nuts are high in monounsaturated approximately 86% fatty acids and oxidizes very fast. Monounsaturated fatty acids have been linked to reduced cholesterol in the blood. They contain antioxidants, vitamins, and minerals with significant health-boosting qualities with potentially high amounts of vitamin B1 and magnesium.

Macadamia oil is good for babies up to a year old but toxic and harmful to dogs, where within twelve hours of eating them, it can cause them serious neurological damage and possible paralysis. The size of the dog and the level of toxicity depends on the weight and size of your dog. The symptoms are muscle tremors, joint pain, and severe abdominal pain. Essential oils blend very well with this oil and is great for dry and old skin.

The oil is used in the cosmetic industry to make soaps, shampoos, and sunscreens.

BIBLICAL

"And Jacob took himself moist rods of trembling poplar and hazelnut, and chestnut, and he peeled white streaks upon them, baring the white that was on the rods." (Genesis 30:37)

"And houses full of all good things that you did not fill, and hewn cisterns that you did not hew, vineyards and olive trees that you did not plant, and you will eat and be satisfied." (Deuteronomy 6:11)

"And the watchers saw a man leave the city. And they said to him, "Show us now the entrance to the city and we will deal kindly with you." (Judges 1:24)

After the death of Joshua, the Israelites asked God "Who shall go up for us first against the Canaanites, to fight against them?" They were nervous to enter the places that were not yet conquered. So, God chooses Judah, he shall go up and claim the land, God trusted the Israelites into the hands of Judah. The tribe of Judah began preparing to go up first to conquer their portion. Judah says to Simeon his brother, "Come up with me into my lot, and we will fight against the Canaanites, and I will also go with you into your lot" Simeon agreed and went with him into war. Judah and his brother Simeon went and fought against the Canaanites, and God gave the Canaanites and the Perizzites into their hands; they attacked ten thousand men in Bezek. Then they smote the Perizzites, where Adoni-bezek fled, they pursued him and when they caught him, they cut off his thumbs and his big toes. Adoni-bezek was shocked and said, "Seventy kings, having their thumbs and their great toes cut off, gathered food under my table; as I have done, so has God punished me."

They brought him to Jerusalem, and he died there, from here we can comprehend the greatness and wealth of the kings of Canaan, Adoni-bezek was not counted as being one of the great kings of Canaan. In Jerusalem, the Canaanites went from there to wage war against Jerusalem, however, Judah fought against Jerusalem and captured it with the edge of his sword; and setting the city on fire throughout. Judah together with Simeon continued to pursue the Canaanites that dwelt in Hebron, Safed, Gaza, Ashkelon, and they drove out all the inhabitants of the mountains; but they could not drive out the inhabitants of the valley, for they had iron chariots. The Midrash says this was due to a punishment they were receiving after they had sinned in the Othniel incident, so they gave Hebron to Caleb as Moses had requested. Caleb then drives out the three large sons of the giant Canaanites from there.

Benjamin did not drive out the Jebusites that inhabited Jerusalem; and the Jebusites dwelt with the children of Benjamin in Jerusalem until this day. There is a section in Jerusalem called Jebuse, which was populated by the descendants of Abimelech who were not driven out because of the oath which Abraham had sworn, until the coming of David. Benjamin, Abraham's grandson was still alive when Abraham had made this oath which he remembered to keep.

Joseph also went up to Beth-El and God helped him defeat Beth-El which fell to their lot, Joseph was smart and decided to send spies into Beth-El before planning his attack. Beth-El's name was formerly called Luz. The spies saw a man leave the city, and they said to him, "Show us now the entrance to the city and we will deal kindly with you." He revealed to them of an entrance to the city through a cave over which one hazelnut bush stood concealing the entrance, making it easy for people to enter the city through the bush. The Hebrew word for hazelnut bush is "Luz," upon which small nuts grow, this is how the spies of Joseph's descendants made their entrance of the city and struck them with the edge of their swords; but the man who gave them the information and his entire family they let go. This man went to the land of the Hittites, and built a city, and called it Luz; this is its name until this day. The tribes of Menasseh, Efraim, Asher, Naftalie, and Dan did not drive out the inhabitants, and the Canaanites dwelt among them, and they became a minority to them.

People have been eating nuts for centuries in the land of Israel, archeologists from the Hebrew University and Bar-Ilan University Researchers say that they found seven types of nut shells, one of which was the pistachio found from around seven-hundred and eighty years ago. In those days all nuts were called "botnim", and this could have meant a large variety of nuts. Israeli researchers have cultivated macadamia trees in Israel among many other fruit trees that were not indigenous to this country.

Neem

Latin Name, Azadirachta Indica

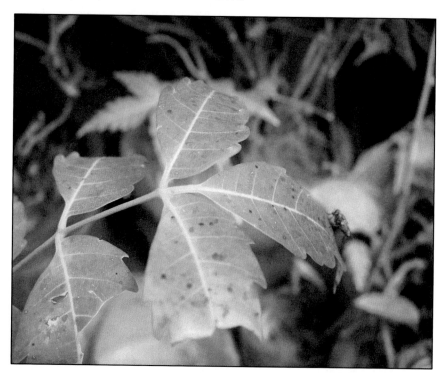

Neem is native to the Indian subcontinent and known as Indian Lilac. You can find them in India, Nepal, Pakistan, Bangladesh, Sri Lanka, and Maldives. This is a great tree to plant in your garden because its leaves are pesticides, it keeps insects and bugs away, it acts as a repellent and protects the other trees in your garden. It grows in tropical and semi-tropical regions and its fruits and seeds are the source of neem oil. The neem tree is totally drought resistance, and its normal habitation are in sub-arid and sub-humid conditions where it thrives. It is a great base oil for skin problems such as eczema and fungus. In India it is used to clean their teeth. This oil was used in India for over two thousand years for its medicinal properties. Neem products are believed by Siddha and Ayurvedic practitioners to be Anthelmintic, antifungal, antidiabetic, antibacterial, antiviral, contraceptive, and a sedative. It is also used for healthy hair, to improve liver function, detoxify the blood, and balance blood sugar levels.

BIBLICAL

"Now no tree of the field was yet on the earth, neither did any herb of the field yet grow, because the Lord God had not brought rain upon the earth, and there was no man to work the soil." (Genesis 2:5)

"And the Lord God caused to sprout from the ground every tree pleasant to see and good to eat, and the Tree of Life in the midst of the garden, and the Tree of Knowledge of good and evil." (Genesis 2:9)

"And the Lord God commanded man, saying, "Of every tree of the garden you may freely eat." (Genesis 2:16)

"But of the Tree of Knowledge of good and evil you shall not eat of it, for on the day that you eat thereof, you shall surely die." (Genesis 2:17)

"Now the Lord God said, "Behold man has become like one of us, having the ability of knowing good and evil, and now, lest he stretch forth his hand and take also from the Tree of Life and eat and live forever." (Genesis 3:22)

"And the Lord Godsent him out of the Garden of Eden, to till the soil, whence he had been taken." (Genesis 3:23)

"And He drove the man out, and He stationed from the east of the Garden of Eden the cherubim and the blade of the revolving sword, to guard the way to the Tree of Life." (Genesis 3:24)

"Fortunate is the man who has found wisdom and a man who gives forth discernment," (Proverbs 3:13)

"It is a tree of life for those who grasp it, and those who draw near it are fortunate." (Proverbs 3:18)

"The fruit of a righteous man is the tree of life, and the wise man acquires souls." (Proverbs 11:30)

"Hope deferred makes the heart sick, but a desire fulfilled is a tree of life." (Proverbs 13:12)

"A healing tongue is a tree of life, but if there is perverseness in it, it causes destruction by wind." (Proverbs 15:4)

There were no trees yet on the earth when the creation of the world was completed it was only on the sixth day just before man was created. We know that God created trees and plants on the third day, when he said, "Let the earth bring forth." However, the plants were created but had not yet emerged, they stood at the entrance of the ground until the sixth day. Simply because there was no man to work the soil, and no man to recognize the benefit of rain, when man came, he instinctively understood that rain was essential to the world. After Adam arrived, he prayed for rain, and rain fell, then the trees and the herbs sprouted. Adam also knew that God was the ultimate ruler and judge over the entire world, and the proof was defined everywhere.

After Adam and Eve disobeyed God by eating fruit from the tree of the knowledge of good and evil, they were driven out of the Garden of Eden. The Midrash says that Adam was not expelled from Paradise until he reviled and blasphemed God, blaming him for giving him Eve, if it were not for her, he would not have eaten from the tree of knowledge.

The Midrash says God was distraught when he expelled Adam from the garden of Eden and said,

"My beloved, this is the Holy One, blessed be He."

"In a fertile corner, in the Garden of Eden."

"He fenced it in with the ten canopies."

"He cleared it of stones, of temptation, until he ate from the tree, and temptation gained entry into him."

"He planted it with the choicest vines, the beginning of his formation was from the place of the altar."

"He built a tower in its midst, and He breathed into his nostrils the spirit of life, from the heavenly beings."

"He hewed therein, a spring flowing, the fountain of wisdom."

"He hoped to produce grapes, that he would thank God and praise God."

"The Garden produced wild berries, putrid things, he reviled and blasphemed."

"Judge now, since the end of the parable comes to say that they too did like him, he asks them the judgment."

"I will inform you, what I decided to do to him, and I did."

"I removed its hedge, I expelled him from amidst his canopies."

"He shall be eaten up; his end will be to die and to be ruled over by wild beasts."

"Breach its wall, I expelled from the enclosure of Paradise."

"I made it a desolation, I made him dwell in desolation, for I did not give the Law in his days."

"It shall neither be pruned nor hoed, they will learn from him neither merit nor good deeds."

"The desolation will come up, temptation ruled over him and his posterity, to perform corrupt deeds."

"I commanded the clouds: I appointed guards over him to guard the way of the Tree of Life."

The tree of life remained in the garden and their access to this tree was forever prevented in the future. There was now a revolving sword at the entrance with a sharp blade to frighten him from re-entering the garden. God no longer trusted or respected Adam, because now he does not know the difference between good and evil. God suspected Adam of being capable of eating from the tree of life and live forever, God said, "and now, lest he stretch forth his hand, if he were to live forever, he would be likely to mislead people to follow him and to say that he too is a deity." God says,

"The house of Israel is to me like that vineyard and the ten tribes were to me like a vineyard producing wine, like an olive orchard, in a fat corner, in a fat land, producing anointing oil for the priesthood, anointing oil for the kingdom, oil for the Menorah, oil for the meal offerings. I fenced them in first with the encirclement of the clouds of glory in the desert and I cleared them of stones. I cleansed them of the transgressors of the generation. I planted them with the choicest vines and gave

*them six hundred and six commandments, and I added for them
to the seven commandments that the children of Noah were
commanded. I built a tower in their midst, my Tabernacle and
my Temple, and also a vat, the altar and the pits."*

The tree of life is associated with wisdom and in Judaism wisdom is very important and more valuable than fine gold and riches. It is associated with calmness, being careful how we speak and guarding our tongues from saying bad things. When the Levites began to ascend the steps, to the holy temple they recited this song. The Psalmist alludes to the steps that ascend are for the righteous, this song is for the one who are destined to make ascents for righteousness in the future from beneath the tree of life to the Throne of Glory. Emphasizing that the tree of life is the path to the Throne of Glory, "And from beneath them thirty steps, one above the other until the Throne of Glory, flying and ascending with the pleasant speech of the song of ascents."

*"A song for ascents. I shall raise my eyes to the mountains,
from where will my help come?"*

"My help is from the Lord, the Maker of heaven and earth."

*"He will not allow your foot to falter; Your Guardian will not
slumber."*

"Behold the Guardian of Israel will neither slumber nor sleep."

*"The Lord is your Guardian; the Lord is your shadow; [He is] by
your right hand."*

"By day, the sun will not smite you, nor will the moon at night."

"The Lord will guard you from all evil; He will guard your soul."

*"The Lord will guard your going out and your coming in from
now and to eternity." (Psalms 121:1-8)*

In Judaism the "tree of life," is a common terminology, it is an expression found in the Book of Proverbs and applies to the Bible. Etz Chaim is also a common name for yeshivas and synagogues as well as for works of Rabbinic literature and even Cemeteries.

Obliphica

Latin Name, Hippophae Goniocarpa

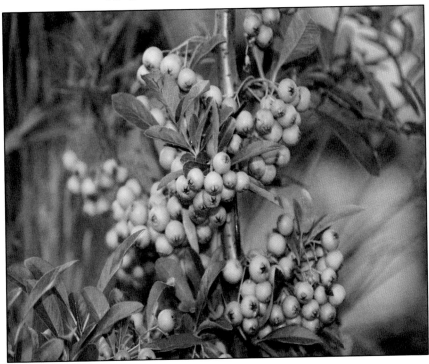

Is a sea-buckthorn whose oil is extracted from the berry of the tree and is a native to a wide area of Europe and Asia. Sea-buckthorn is known for its benefits of both internal and external use, its oil being rich with carotene, vitamins E and F. This oil is responsible for skin and body regeneration as well as metabolism. Applying sea-buckthorn oil strengthens the hair follicles and makes the hair thick and healthy. It is also indispensable for dry and aging skin due to its moisturizing and regenerating effects. Sea-buckthorn based face creams and masks smooth and tone up the skin, bleach freckles and pigment spots. Obliphica also relieves itchiness and is used as part of a base formula for eczema and hemorrhoids.

BIBLICAL

"And He said, if you hearken to the voice of the Lord, your God, and you do what is proper in His eyes, and you listen closely to His commandments and observe all His statutes, all the sicknesses that I have visited upon Egypt I will not visit upon you, for I, the Lord, heal you" (Exodus 15:26)

"See now that it is I! I am the One, and there is no Godlike Me! I cause death and grant life. I strike, but I heal, and no one can rescue from My Hand!" (Deuteronomy 32:39)

"And he fenced it in, and he cleared it of stones, and he planted it with the choicest vines, and he built a tower in its midst, and also a vat he hewed therein; and he hoped to produce grapes, but it produced wild berries." (Isiah 5:2)

"But by the stream, on its bank from either side, will grow every tree for food; its leaf will not wither, neither will its fruit end; month after month its fruits will ripen, for its waters will emanate from the Sanctuary, and its fruit shall be for food and its leaves for a cure." (Ezekiel 47:12)

"Heal me, O Lord, then shall I be healed; help me, then I shall be helped, for You are my praise!" (Jeremiah 17:14)

"For I will bring healing to you, and of your wounds I will heal you, says the Lord, for they called you an outcast, that is Zion whom no one seeks out." (Jeremiah 30:17)

God promised the world that he will not visit upon its sickness unless he provides the cure saying, "for I, the Lord, am your Physician." We see in the bible God repeats this many times, stating that all the answers are in the bible. The scripture says, "it shall be healing for your navel," interpreted as, for every disease there is a cure, and God takes this a little further by saying, "an act of good deeds saves us from illnesses." God wants his people to believe in him and grasp onto his faith and draw it close, and in return as an oath and with unconditional love, he still promises to heal even if nobody believes him. It is usually only when people get sick, that they suddenly remember God and pray to him to be healed, they make a pact with God saying if he heals them, they we will openly recognize him. "I praise myself and boast with you, saying that You are my Savior." Sadly, it is only after God has healed us will we dedicate time to do charity. God doesn't want us to take any of the miracles of our life for granted, God is our constant reminder that we are mere mortals. We may feel we are in control of our lives, which we can be once we recognize and appreciate all that God has given to us. God says,

"It is I who can bring someone down, and I am the only one who can lift someone up. A nation who lacks law and guidance and are devoid of sound counsel, their enemies will sit in judgment."

Obliphica is a cure for all and if there is an oil that can cure almost anything it is this. The Jewish philosopher Maimonides from the twelfth Century, also known as the Rambam, Rabbi Moses Ben Maimon, said "Any illness which can be cured by nutrition should not be treated by any other means." Maimonides" believed in alternative healing over conventional medicine.

When God made Abimelech king, by the plain of stones in Shechem, Jotham went up and stood on the peak of Mount Gerizim he raised his voice, and called, "Listen to me, you men of Shechem, that God may listen to you."

So, the trees went forth to anoint a king over them,

"And they said to the olive tree, "reign over us," but the olive tree said to them, "should I leave my fatness, wherewith by me they honor God and men, and go to wave over the trees?"

"And the trees said to the fig tree, "go you, and reign over us," but the fig tree said to them, "should I leave my sweetness, and my good fruitage, and go to wave over the trees?"

"And the trees said to the vine, "go you and reign over us."

"And the vine said to them, "should I leave my wine, which causes God and men to rejoice, and go to wave over the trees?"

"Then all the trees said to the thorn, "come you, and reign over us."

"And the thorn said to the trees, "if in truth you anoint me king over you, then come and take refuge in my shade, but if not, let fire come out of the thorn, and consume the cedars of Lebanon."
(Judges 9:8-15)

Olive

Latin Name, Olea Europaea

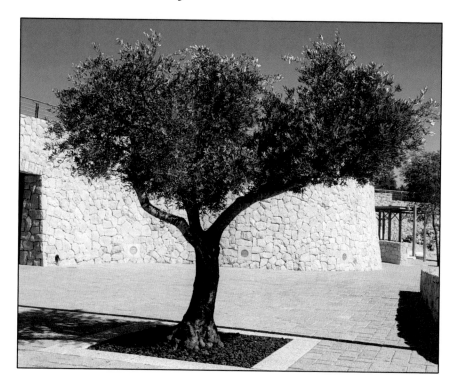

Olive trees grow in groves and hills all around Israel, some being centuries old, and others up to over two-thousand years. The Intriguing Qualities of Olive Oil has been known and recognized for centuries since biblical times. Today, the olive remains a popular food and its golden oil is a coveted commodity worldwide. Moreover, olive oil has become more popular since the discovery of its ability to lower cholesterol and skin health, it is used for many skin care products such as cleansers, moisturizers, and antibacterial creams. Olive oil contains several types of polyphenols, mainly tyrosols, phenolic acids, flavanols and for black olives, anthocyanins.

Olive oil qualities are acknowledged both for its religious rituals and medicinal properties. Olive Oil was then used as fuel in oil lamps, and Olive Oil was also the main ingredient in soap-making, and skin care application. Olive oil that is dark yellow in color and has a nutty flavor is an indication of its good quality, it also contains low amounts of vitamin E and is advisable to store it in a dark bottle. The Olive trunk's wood has light and dark grains and is popular for small decorative items, while the olive branch persists as a symbol of peace.

BIBLICAL

> "And the dove returned to him at eventide and behold it had plucked an olive leaf in its mouth; so, Noah knew that the water had abated from upon the earth." (Genesis 8:11)

> "And you shall place it in front of the dividing curtain, which is upon the Ark of Testimony, in front of the ark cover, which is upon the testimony, where I will arrange to meet with you." (Exodus 30:6)

> "And of cassia five-hundred-shekel weights according to the holy shekel, and one hin of olive oil." (Exodus 30:6)

> "And his offering was one silver bowl weighing one hundred and thirty shekels, one silver sprinkling basin weighing seventy shekels according to the holy shekel, both filled with fine flour mixed with olive oil for a meal offering." (Numbers 7:13)

> "When you beat your olive tree, you shall not de-glorify it by picking all its fruit after you; it shall be left for the stranger, the orphan and the widow." (Deuteronomy 24:20)

> "And of Asher he said: "May Asher be blessed with sons. He will be pleasing to his brothers and immerse his foot in oil." (Deuteronomy 33:24)

> "And gleanings shall be left in it like the cutting of an olive tree, two or three berries at the end of the uppermost bough; four or five on its branches when it produces fruit, says the Lord, God of Israel." (Isaiah 17:6)

Olive symbolizes continuity, its gnarled barks of the ancient olive trees on Israel's terraced hillsides seem to exude a wisdom accumulated from witnessing centuries of human history. In ancient times, olive oil was used to cook, to light lamps and as soap and skin conditioner and is the sixth fruit of the seven species of Israel. Hezekiah and his team, who were based inside Jerusalem were some of the people who were involved in the gleanings of olive vineyards, and were experienced olive tree cutters, they always left over two or three berries to each of the top branches. Just like the cutter of an olive tree, the tradition is the one who cuts olives will pick them from the tree, "and the thickets of the forest shall be cut off." The glory of an olive tree is its fruit, meaning "you shall not take its glory from it," and not to remove all its fruit. The Midrash derives from this that in addition to olives, it includes the harvest of grains and produce and in all fruit, bearing trees, one must leave behind a portion of their fruits at the end of the harvest. In sensitivity to poor people, the "forgotten fruit" of fruit bearing trees, must left for the poor to collect without being shamed.

Among all the twelve tribes, we will not find one that is more blessed with sons than the tribe of Asher. There are a few different explanations why this could be, Asher used to please his brothers with the oil of unripe olives from his orchard, which they used for anointing their skin and to cook tasty dishes, and they would please him by repaying him with grain. Another explanation for this was, "he will be pleasing to his brothers," because the women who came from Asher were very beautiful and were sought after for marriage. Malchiel, Asher's grandson, was literally called "olive-child," Asher's daughters were all married off to High Priests and kings, all of whom were anointed with his olive oil. The Midrash says, his land flowed like a spring with oil. Once the people of Laodicea needed olive oil, and they sent an agent from place to place, until he found an olive farmer. The farmer brought this agent to his home, and there, the agent watched the olive farmer wash himself and then dip his hands and feet in the oil, "And dip his foot in oil." He then supplied the agent from Laodicea with one million, one hundred and eighteen thousand portions of olive oil.

Olive oil is the base oil used in the holy Temple to make the Ketoret and the Anointing oil. The Sages of Israel differ concerning how the Anointing oil was made, some say that whoever made the blend boiled the roots in it the oil of the anointment. Others say that it could not be so because the anointment oil did not even suffice to anoint the roots, so they certainly couldn't boil the spices in the oil. Rather, they soaked the spices in water first so that they would not absorb the oil, and then poured the oil on them until they were saturated with the scent, after which they wiped the oil off the roots. Their conclusion being that any substance mixed with different substance until one becomes permeated from the other with either scent or taste which is called pharmacy.

This became the original Anointing Oil, also known as, "Oil of Messiah," it was first prescribed for the High Priest of the Temple, known as the Kohen Ha Gadol. The high priest of the Temple of Jerusalem, Israel was instructed to put the Anointing Oil on himself before he blessed the children of Israel. Later this same Anointing Oil was used by the Kings of Israel to anoint kings and prophets. Today we use the oil to symbolize a priestly, regal, and higher self within ourselves, allowing us to connect and identify with God.

Palm

Latin Name, Arecaceae

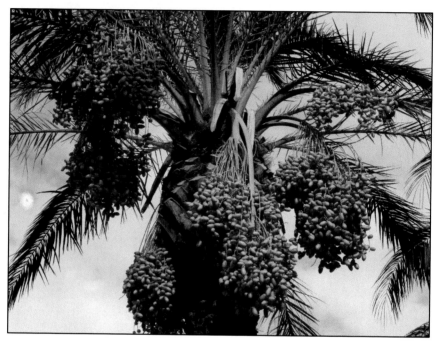

This is another edible oil, though it is not good to eat too much of it. It increases blood levels of low-density lipoprotein and total cholesterol, and so increases risk of cardiovascular diseases. It is yellowish in color and contains beta carotene, linoleic acid as well as Vitamins A and E. This composition gives this plant the power to be a complete treatment all on its own. A great oil for the digestive system, and many skin problems.

BIBLICAL

"Bring the Tribe of Levi near and present them before Aaron the Priest that they may serve him." (Numbers 3:6)

"Now Deborah was a woman prophetess, the wife of Lappidoth; she judged Israel at that time." (Judges 4:4)

"And she sat under the palm tree of Deborah, between Ramah and Beth-el, in the mountain of Ephraim; and the children of Israel came up to her for judgment." (Judges 4:5)

"I arose a mother in Israel;" arose with a sword and a word and without her they could not move (Judges 4:7)

"The righteous one flourishes like the palm; as a cedar in Lebanon, he grows." (Psalms 92:13)

"Planted in the house of the Lord, in the courts of our God they will flourish." (Psalms 92:14)

"This, your stature, is like a palm tree, and your breasts are like clusters of dates." (Song of Songs 7:8)

"I said, let me climb up the palm tree, let me seize its boughs, and let your breasts be now like clusters of the vine and the fragrance of your countenance like that of apples." (Song of Songs 7:9)

Our forefather Abraham lived with his wife Sarah in Beer-Sheba, deep in the desert for as far as the eye could see. They had a huge house with four main entrances, one on each of the four sides of their home. This was done so that they could welcome travelers from any direction and would run out to greet them. They had a very tall and large palm tree in their garden, and it is said that it would spread out its branches and offer welcome shade if the traveler was a good person. Abraham and Sarah welcomed all their guests into their home and treated them like honored dignitaries. They gave their visitors baths, provided them with clean and new clothing and with an abundance of high-quality home delicious, cooked food, like a banquet fit for kings.

We learned from Abraham and Sara the valuable lesson of "Hachnasat Orchim" which is hospitality of the highest level. Many Jews go to the synagogue on the Sabbath and bring home guests that have no place to eat the Sabbath meal. In fact, people who have no place to go to on the Sabbath know to go to the synagogue where they are likely to be hosted with generosity and kindness. For this quality the palm tree is blessed, it produces fruit, and we see how God complements its beauty and its stature, comparing the braveness of that of the Israelites in the days of Nebuchadnezzar. When all other nations were kneeling and falling before the image, the Israelites stood as erect as this palm tree.

Jethro was Moses's father-in-law, he went up from the city of date palms, with the children of Judah into the wilderness of Judah, which is south of Arad and lived there with the people. The city of date palms was another name for the city of Jericho. They were given the generous pasture grounds of Jericho to live on until the Temple would be built. This portion of land would belong to the Temple so that all Israel could have a portion in the Temple, since Temple would not be built upon the private property of any tribe, it was given to the descendants of Jethro for four-hundred and forty years.

Once the Temple was built, Torah students left and went to Othniel, in the desert of Judah, south of Arad, to study Torah. Later Deborah the Prophetess who lived in the Mountains of Ephraim, between Ramah and Beth-El. It was said, she was living at a time of the sin and idolatry, however, Deborah remained true to God and the bible. She was a very wise and God-fearing lady, and the people flocked to her for advice and help. Deborah would sit beneath a palm tree, in the open air. There, where everyone could hear her, she warned the Jewish people and urged them to leave their evil ways and return to God. The entire Jewish nation respected this great prophetess.

Peach

Latin Name, Prunus Persica

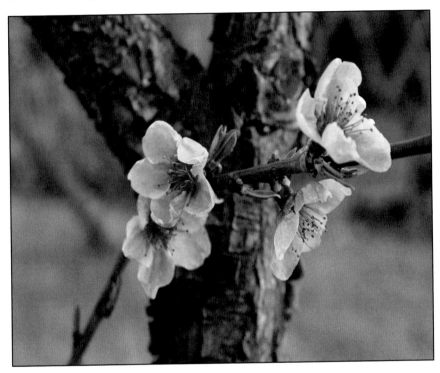

The Peach tree belongs to the Prunus family which includes the cherry, apricot, almond and plum, it also includes the rose in this family. Its flowers blossom beautiful pink flowers with five petals. Peach trees are native to the Middle east and were one of the fruits that the Israelites grew in their fields and orchards. "And from beneath them thirty steps, one above the other until the Throne of Glory, flying and ascending with the pleasant speech of the song of ascents."

It's essential oil is a monosaturated fatty acid oil and is very gentle and light. It is great for sensitive skin and for babies. Peach kernel oil is a light textured oil, with a clear orange tint and it has a delicate aromatic scent.

Peach oil has strong anti-aging properties containing vitamins A and E as well as a variety of B-group vitamins. Its vitamin E is an antioxidant and eliminates free radicals associated with some cancers. Peach kernel oil delays the aging process by maintaining the elasticity of your skin. Its lightness allows it to absorb easily into your skin without leaving that greasy feeling.

BIBLICAL

"And the festival of the harvest, the first fruits of your labors, which you will sow in the field, and the festival of the ingathering at the departure of the year, when you gather in the products of your labors from the field." (Exodus 23:16)

"The choicest of the first fruits of your soil you shall bring to the house of the Lord, your God. You shall not cook a kid in its mother's milk." (Exodus 23:19)

"I will give your rains in their time, the Land will yield its produce, and the tree of the field will give forth its fruit." (Leviticus 26:4)

"The tree grew and became strong, and its height reached the sky, and its appearance was seen to the end of all the earth." (Daniel 4:8)

"Its branches were beautiful, and its fruit was plentiful, and on it was sustenance for all. Under it, the beasts of the field took shade, and in its branches dwelt the birds of the heavens, and all flesh was nourished from it." (Daniel 4:9)

"Crying out loudly, and so he said, "Cut down the tree and cut off its branches, shake off its branches and scatter its fruit; the beasts shall wander away from beneath it and the birds from its branches."
(Daniel 4:11)

"But leave its main roots in the ground, and in fetters of iron and copper in the grass of the field, and with the dew of the heavens it shall be drenched, and with the beasts shall be its lot in the grass of the earth." (Daniel 4:12)

"And whose branches were beautiful, and whose fruit was plentiful, and on which was sustenance for all, under which dwelt the beasts of the field, and in whose branches dwelt the birds of the heavens."

(Daniel 4:18)

"I made myself gardens and orchards, and I planted in them all sorts of fruit trees." (Ecclesiastes 2:5)

The prophet Daniel was a prince as well as a brilliant interpreter of dreams who was exiled to Babylon after the destruction of the Holy Temple by the evil Nebuchadnezzar. He was well known because of his interpreting and the averting of an evil royal decree to slay all the wise men of Babylon, and because of his survival of the lion's den. Daniel being from the tribe of Judah, was a natural born warrior and became a gifted scholar at a very young age who had built up quite a following of loyal students.

Daniel dreamed with the vivid visions of his mind that he had while lying in bed, it played for him like a movie. "I was looking and behold there was a tree amid the earth, and its height was tremendous. This tree grew stronger until its height reached the skies and was able to be seen from all parts of the earth. It was a beautiful tree with plentiful fruit and all the beasts enjoyed its shade. Suddenly an angel who is forever awake and holy was standing on his bed, crying loudly, cut down the tree and bring it down so all the beasts shall wander away from beneath it." The angel warned that the roots should not be destroyed, he shall place his feet in iron fetters as is done to a horse that is left in the meadow. "So shall you chain the beast with fetters. The beast shall stay there drenched for seven years, and all the living should know, since they must take counsel from God, before Nebuchadnezzar issues his decree."

The bewildered Daniel woke up and told himself that he should not be alarmed, he remained in thoughtful silence because he was afraid to interpret the dream. He raised his eyes to God and said, "May this dream be fulfilled upon your enemies." Daniel interprets that the beautiful tree in his dream was God, who Nebuchadnezzar wishes to banish from mankind. The drenched dew of the heavens will immerse God, and seven periods shall pass over, which we may say that this is the recompense for the Temple, which Nebuchadnezzar destroyed, and was re-built with-in seven years. Perhaps there will be time for your tranquility, that the evil should not come swiftly, what did Daniel see to give Nebuchadnezzar good advice? He saw the Jews poor and humbled by the exile, going from door-to-door begging for food, and he recommended that Nebuchadnezzar deals mercifully with them. He said to him, "These poor people whom you exiled are hungry, so nourish them," which he did. He opened his storehouses and fed them for a full twelve months. After twelve months Nebuchadnezzar the heard poor people coming to his door and crying for food. He asked his servants, "What is the sound of this multitude in my ears?" His servants said to him, "These are the poor for whom you arranged a time to feed." Nebuchadnezzar got irritated and said, "is this not the great Babylon, if I had squandered my storehouses, from where would I have built all these palaces? From now on, I shall not feed them."

So, God's decree was executed upon him, hair grew over his entire body like eagles' feathers and his nails became like a bird's talons. Finally, at the end of the days that were set for him; at the end of the seven years. Nebuchadnezzar cries out to God and says, "my understanding was restored to me, and I praised and glorified God to eternity." At this time once Nebuchadnezzar understood the power of God, he is allowed to return to the glory of his kingdom and the splendorous features of his face. He returns to his leaders and his dignitaries are once again seeking him, his advisers and his princes missed him and were hoping for his return. Nebuchadnezzar was established, and excessive greatness was added to him, even more intensity than the earlier. Kings were connected to him; he even rode astride a lion and tied a serpent to its head. His ways are just, the man who once walked with arrogance is now humbled.

The first best and most choicest fruits of the tree was brought to the Holy Temple. Today we don't have a Holy Temple so we cannot do that anymore, but to commemorates this tradition, we are not permitted to eat the fruits of a tree until it is three years old. Once a tree is planted in the ground in Israel, we are not permitted to uproot it. Modern day Israeli law applies this biblical law seriously to protects its trees. In Israel it is illegal to uproot an old tree, you may cut it down to a stump but must leave its roots free in the ground.

Pomegranate

Latin Name, Punica Granatum

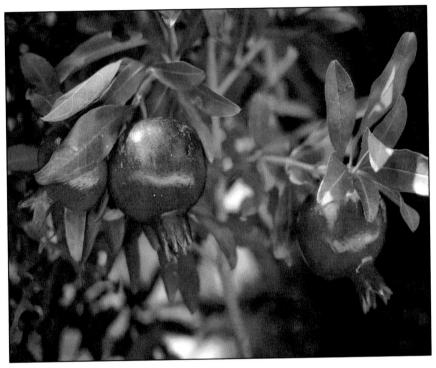

The pomegranate tree is a shrub and is indigenous of the Middle Eastern region. Its name in English starts with Pomum stemming from apple in French and Granatum meaning seeded. The fruit is a large reddish-purple grenade shaped fruit which is mentioned in the Bible many times. When it comes to pomegranate oil, there is no comparison. It is red and is reputed to be a wonderful blood cleanser and an antioxidant. It contains vitamin C and K, and its seeds are a rich source of dietary fiber and known to be a curer of all ills. Pomegranate oil is prepared from the seeds making a very rich high-quality oil with a unique hormone producing skill which affects and stimulates estrogen hormones. It is also used to prepare cosmetics and moisturizing body lotions, safeguarding most forms of skin damage. Pomegranate supplies iron to the blood helping to decrease symptoms of anemia, such as exhaustion, dizziness, and weakness.

BIBLICAL

"And on its bottom hem you shall make pomegranates of blue, purple, and crimson wool, on its bottom hem all around, and golden bells in their midst all around."

"A golden bell and a pomegranate, a golden bell and a pomegranate, on the bottom hem of the robe, all around."
(Exodus 28:23-24)

"And they made on the bottom hem of the robe pomegranates of blue, purple, and crimson wool, twisted."

"And they made bells of pure gold, and they placed the bells in the midst of the pomegranates all around on the bottom hem of the robe, in the midst of the pomegranates."

"A bell and a pomegranate, a bell and a pomegranate, all around on the bottom hem of the robe, to serve as the Lord had commanded Moses." (Exodus 39:24-26)

"A land of wheat, and barley, and vines, and fig trees and pomegranates; a land of oil producing olive and honey."
(Deuteronomy 8:8)

"And they came unto the valley of Eshkol, and cut down from thence a branch with one cluster of grapes, and they bore it upon a pole between two; they took also of the pomegranates, and of the figs." (Number 13:23)

"Thy lips are like a thread of scarlet, and thy speech is comely, thy temples are like a piece of a pomegranate within thy locks."
(Song of Solomon 4:3)

The Pomegranate is a very beautiful and majestic fruit with a crown on its head. It is the fifth fruit of the seven species of Israel and is mentioned and referred to in the Bible many times. It is also included in coinage and various types of ancient and modern cultural works of art. Pomegranates were one of the fruits the scouts brought back to Moses and the people of Israel, when they returned from their mission of checking out the fertility of the promised land. The robe worn by the high priest, had pomegranates embroidered on his hem and alternated with golden bells. The pomegranates were round and hollow, shaped like hens' eggs, and the golden bells had clappers inside them. It was by these bells the Kohen could be heard as he entered and left the Holy of Holies. In the Books of Kings, it describes the capitals of the two pillars Joachim and Boaz, that stood in front of Solomon's Temple in Jerusalem engraved with pomegranates.

They weavers made tunics, very high glorious caps, and pants all fine twisted with linen. Their wide sashes were made of the same twisted fine linen, with blue, purple, and crimson wool, and intricate embroidery work exactly as God had directed to Moses. The show plate and the holy crown, were designed of pure gold, with an inscription of a seal engraved on them saying, "Holy to the Lord." A beautiful blue corded wool was placed upon the cap, from above also as God had commanded Moses.

All the work of the Temple and the Tent of Meetings were completed by the Israelites also exactly as God had commanded Moses. Once it was ready, they brought the Mishkan to Moses, together with the tent and all its furnishings, its clasps, its planks, its bars, its pillars, and its sockets. They were not able to erect it and since Moses had done no work in the preparation of the Temple, God left for Moses the important task of constructing it. No human being would be able to assemble the Temple because of the pure heaviness of the planks; no human was strong enough to do this, except Moses. Moses said to God, "How is it possible for a human being to erect the Temple?" God replied, "You work with your hands." Then Moses appeared to be assembling the Temple, however the pieces arose and fit to each other by themselves, this is why the Midrash says, "the Mishkan was set up" Moses saw the entire work, being done for him and so, as it is said, they were done as God had commanded, and Moses blessed them by saying, "May it be His will that the Holy Presence should rest in the work of your hands and may the pleasantness of the Lord our God be upon us."

It is traditional for Jews to eat pomegranates on Rosh Hashana, the Jewish New Year because of its numerous seeds which symbolizes fruitfulness. The commentaries say that the pomegranate has six-hundred and thirteen seeds corresponding with the six-hundred and thirteen commandments in the Torah.

Rosehip

Latin Name, Rosa Canina

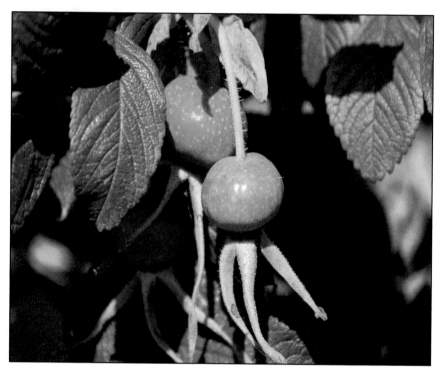

Rose hip is the accessory fruit behind the rose, its colors range from orange to pink and from purple to black depending on its species. The rose "hip" contains small seeds called achenes that germinate the rose. The essential oil is usually used as part of a formula and is extracted from the seeds. It is an orange plant and contains Carotene, Vitamins A and E, it is great for skin pigmentation and wrinkles and has been compared to Botox in its capabilities. Rose hip fruits are very rich in vitamin C, it also contains carotenoids beta-carotene, lutein, zeaxanthin, and lycopene. It has the potential for its extracts to reduce arthritis pain, though rose hips is not considered an effective treatment for knee osteoarthritis.

BIBLICAL

"The king of Tirzah, one; all the kings thirty-one." (Joshua 12:24)

"My beloved has gone down to his garden, to the spice beds, to graze in the gardens and to gather roses." (Song of Songs 6:2)

"I am my beloved's, and my beloved is mine, who grazes among the roses." (Song of Songs 6:3)

"You are fair, my beloved, as Tirzah, comely as Jerusalem, awesome as the bannered legions." (Song of Songs 6:4)

"Turn away your eyes from me, for they have made me haughty; your hair is like a flock of goats that streamed down from Gilead." (Song of Songs 6:5)

Anything to do with roses in the Bible is usually connected with King Solomon, the rose of Sharon mentioned in the Bible are not roses as we know them today, but the hibiscus flower. King Solomon was the focal fantasy of all the women in Israel at that time, and he in turn loved to swoon all women. The love story mentioned in the Song of Songs, of a young man whose betrothed is dear and sweet to him, and her eyes are comely, and he says to her, "Turn away your eyes from me, for when I see you, my heart becomes haughty and proud, and my spirit becomes arrogant, and I cannot resist." But most times love is painful, because the pride is toil and pain, "You are fair, my beloved, as Tirzah," Tirzah was a beautiful town in the hills of Samaria Northeast of Shechem, there she had a king whom the Israelites defeated. King Solomon who composed the Song of Songs, describing a lover who compares his beloved's beauty to that of Tirzah.

During the reigns of Baasha, Elah, Zimri and Omri, Tirzah was the capital of the northern kingdom of Israel, then Zimri set fire to Tirzah before he surrendered to Omri. Omri remained the King of Tirzah for six years after his victorious conquering of the city, then decided to move to Samaria the then capital of Israel. The allegorical meaning is as follows, God says, "In this Temple, it is impossible to restore to you the Ark, the Ark cover, and the cherubim, which made Me proud in the First Temple, to show you great affection, until you betrayed Me." Only an ewe is entirely devoted to holiness: its wool is used for the blue thread, its flesh for a sacrifice, its horns for the Shofar, its thighs for flutes, its intestines for harps, its hide for a drum; but the wicked were likened to dogs, for they have nothing to offer to holiness. Like a flower that blooms in the late summer that is very pungent and splendid, known simply as one of the many flowers of the field here in the Land of Israel.

"And Menahem the son of Gadi went up from Tirzah and came to Samaria; and he struck down Shallum the son of Jabesh and slew him and reigned in his stead. And the rest of the deeds of Shallum and his revolt that he revolted, are written in the book of the chronicles of the kings of Israel. Then Menahem attacked Tiphsah and all those therein and its boundaries from Tirzah; since he did not open, he attacked it; he ripped open all its pregnant women." (II Kings 15:14-16)

In Hebrew Tirzah is also a woman's name meaning "she is my delight," she is mentioned in the bible as one of the daughters of Zelophehad. After the death of their father, who left five sisters and no sons. The five girls, Tirzah being one of them, approached Moses and asked him to review their hereditary rights. Moses brought their plea to God, and it was granted making this a new revolutionary situation, this is the first encounter where women have the right to inherit properties and Israelite women continued to have the right to inherit property. However, the girls married their cousins from the tribe of Menashe, son of Joseph, and their inheritance remained with the tribe of their father's family, and they were married in the order they were born. This was done by the ordinance of God, through Moses in the plains of Moab, by the Jordan river, Jericho.

Joseph cherished the Land of his tribe, it was so important to him to be buried there that Moses took Joseph's bones with him to Israel and said, "God will surely remember you, and you shall bring up my bones from here with you." As did the daughters of Zelophehad by their not being willing to give it up, being Joseph's unified family in spirit.

Sesame

Latin Name, Sesamum Indicum

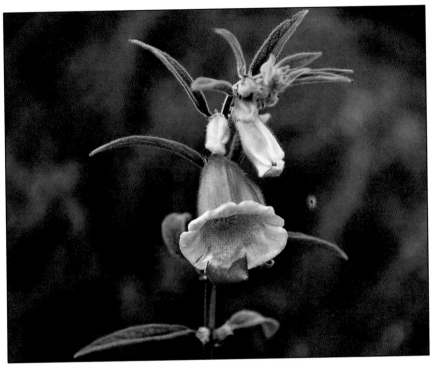

Sesame seed is one of the oldest oilseed crops known to man and was domesticated well over three-thousand years ago. It grows mainly in the wild and is a native of Africa and India. It has a rich, nutty flavor and is a common ingredient in cuisines across the world. Sesame seeds and sesame oil may cause serious allergic reactions to some adults and infants. Its oil is a natural pain killer and acts as an anti-inflammatory, use on cramped muscles after workouts, it works by warming up the muscle and soothing the pain. Apply on clean skin, after workouts and best not to eat for two hours after application, to allow the oil to be absorbed into the digestive tract. Some research has shown that Sesame consumption produced small reductions in both systolic and diastolic blood pressure. Sesame oil studies also reported a reduction of oxidative stress markers and lipid peroxidation.

BIBLICAL

"And unleavened bread and unleavened loaves mixed with oil, and unleavened wafers anointed with oil; you shall make them out of fine wheat flour." (Exodus 29:2)

"And one loaf of bread, one loaf of oil bread, and one wafer from the basket of matzoth that stands before the Lord." (Exodus 29:23)

"The first portion of your dough, you shall separate a loaf for a gift; as in the case of the gift of the threshing floor, so shall you separate it." (Numbers 15:20)

"And you shall bathe and anoint yourself and put on your clothes and go down to the threshing-floor; do not make yourself known to the man until he has finished eating and drinking." (Ruth 3:3)

"And when each maiden's turn arrived to go to King Ahasuerus, after having been treated according to the practice prescribed for the women, for twelve months, for so were the days of their ointments completed, six months with myrrh oil, and six months with perfumes, and with the ointments of the women." (Esther 2:12)

Sesame is referred to in the Mishna as an oil for cosmetics and was among the list of Maimonides collection of first aid medications, amongst sesame oil there were dill, fennel, fenugreek, finger, hyssop, beet juice, borax, celery, cinnamon, quince, saffron, sesame, licorice, and pine nuts. The bible refers to three types of matzahs, which is basically scalding the dough to make loaves and wafers. The unleavened bread is also called "loaf of oil bread," because Moses would put as much oil into the scalded dough for the loaves and the wafers, and of each of the types of unleavened bread referred to in the bible, ten loaves in total were brought to the Temple. Whether it was the bread mix just was the flour, Moses would pour oil on them and mix them, after they were baked, he would anoint them. In today's tradition we bake "challah," for the Sabbath meal and some are sprinkled with sesame seeds. The Gemara also proves that sesame was used in the times of Moses,

"Come and hear, in the case of matza that one seasoned with black cumin, with sesame, or with any type of spice, it is fit to

be eaten during the festival of Passover, as it is considered matza, but it is called seasoned matza. The Gemara comments: It enters your mind to explain that this is a case where there were more spices than the matza itself."

Another interesting fact about sesame is about where the term "Open Sesame" originated from. We have all heard it and probably shouted it many times when we were kids. It is the magical idiom of the story of "Ali Baba and the Forty Thieves", The thieves call out "Open Sesame," or "Open, O Simsim," which opens the mouth of the cave where the forty thieves kept their hidden treasures. This replicates the way sesame seeds grows and develops in a pod that splits open when it reaches maturity, and the phrase "open sesame" was associated to the unlocking of treasures.

The word "sisma" which means password in Hebrew is also said to originate from sesame. Sesame is an effigy originating from the Hebrew word, shem meaning "name," which is the term used in Judaism when referring to God, saying "Hashem," meaning "the name." It originated from the kabbalah which represents the Talmudic term, "shem-shamayim," meaning "name of heaven." Today sesame is the main ingredient for two main Israeli foods, Halva and Tahini, Halva is a dense and very sweet desert originating in the Middle East and adopted into Israeli culture. Tahini is a Mediterranean condiment served as a dip, a salad dressing or simply eaten with Pita bread.

Shea Butter

Latin Name, Vitellaria Paradoxa

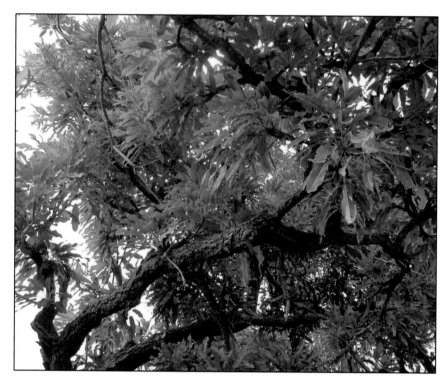

Shea butter is a fat extracted from a nut tree in Africa called the Karitae, Vitellaria paradoxa. Usually, the Chieftain of the tribe had a chain made from this tree. It is a large nut tree with a very dominant scent and is very often used as a base for medicinal ointments. The fat which is known as butter is yellow when it is raw, but once refined Shea butter becomes very white. The butter is a triglyceride type fat which originates from Stearic Acid and Oleic Acid and is used in cosmetics as a moisturizer. Some of the isolated chemical constituents are reported to have anti-inflammatory, emollient, and humectant properties and is very safe for babies. This oil contains Omegas 3, 6 and 9. Omega 6 is a good sunscreen and heals acne. It is an antioxidant, anti-cancer and has been used to treat melanomas. Shea butter has been used as a sun blocking lotion because of its components "have limited capacity to absorb ultraviolet radiation." It blends well with Vitamin E and Cannabis Oil, an oil certainly worth having.

BIBLICAL

"So, Israel, their father, said to them, "If so, then do this, take some of the choice products of the land in your vessels, and take down to the man as a gift, a little balm and a little honey, wax and lotus, pistachios and almonds." (Genesis 43:11)

"For you are a holy people to the Lord, your God: The Lord your God has chosen you to be His treasured people, out of all the peoples upon the face of the earth."

"Not because you are more numerous than any people did the Lord delight in you and choose you, for you are the least of all the peoples. (Deuteronomy 7:6-7)

"The beasts of the field shall honor Me, the jackals and the ostriches, for I gave water in the desert, rivers in the wasteland, to give My chosen people drink." (Isaiah 43:20)

"I went down to the nut garden to see the green plants of the valley, to see whether the vine had blossomed, the pomegranates were in bloom." (Songs of Songs 6:11)

There were many nuts around with shells in Biblical times, such as Almonds, Walnuts and Pistachio, all of which come in shells, just like the Shea Nut. The Bible compares the Israelites to a nut, it comes from an ancient commentary that says, "Just as with a nut at first all you see is just wood, and what is inside is not discernible. Once it is cracked open it is found to be full of sections of edible food. So are the Israelites modest and humble in their deeds and the students among them are not discernible, but if you examine him, you find him full of wisdom." The Israelites do not boast or proclaim self-praise, even if they are full of wisdom. Being modest and humble about successes is an attractive trait, speaking to peers, as is said in Israel "with four eyes," it is looking into people's eyes and being sincere. An additional interpretation is if a nut falls into the mud, its interior does not become dirty or damaged, just as what God expects of the Israelites, even when we are hit with many blows their deeds do not get corrupted.

The Israelites described Israel as a place that is desolate and a habitat of the beasts of the field only, for the jackals and for the ostriches. They forgot that God had promised them, "in a desolate land I will place a settlement."

God chose the Israelites so that they would recite his name in praise, but they did not, instead they chose to turn towards idol worshipping. God told Jacob, *"Your people quickly got wearied of worshipping me. They found themselves overworked by having to prepare the highest quality meal offerings which I deserve. Even that I did not ordain upon you to sacrifice as an obligation but as a free-will offering."* The Israelites were not even expected to have to purchase expensive spices, because God had given them lavish spices to grow naturally in abundance in the land, cinnamon's natural habitat is Israel, goats and deers eats it. Yet after all that, God had still gone to conquer the whole world under the domination of Nebuchadnezzar to save his people. He is the God that erases his people's transgressions and forgets their sins for his own sake, even till today.

The Midrash explains that God chose the Jewish people not because they are great, God says, "because you do not boast yourselves when I shower good upon you, this is why I delighted in you, because you humble yourselves." It was Abraham, who said, "For I am dust and ashes." Then it was also Moses and Aaron, who said, "but of what significance are we?" completely unlike, Nebuchadnezzar, who said, "I will liken myself to the Highest," or Hiram, who said, "I am a god, I have sat in a seat of God"

> *"Your holiness stems from your forefathers, and, moreover, "the Lord has chosen you."*

Stellaria Media

Latin Name, Common chickweed

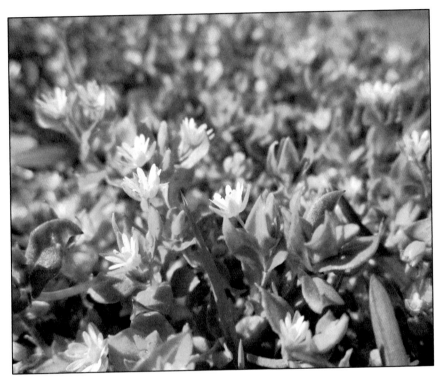

Stellaria Media is a plant also known as chickweed and from the carnation family, it likes to live in open meadows and fields grows wild across the countryside. It blankets whole ground areas with white quickly taking control. It is a green plant with white flowers of which the center is a square and is indigenous of North America, Europe, and Asia. It is a nutritious and edible plant that can be eaten raw in salads. Its oil is light and silky Mainly used for skin inflammation, acne, and all sorts of scars. When used internally as a tea, it raises the HDL the good cholesterol and helps diabetes. Its name Stellaria means star and is also known as star weed due to its star shaped flowers as well as the Star of Bethlehem.

Herbalists prescribe it for iron-deficiency anemia for its high iron content, as well as for skin diseases, bronchitis, rheumatic pains, arthritis, and period pain.

BIBLICAL

"And to all the beasts of the earth and to all the fowl of the heavens, and to everything that moves upon the earth, in which there is a living spirit, every green herb to eat," and it was so." (Genesis 1:30)

"And he made the menorah of pure gold; of hammered work he made the menorah, its base and its stem, its goblets, its knobs, and its flowers were all one piece with it." (Exodus 37:17)

"And the cedar of the house within was carved with knobs and open flowers; all was cedar; there was no stone seen." (I Kings 6:18)

"And all the walls of the house he surrounded with figures, carved figures of cherubim and palm trees and open flowers; from within and for the one without." (I Kings 6:9)

"It was all overgrown with thorns; Its surface was covered with chickweed, and its stone fence lay in ruins." (Proverbs 24:16)

Israel is blessed with many wildflowers; Chickweed is found in the Upper and Lower Galil and Kinneret areas. Jonathan, son of Solomon used open petalled open flowers in the form of chains decorating the Cherubs in the Holy Temple of Jerusalem, and they resembled chickweed. The six leaf petals of the Chickweed and serves as the inspiration to symbolize the Star of David. "Star of David," which since became the symbol of Judaism. The two interlaced triangles were the shape of the signet ring worn by King Solomon, known as the Seal of Solomon, the ring empowered Solomon to command demons, genies, spirits, and to even to speak with animals. Chickweed resembles stars, shining on green grass surface, just like the stars shine in a blue surface of the skies.

When God created vegetation on the third day of creation, he planned it so that when animals were created on the fifth day, they also had food. In God's equation, he regarded cattle and beasts equal to man regarding the food chain that they were permitted to eat. God did not permit Adam and his wife to kill a creature and to eat its flesh; they were however given every green herb, which they were all permitted to eat equally.

Wheat

Latin Name, Triticum Aestivum

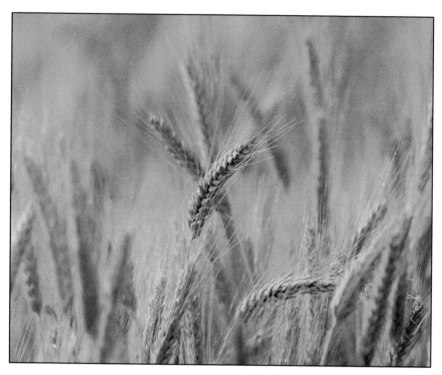

Wheat oil is taken from the seed, which is the sperm of the plant, land the germ of a cereal is the reproductive part that germinates and grows into a plant. In fact, it is the embryo of the seed that produces refined grain. Wheatgerm has several essential nutrients, including vitamin E, folate which is folic acid, phosphorus, thiamin, zinc, and magnesium, as well as essential fatty acids and fatty alcohols. Wheat germ oil helps people suffering from diabetes, high blood pressure, obesity, hair loss, dandruff, dry skin, wrinkles, premature aging, dementia, memory loss, acne, fatigue, psoriasis, and various other health conditions.

BIBLICAL

"And he named him Noah, saying, "This one will give us rest from our work and from the toil of our hands from the ground, which the Lord has cursed." (Genesis 5:29)

"These are the generations of Noah; Noah was a righteous man he was perfect in his generations; Noah walked with God." (Genesis 6:9)

"And you shall make for yourself a Festival of Weeks, the first of the wheat harvest, and the festival of the ingathering, at the turn of the year." (Exodus 34:22)

"A land of wheat and barley, vines and figs and pomegranates, a land of oil producing olives and honey," (Deuteronomy 8:8)

"And it will be, when you come into the land which the Lord, your God, gives you for an inheritance, and you possess it and settle in it," (Deuteronomy 26:1)

"That you shall take of the first of all the fruit of the ground, which you will bring from your land, which the Lord, your God, is giving you. And you shall put [them] into a basket and go to the place which the Lord, your God, will choose to have His Name dwell there." (Deuteronomy 26:2)

"The cream of cattle and the milk of sheep, with the fat of lambs and rams of Bashan and he goats, with kidneys of wheat, and the congregation of Israel would drink the blood of grapes which was as the finest wine." (Deuteronomy 32:14)

Wheat is the first fruit of the seven species of Israel with which the Land of Israel is blessed. In the beginning, the Land of Israel was cursed because of Adam and Eve, even when they sowed land it only produced thorns and thistles instead of wheat. God's great anger with the first man Adam who he threw out of the garden of Eden lasted all the way to Noah. God said when Noah was born that this one will give us rest from the toil of our hands. God says, "he will comfort us," but from the root Hebrew root of his name it would have to mean, "comfort." With God's intentions, his name probably should have been "Menachem," meaning "this one will console us," the true meaning of Noah's name is comfortable.

The curse broke when Noah arrived, and all the difficult conditions subsided. God loved Noah very much because he saw he was a hard worker, Noah listened and obeyed God, and so his deeds brought blessing to the Land. Before Noah came, they did not have plowshares and the land was still producing thorns and thistles when he sowed wheat. Noah worked hard on the land and became an experienced gardener; he took the initiative of preparing ploughing tools to help him work the land. Noah knew when it came to planting crop, that in a field beset with thistles he sowed wheat, and in a field beset with weeds, he sowed barley.

In the days of Noah there existed Nephilim, who were large mysterious beings, their names translate into, "the fallen," because they fell to earth thus causing the world to fall. These were the fallen angels, when the ocean rose up and inundated a third of the world and the generation of the flood did not humble them, and their destruction made the world desolate again. God regretted that he created Enosh and the children of Cain, but it was a consolation to him that he had created earthly beings, such as Noah. God mourned the destruction of his handiwork, but he rejoiced over his son Noah and if you ask any father, "was a son ever born to you?" Like any father, who rejoices and made everyone rejoice at the birth of his son, even though he knows his son is destined to die. This is why it is said, "At the time of joy, there is also a time of mourning." So, God revealed that even though he knows that man will ultimately sin, and he could destroy them for this, he still did not refrain from creating man, at the credit of the few righteous men who were destined to arise from them, such as Noah.

God says about Noah, "The mention of a righteous man is for a blessing." why are the names of the children of Noah are not mentioned immediately following saying, "These are the generations of Noah." The main lesson here is that the main generations of biological offspring are not the focus of a man's worth, but of his righteous good deeds. The Midrash says that Noah was a righteous man of his time, however, had he been living in Abraham's generation, he would not have been considered of any importance.

"Noah walked with God, but Abraham strengthened himself and walked in his righteousness by himself."

Essential Oils

Mixing Essential Oils

As mentioned above, every blend must contain a base oil to keep safe, essential oils must not be underestimated for their potency. There are only a few exceptions of oils that may be used directly onto the skin, but in general it is always best to use a base oil for all oils.

Synergy Blends

Since Essential oils are not to be used directly onto your skin unless it is a synergy blend. These unique blends of essential oils recipes with equal amounts of each, 1:1 Synergy blends uses a combination of many different oils that complement each other and allowing them to work together for a specific purpose. Synergetic oils work harmoniously together, and their therapeutic benefits being greater.

Some essential oils also have an additive or antagonistic effect, the synergy occurs between two oils, one dominating and the other more passive, when blended they act together and significantly increase the whole oil's activity. Use a synergy blend directly on the skin or in the mouth without a base oil, unless it is a young baby or a person with sensitive skin.

Acacia

Latin Name, Acacia Penninervis
Aroma, Deep honey, floral, balsamic

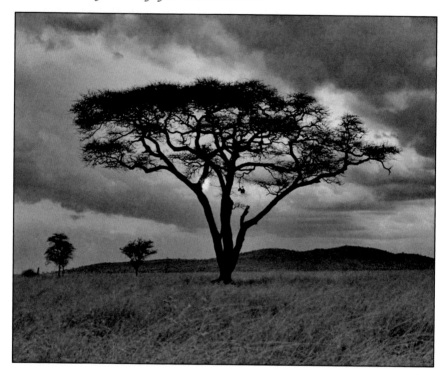

PHYSICAL

Acacia is also known as Wattles who are large shrubs and trees that can be found all over Southern Israel today. All Acacia species are pod-bearing, with sap and leaves often bearing large amounts of tannins. Many of these trees are yielded for their gum and seeds, the gum is used in a wide variety of food products and soft drinks. Acacia oil is an astringent and used as medicine, the tannins are obtained by boiling the wood by evaporating the solution to get the extract. Acacia's thick tree stump is high quality wood and is used to make furniture that is still left with a beautiful and fragrant timber. Many people use Acacia to make ornaments, carvings, and animal statues.

Acacia oil is a pain killer, it reduces irritation and inflammation and eases throat or stomach discomfort. It may help promote weight loss because it is an excellent source of soluble fiber by helping you feel full and stops you reaching for unhealthy snacks. It dramatically heals wounds and helps treat various skin diseases including acne and skin irritations and cleanses pores of the skin that may cause Acne. Acacia is also used for oral hygiene and can be used as a mouthwash. It is an ingredient used in total body detox or cleansing procedures.

EMOTIONAL

Acacia oil relieves stress, nervous exhaustion, its oil is extracted from its small yellow flowers and is used primarily to treat emotional conditions such as stress, anxiety, and depressed moods. This is oil has overall a very grounding, calming and uplifting qualities together with its stress relieving and anti-depressant abilities, this makes it an amazing oil.

BIBLICAL

"Ram skins dyed red, tachash skins, and acacia wood;"
(Exodus 25:5)

"They shall make an Ark of acacia wood, two and a half cubits its length, a cubit and a half its width, and a cubit and a half its height." (Exodus 25:10)

"And you shall make the planks for the Mishkan of acacia wood, upright. (Exodus 26:15)

"And he made poles of acacia wood and overlaid them with gold." (Exodus 37:4)

"So, I made an Ark of acacia wood, and I hewed two stone tablets like the first ones, and I ascended the mountain, with the two tablets in my hand." (Deuteronomy 10:3)

"I will plant in the wilderness the acacia tree, and the myrtle and the Etz Shemen "Oil Tree" I will set in the Arava cypress, maple and box-tree together." (Isaiah 41:19)

There are many references of this tree in the Bible, valuable for its wood as well as its aroma to make fragrant balms. The Acacia tree was used to build Noah's ark and the Holy Ark of the Temple of Jerusalem. The ark was designed like a chest made without feet, made like a sort of trunk or box resting on a base without being raised off the floor by the attachment of legs. The Israelites built three arks, two of gold and one of wood, each one had four walls and a bottom, and were open on the top. The wooden one was placed inside the larger golden one and the second golden chest was placed inside the wooden one. The upper rim was coated with gold, so that the wooden chest was also overlaid from inside and from outside with gold.

God asked the Israelites to make planks that were to stand and be ready, designated for the purpose of being without a specific use, just in case. "See that they should be ready in your hands. They should stand upright, perpendicular and the length of the planks shall be perpendicular to each other inside the walls of the Mishkan. You shall not make the walls of horizontal planks, so that the width of the planks will be along the height of the walls, one plank lying upon the other." Jacob foresaw with his divine prophesy that the Israelites were destined to build a Mishkan, the Holy Ark in the desert so he took the initiative to plant cedars in Egypt. When he was dying, he commanded his sons to deliver them to Israel when they left Egypt. He told them that God needed them, he was planning to design a Mishkan of acacia woods in the desert with specific instructions for Moses. In the bible the acacia is called the shittah tree, which had the honor to be the main tree used in the construction of the holy Ark of the Covenant.

"God's voice flew to the planting of the quickened ones, the cedar beams of our houses, for they hurried to have the cedars ready in their hands prior to this moment, of the command to build the Mishkan."

God promised to plant trees in the desert for all kinds of civilizations, giving trees the privilege all kinds of wisdom, goodness, and peace. Firs and cypresses are trees that were not created to produce fruit and destined to be used for building.

Angelica

Latin Name, Angelica Archangelica
Aroma, Earthy Herbal Green

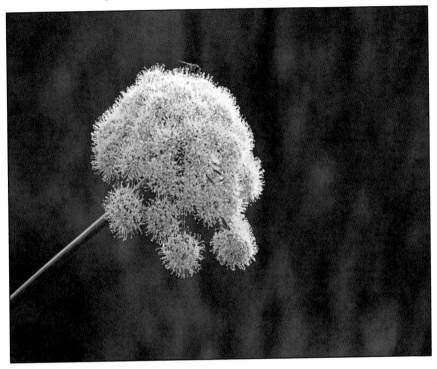

PHYSICAL

This Angelica is a native of Northern European countries and its appearance is similar to the poisonous species, Conium and Heracleum. Do not consume unless you have positively identified the Angelica with absolute certainty. It is a relaxant with quite a dominant aroma, and so relieves muscle spasms because it interacts directly with our nervous system. Its oil is made from the root of the plant and because of this it has an earthy scent and is used for base chakra treatments. This oil helps people to see the simple meanings that are a delight to the sight of the eyes, making the heart happy. Angelica is great also for heart problems such as angina, it helps the recovery process after heart by-pass surgery, take a few drops and spread them across your sternum. Other uses of this oil are to lower Blood Pressure, Vitiligo and rids the body of toxins.

Warning, this oil must not be used if you will be in direct sunshine and may cause pigmentation.

EMOTIONAL

It is used for relaxation because of its effect on the heart when dealing with a trauma. This oil blends beautifully with Patchouli and Ylang Ylang because of their basal earthy yet flowery fragrance. Angelica encourages strength and stamina; it comforts while at the same time helping to focus. This oil has a solid personality, by grounding and forcing inward reflection.

Angelica oil is graceful, light and ethereal, this angelic oil brings out the inner angel spirit. It is through its amazing fragrance that stimulates the "angel" about, protecting from inner vulnerable thoughts.

BIBLICAL

"And when these days were over, the king made for all the people present in Shushan the capital, for everyone both great and small, a banquet for seven days, in the court of the garden of the king's orchard." (Esther 1:5)

"And they gave them to drink in golden vessels, and the vessels differed from one another, and royal wine was plentiful according to the bounty of the king." (Esther 1:7)

"And the drinking was according to the law with no one coercing, for so had the king ordained upon every steward of his house, to do according to every man's wish." (Esther 1:8)

"And the Jews who were in Shushan assembled on the thirteenth thereof and on the fourteenth thereof, and rested on the fifteenth thereof, and made it a day of feasting and joy."

"Therefore, the Jewish villagers, who live in open towns, make the fourteenth day of the month of Adar a day of joy and feasting and a festive day, and of sending portions to one another." (Esther 9:18-19)

"Then the work of the House of God, which was in Jerusalem, was stopped, and it was suspended until the second year of the reign of Darius, the king of Persia." (Ezra 4:24) "

I said to myself, "Come now, I will mix wine with joy and experience pleasure"; and behold, this too was vanity."

"Of laughter, I said, "It is mingled"; and concerning joy, "What does this accomplish?" (Ecclesiastes 2:1-2)

"On joyous occasions, a feast is made, and wine gladdens the living, and money answers everything." (Ecclesiastes 10:19)

"And he said to them, "Go, eat fat foods, and drink sweet drinks and send portions to whoever has nothing prepared, for the day is holy to our Lord, and do not be sad, for the joy of the Lord is your strength." (Nehemiah 8:10)

At the time of Purim in Shushan the Capital of Persia, the Israelites were celebrating and drinking gin, specifically told by God to drink, act frivolous and be happy. The custom is to dress up in costumes and celebrate Queen Esther saving the Jews. The work of the building of the Second Temple which was to be built in Jerusalem, was suspended until the second year of king Darius's reign of Persia. Darius reigned after Ahasuerus and was the son of Ahasuerus and Esther and heir to the crown. Eighteen years into Darius's rule was exactly seventy years since the destruction of the first Temple of Jerusalem. The destruction of the Temple happened from when Zedekiah was exiled, until the first year of king Cyrus's rule in Persia. This took a total of seventy years between the destruction of the first and second Temple. Darius was in his second year of rule from when they commenced to build the Temple until they completed it.

At weddings we expect to have joy and musical entertainment, we expect a grand feast calling for bread and wine to drink and create a celebration that gladdens life. The bible understands that if there is no money, there can be no feast; therefore, a person should not their neglect work to earn a good living, so they have enough money to spend on the enjoyment of life. However, on the contrary, drinking too much will refrain a person from using wisdom, and the constant engagement in drinking and the mixing of wines, especially the mingling of wine with water to improve it. Some even mingle the wine with spices for conditum, and it doesn't take a prophet to foresee that many misfortunes can come about through drunk laughter. There will be mixed laughter with weeping and sighs and behold, its end is usually grief. It is good to eat and drink and enjoy life, but we must be careful to notice how much we are drinking. Appreciation of our hard-earned enjoyment should be with wisdom and comprehension in order to rejoice in our portion of eating, drinking, and having clean clothing and a roof over our heads. We should not toil all our lives only to have someone else take away the fruits of our labor.

Angelica roots are the ingredients used in the distillation of gin together with Juniper berries and coriander. All these condiments are used and mentioned frequently in the Bible. Just like in Purim when we are commanded to be happy, and to train to always see the beauty of nature, so Angelica cleanses the sadness's of the heart.

Anise Star

Latin Name, Pimpinella Anisum
Aroma, Spicy Sweet

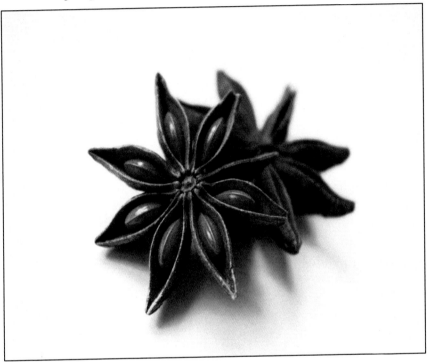

PHYSICAL

Anise is a tree with brown flowers that have a spot on each petal, this is the fruit of the tree. These "spots" are harvested and used for teas and remedies. Anise eases coughs, opens the bronchioles, and softens the phlegm that has built up and stagnated in the lungs during an illness. It gets into the lungs and dislodges the phlegm, causing an efficient cough to clear the system.

It assists in the contractions of the diaphragm, the performance of the digestive and respiratory system. Just one drop of this oil on the tongue will help with difficulty breathing, ease digestive problems like a gassy stomach and ease PMS symptoms. This oil is great for adults and kids, it helps lower sugar levels and balance diabetics.

EMOTIONAL

Anise is harmony and balance while releasing stress and mental pressure, it encourages uplifting stimulation, helping strive for fearlessness and dispels timidity. If a person doesn't like this scent, this may indicate that they were raised very strictly. This oil brings out the defiance in a person, it insists that in staying true to self. It teaches how to travel the highway of life and clarifies journeys. Anise oil smoothens out all confusions and conflicting thoughts, helping to make calm decisions to help achieve and complete goals.

BIBLICAL

"And she came to Jerusalem with a very large retinue, with camels bearing spices and very much gold and precious stones; and when she came to Solomon, she spoke with him all that was in her heart."

"And Solomon answered all her questions; nothing was hidden from the king that he did not tell her."

"And when the Queen of Sheba had seen all Solomon's wisdom and the house that he had built."

"And the food of his table, and the seating of his servants and the station of his attendants and their attire and his cupbearers and his ascent by which he would go up to the Temple of the Lord, she was breathless."

"And she said to the king; "It was a true report that I heard in my country of your deeds and of your wisdom."

"However, I did not believe the words until I came and saw with my own eyes, and I have beheld that not even a half had been told to me. You have wisdom and goodness in excess of that which I have heard."

"Fortunate are your men; fortunate are these your servants who always stand before you and listen to your profound wisdom." (I Kings 10:2-8)

"And the queen of Sheba heard of Solomon's fame, and she came to test Solomon with riddles in Jerusalem with an exceedingly large retinue, with camels bearing spices and gold in abundance and precious stones; and she came to Solomon and spoke with him all that was in her heart." (II Chronicles 9:1)

"And Hezekiah rejoiced over them, and he showed them his entire treasure house, the silver, the gold, the spices, and the good oil, and the entire house in which he kept his vessels, and everything that was found in his treasures; there was nothing that Hezekiah did not show them in his palace and in his kingdom." (Isaiah 39:2)

"Judea and the land of Israel-they are your peddlers; with wheat of Minnith, balsam trees, honey, oil, and balm, they gave your necessities." (Ezekiel 27:17)

Anise is one of the oldest known spices and this medicinal plant and is mentioned in the Bible several times. It was used in Israel during biblical times, originating in the Middle East and is indigenous to the general Mediterranean area. The queen of Sheba heard many rumors about king Solomon's wisdom, and she travelled to Israel to see for herself whether what she had heard about his wisdom was true, and she came with the intention to test him. King Solomon gave the queen of Sheba all the wishes she requested and teaching her much wisdom. She saw that he was open and honest with her, he revealed to her everything that she asked of him, and nothing was hidden from her, she had to admit that the all the reports she had heard about him were true. The queen of Sheba gave the king one hundred and twenty talents of gold and very many spices and precious stones; there had never arrived such an abundance of spices like those which the queen of Sheba brought to king Solomon. The king in turn gave her many gifts and delicacies that are found Israel and were rare in her own country.

"Solomon's wisdom was greater than the wisdom of all the children of the east, and all the wisdom of Egypt."

The food at the king's table were laid with many kinds of delicacies and were served in abundance. The royal servants had their own seating arrangements each recognizing their own place at the table, and no one was allowed to sit in another's place all the days of his life. Those servants who faced the king regularly would retain his station and his position for life and never change while their attire would change daily. There was a special stairway for the king by which he ascended from his palace to the Temple and at the sight of him, the queen was suddenly breathless. As a queen she became aware that unlike king Solomon, there was no such wisdom existing in any of her kingdoms. In her own country the equivalent of wise men were stargazers, her country being in the east while Israel is in the west of Babylon. It is said that the wise people who migrated from the east of Egypt were sorcerers, necromancers, and astrologers, their wisdom and divination being bogus.

Aside from his lessons of wisdom he gave her according to his ability, she returned to her land with her servants. The Midrash says that king Solomon had relations with her and out of that union Nebuchadnezzar was born to her. He was the wicked ruler who later destroyed the Temple that had stood four-hundred and ten years in the territory of the twelve tribes. The drink Arak is a Levantine Middle Eastern alcohol spirit which is anise flavored and has now become the traditional and a favored drink of the Middle East.

Basil

Latin Name, Ocimum Basilicum
Aroma, Fiery and peppery

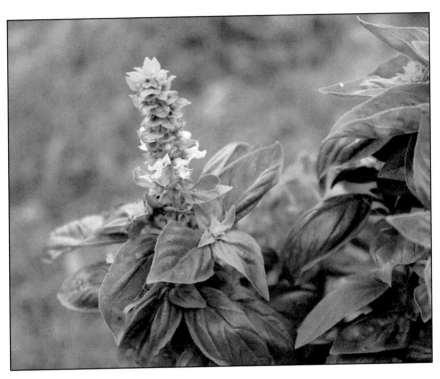

PHYSICAL

Originates in Africa and Southeast Asia, this oil is also called St. John's Wort and is an herbaceous plant. Basil is used in culinary cuisines all over the world now and used in a wide variety of dishes, depending on culture. It was also known as Holy Basil, this Bohemian oil is an Indian oil used for its leaves, branches, and roots. Basil tea at night will help sleep as it is a relaxant and affects the nervous system. Its other qualities are anti-fungal, anti-spasmatic and an anti-depressant. It is also used as a blood thinner and painkiller and is a strong anti-bacterial oil. Italians like to use this oil to help themselves metabolize after a very full meal. Italians like to eat dough and pasta, and they usually eat it with Pesto, where basil is the main ingredient. Basil does not allow food to stagnate in the digestive tract and keeps the food moving. It does this by calming gassy stomachs and encourages digestion to secrete enzymes to relax the stomach and digest.

The adrenal gland and the thyroid glands are assisted by basil's anti-spasmodic, digestive tonic and relaxing quality. It helps by releasing stress and fatigue caused by hypo or hyper thyroids and it balances the hormones. Basil eases PMS symptoms use it by rubbing it onto the stomach with a base oil.

Warning do not use this oil if you are nursing because it will dry up your milk, unless you want to of course.

EMOTIONAL

Because basil is used to balance thyroids and adrenal glands, which are hormonal, it is also used to help people who are despondent or fed up. Use in tea as an anti-depressant, this oil will definitely cheer you up. Basil encourages positivity and purposefulness, as well as enhancing concentration and assertiveness, being a straightforward oil, it is trustful, full of integrity and enthusiasm.

Basil is enlightenment and combines your physical and spiritual awareness into one grounding and balancing action. This oil enhances subconscious thoughts and helps the mind soar through all realms and because of its name Holy Basil, Krishna believes it protects and guards the spirit, and the spirit of the family. Basil can adjust DNA, therefore it must not be taken when pregnant, it can cause a mutation by changing the fetus's DNA too, so please be careful.

BIBLICAL

"And God said, "Let the earth sprout vegetation, seed yielding herbs and fruit trees producing fruit according to its kind in which its seed is found, on the earth," and it was so."
(Genesis 1:11)

"And the earth gave forth vegetation, seed yielding herbs according to its kind, and trees producing fruit, in which its seed is found, according to its kind, and God saw that it was good." (Genesis 1:12)

"And one went out to the field to gather herbs; and he found a vine in the field and gathered from its wild mushrooms his

garment full; and he came and diced them into the pot of stew, for they did not know." (II Kings 4:39)

"Now who can abide the day of his coming, and who will stand when he appears, for it is like fire that refines and like fullers' soap."

"And he shall sit refining and purifying silver, and he shall purify the children of Levi. And he shall purge them as gold and as silver, and they shall be offering up an offering to the Lord with righteousness." (Malachi 3:2-3)

"But for naught I cleansed my heart and bathed my hands with cleanliness." (Psalms 73:13)

When God said "let the earth bring forth herbs" he wanted various species, and each one to be unique. They will form the earth's covering and when it is filled with vegetation and herbs, their seeds should grow within them. Basil grew in Israel in the times of the bible, and it still grows naturally in Israel today, most people grow them in their herb gardens. The bible says, whoever can be like soap and remove entire stains, will be able to remove all wickedness. There are herbs which removes stains, and in these contexts the stain signifies not only to clean physically but to purify spiritually, "to the pure of heart." How does God know what is in our hearts? is always asked, the answer is by our actions, for nothing goes unnoticed or in vain, actions come after thought.

God wants his people to keep his commandments, this has never changed, although he restrains his anger for a long time, he never changed his mind about the way it was originally, to love evil and to hate good. God says to the sons of Jacob, "although you die in your evil, and I have not requited the wicked in their lifetime." God warns, "you have not reached the end and I have not finished with you, for the souls to be requited still remain in hell." Those who think that when they die from this world, his verdict has ended, and God's verdict has been nullified and will no longer be punished. The Sages explain this as, God did not strike a nation and repeat the blow to it, because once it was struck it no longer existed. However, God maintains his love for his people even after much punishment, but once God's arrows of anger have ended, his people are still his people. When the sun comes in the mornings, is an expression God uses and the Sages say that it means, that there will be no hell in the future, because God will punish the wicked and heal the righteous. That is the intention the statement, "And the sun of mercy shall rise with

125

healing in its wings for you who fear My Name. Then will you go forth and be fat as fatted calves." Then God will come to make peace in the world.

Basil was used in Egypt for embalming and preserving mummies in their tombs, and that it corresponds with Biblical times. The Jews were slaves in Egypt for approximately two-hundred and ten years though they were supposed to be enslaved for four-hundred years. During that time, they were obviously exposed to Egyptian culture and cuisine and knew about Basil and it's amazing and purifying qualities.

Benzoin Resin

Latin Name, Styrax
Aroma, Sweet, chocolatey vanilla

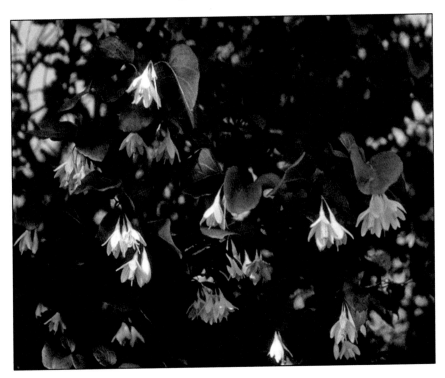

PHYSICAL

Benzoin is a balsamic resin taken from the bark of several species of Styrax. It is used in perfumes, incense, as a flavoring, and in the medicinal industries. Benzoin has a sweet vanilla type aroma and there are two common kinds of benzoin, benzoin Siam and benzoin Sumatra. Sumatran benzoin contains cinnamic acid as well as benzoic acid.

In perfumery, benzoin is used as a fixative, slowing the dispersion of essential oils and other fragrance materials into the air. Benzoin is used in cosmetics, veterinary medicine, and scented candles. It is used as a flavoring in alcoholic and nonalcoholic beverages, baked goods, chewing gum, frozen dairy products, gelatins, puddings, and soft candy. It is an antiseptic, anti-depressant, and an expectorant, and can cause some skin irritation to sensitive skin.

Warning do not administer to Pregnant Women.

EMOTIONAL

Benzoin encourages and comforts with high quality emotional healing abilities. It knows how to elevate the spirit and give inner peace and confidence. It transmits determination while at the same time soothes, cushions, and protects. It guides and helps to comprehend and clear all confusions, guiding true decision choices from deep in one's own heart. As personal growth develops through a full lifetime, Benzoin demonstrates how the inner soul can be the hero from within.

Benzoin is persuasive and direct; it will open the heart and mind to receiving gifts which have yet been denied. When the spirit allows acceptance to receive that in turn enables receiving physically. Only truly believing and being convinced that receiving whatever one desires is possible, will one feel that the spiritual path of receiving open, and so the spirit will receive. Learning to see the messages behind the difficult messages and learning to accept what is sometimes hard to understand, getting older makes everything suddenly clearer, and learn what is inner peace and true enlightenment.

BIBLICAL

"And the Lord said to Moses, "Take for yourself aromatics, balsam sap, onycha and galbanum, aromatics and pure frankincense; they shall be of equal weight." (Exodus 30:34)

"They sacrifice upon the mountaintops and burn incense upon the hills, under oaks and styraxes and elms, because its shadow is good; therefore, your daughters commit harlotry, and your daughters-in-law commit adultery." (Hosea 4:13)

"And Hezekiah listened to them, and he showed them his entire treasure-house, the silver, the gold, the spices, and the good oil, and the entire house in which he kept his vessels, and everything that was found in his treasuries; there was nothing that Hezekiah did not show them in his palace and in his kingdom."

"And Isaiah the prophet came to King Hezekiah and said to him, "What did these men say, and whence did they come to you?" And Hezekiah said, "They have come from a distant country- from Babylonia." And he said, "What did they see in your palace?"

"And Hezekiah said, "They saw everything that is in my palace. There was nothing that I did not show them in my treasuries."

"And Isaiah said to Hezekiah, "Hearken to the word of the Lord."

"Behold a time will come when everything in your palace and what your forefathers have stored up, will be carried off to Babylonia; nothing shall remain," said the Lord."
(II Kings 20:13-17)

Hezekiah became king at the age of twenty-five years, and he reigned twenty-nine years in Jerusalem, he was actually a very good king and was proper in the eyes of God, just as David had done. Right from the very start of his reign he opened the doors of the House of God and reinforced them, exactly the opposite of his father Ahaz. He summoned the priests and Levites and ordered them to sanctify themselves and to remove all the uncleanliness out of the Temple, and he destroyed the numerous idols in the kingdom. Once the Temple itself was completely cleansed and renovated to its original glory the people were then able come to Jerusalem to bring their offerings to God.

He was one of the three men whom God tested and found them to be a vessel of dense water. God tested Cain, Balaam, and Hezekiah. Cain said "I know not. Am I my brother's keeper?" when he should have said, "Lord of the Universe! Are all hidden things not revealed to You?" Balaam answered God when he asked him, "Who are these men with you?" he should have said, "O Lord God, you know!" Yet he retorted arrogantly, "Balak, son of Zippor, king of Moab, sent them to me." Hezekiah had said to God, "many people seek me." When he should have replied to the prophet Isaiah, "You are the prophet of the Omnipresent, yet you ask me?" Instead, Hezekiah commenced to become haughty, and said, "they have come to me from a distant land." Therefore, he was punished, for both reasons, firstly for his rude answer and secondly because he rejoiced over them and served them at his table.

Isaiah told him that nothing shall remain, and he will be paid in kind, corresponding to his answer, "There was nothing." Your future sons, Hananiah, Mishael, and Azariah, will be taken from you and they will be officers in the palace of the king of Babylonia. Hezekiah, who was a good man, said to Isaiah, "the word of the Lord that you have spoken is good." But he was really thinking, how can it be true, is there not peace and truth right now in my days. The Sages say that Cain was blamed for his weakness during the days of the flood, but he was rectified and strengthened through the reincarnation of Hezekiah, the translation of Hezekiah from Hebrew means "strength."

Benzoin also known as Nataf is a balsam sap that drips from balsamic trees and was another component of the ingredient for the Ketoret the incense in the Holy Ark of the Temple of Jerusalem. Some Sages interpret this as the anointing oil and others interpret it as balsam oil, which is found in Israel, Pannag is another balsam that grows in Jericho, this is the reason for its name, because Jericho means aroma, from all the beautiful trees that naturally grow in that area. It is known that the Israelites were familiar with the ancient art of perfumery of the Egyptians from whom they had just been liberated. Benzoin also called styrax was amongst the only materials most certain to have been used in ancient Egypt. It grew in abundance in the countries bordering the Mediterranean with which Egypt had affinity.

Bergamot

Latin Name, Citrus Bergamia
Aroma, Sweet, Fruity and Citrus

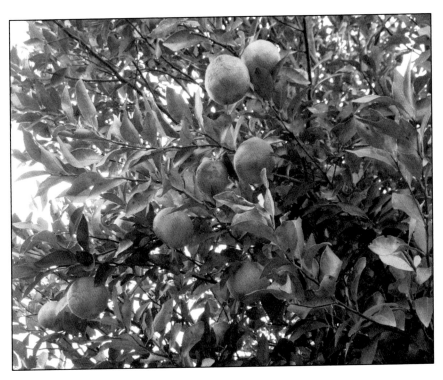

PHYSICAL

This oil comes from an orange tree in Italy, it has an amazing aroma which also affects our neuro system. It is an antiseptic, an anti-spasmodic and an anti-depressant, and can also be taken in your tea. Bergamot can help skin problems such as psoriasis, using its relaxing qualities to prevent attacks. It is very gentle on your skin, but it is phototoxic and should not be used in the sun. It is an anti-depressant, a pain reliever and relaxant. Bergamot also helps ADD and ADHD sufferers, reduces aggression, hysteria, and shouting.

EMOTIONAL

Bergamot lightens the shadows of the mind generating happiness. It helps to enlighten and emphasize that problems must not be the focus even when they are overwhelming. Putting problems aside to focus on the good things, helps to put them into perspective. This oil provokes super confidence, strength, and motivation to gain inner strength to feel real happiness and joy. With this oil a good mood is easy to accomplish giving a sense of harmony and self-confidence.

The shouting and crying from deep inside with an aching heart and self-hate, Bergamot will for sure help to see the lighter side of life and dispel destructive feelings. Bergamot works on a high frequency field and has a powerful aura that amplifies and magnifies as it gets closer to the body. It dusts out the shadows and cobwebs that have built up over the years and brightens and illuminates the soul. It is said that Bergamot brings eternal youth and happiness, even to those who seem to be suffering more than most. It releases one's own personal guardian angel, all one has to do is reach out for it.

BIBLICAL

"As an apple tree among the trees of the forest, so is my beloved among the sons; in his shade I delighted and sat, and his fruit was sweet to my palate." (Song of Songs 2:3)

"Who is this coming up from the desert, embracing her beloved?" "Under the apple tree I aroused you; there your mother was in travail with you; there she that bore you was in travail." (Song of Songs 8:5)

"Solomon had a vineyard in Baal-Hamon; he gave the vineyard to the keepers; each one brought for the fruit thereof one thousand pieces of silver."

"My vineyard, which is mine, is before me; you, O Solomon, shall have the thousand, and those who watch its fruit, two hundred." (Song of Songs 8:11-12)

"You, who sit in the gardens the friends hearken to your voice; let me hear it."

"Flee, my beloved, and liken yourself to a gazelle or to a fawn of the hinds on the spice mountains." (Song of Songs 8:13-14)

Even when a fruit tree is among trees in an orchard that do not bear fruit, its tree's fruit is good in both taste and fragrance. Orange trees are a native of the Middle East, probably came to Israel because of its citrus cousins, the Lemon, Pomelo, Grapefruit, Mandarin, and the Etrog. The love song written by king Solomon about a girl attached to her beloved, admitting that she is his companion and clinging to him in union. She says to him in the request of the affection of her beloved, "under the apple tree I aroused you." Which is an expression of desire the wife has of her youth, who arouses her beloved at night when he is asleep on his bed and embraces him and kisses him. Then she matures and becomes like your mother struggling with birth the pangs of a woman in confinement and if he was an unwise son and never learned from his mother, he will lose out and he shall not stand at the birthstool of his children's birth.

King Solomon ruled over Jerusalem at a time in which the populous had a multitude of people. Solomon gave away his vineyards into the hands of some harsh masters of Babylon, Media, Greece, and Edom. The Midrash says that these people were the keepers of their kingdoms. Each one brought the fruits of the trees or whatever they could collect from their people, as head taxes, tithes, and illegal foreclosures, they had the license to collect everything from them to bring into their homes. God promised he will bring them to justice saying, "my vineyard, even though I delivered it into your hands, it is mine, and before me is all that you seized for yourselves, its fruit. And that which you collected from them is not hidden from Me." Then the keepers will return the thousand pieces of silver they earned from them and will return everything to Solomon with interest, "Instead of copper I will bring gold." Two-hundred Torah scholars were paid to watch the fruits of the orchards, as the Midrash says, those who watch its fruit according to the law, is a person who derives benefit from sanctified commodities.

God says to the people of Israel, those who sits in the gardens of strangers and are scattered in exile, while you sit in synagogues and study halls, speak to your friends so they listen to your voice as though you are a commissioned angel. Tell your friends, that they are the children of God and about their land, speak to them in a way that afterwards they will declare God's sanctity, "when the morning stars sing together," these are the Israelites, after which, "and all the angels of God will shout." God's desire is that all the Israelites flee from exile and live together and like a gazelle, to hasten the redemption and to cause God to rest on the spice mountains of Moriah and the Temple. Sweet Oranges can be dated in Israel for sure after the fifteenth Century when they came over from European countries like Portugal and were first grown by Arab farmers in Israel, then named Palestine by the Romans in the mid-nineteenth century. They started growing orange orchards in Jaffa which is now producing exported fruits all over the world.

Bishops Weed

Latin Name, Amni Visnaga
Aroma, faintly grassy

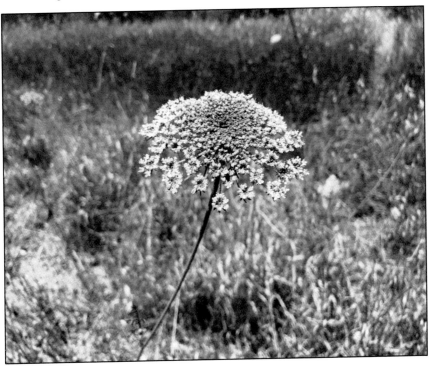

PHYSICAL

It has a black flower in the center and it's the many little flowers around it that form a mushroom like shape also known as toothpick weed. This plant grows in abundance all over Northern Israel, it is a beautiful plant and stays attractive well into the winter. This plant belongs to the carrot family and originates in Europe and the Middle East. In tea form, it is used to dissolve kidney stones and is great for angina, palpitations and lowers high blood pressure. Ammi Visnaga is used for respiratory conditions including asthma, bronchitis, cough, and whooping cough. It is a great oil for kids and can be used in a cold humidifier with Ventolin. Put a drop of Ammi Visnaga on of your child's palm or sole of foot to help him or her breathe. The oil opens the bronchioles and can be used together with respiratory related steroids.

EMOTIONAL

This plant is very relaxing because it knows how to lower your blood pressure and it helps sleep and breathing at night. This plant should not be used for long periods since it can be addictive.

BIBLICAL

"He shall be as a tree planted beside rivulets of water, which brings forth its fruit in its season, and its leaves do not wilt; and whatever he does prospers." (Psalms 1:3)

"And the Lord God planted a garden in Eden from the east, and He placed there the man whom He had formed." (Genesis 2:8)

"The name of one is Pishon; that is the one that encompasses all the land of Havilah, where there is gold." (Genesis 2:11)

"Go to Pharaoh in the morning; behold, he is going forth to the water, and you shall stand opposite him on the bank of the Nile, and the staff that was turned into a serpent you shall take in your hand." (Exodus 7:15)

The river Pishon Nile is the river of Egypt, and the bible says its waters are blessed, they rise and water the land, another reason it is called Pishon because it causes flax to grow and the land is said to be good, where there is gold, crystal the onyx stones. Moses and Aaron came to Pharaoh as God had commanded them, to ask him to let the Israelites free. Aaron cast his staff in front of Pharaoh and his servants, and suddenly it became a serpent. Still Pharaoh was unimpressed and refused their plea, he demonstrated he himself could have his magician perform similar acts. God instructed Moses to meet Pharaoh at the river Nile, Pharaoh would go there to relieve himself, for he had deified himself and said that he did not need to relieve himself; so, early in the morning he went out to the Nile and there he would perform his needs. There Moses's staff turned into a snake and said to him,

"The Lord God of the Hebrews sent me to you, saying, "Send forth My people, so that they may serve Me in the desert," but behold, until now, you have not hearkened. and he still refused."

Until you hear from me is the announcement of a threat which Pharaoh did not catch on to, it was the ultimate plague of the killing of the firstborns. As God had instructed, Moses struck the river with the serpent and started the deadly havoc on Pharaoh and the river turned to blood. Since there is no rainfall in Egypt, and the Nile ascends and waters the land, so it was natural for the Egyptians to assume to worship the Nile. God smote first their deity and then God smote them the people, the result of the bloody river was that all the fish died, the river became putrid, and the Egyptians could not drink the water. Pharaoh being a very stubborn man, he simply turned and went home, and he paid no heed even to this and it would take another seven plagues to ravage him and his people for him to take the God of the Israelites seriously.

Ammi originates from the Nile delta and may have been one of the weeds that concealed Baby Moses in his basket. This plant was used by the Egyptians as a tea because it is so therapeutic, it was also used in folk medicine to treat urinary calculi and bladder stones, it has always been a native to the Mediterranean markets in the Middle East.

Bitter Orange

Latin Name, Trifoliate Orange
Aroma, Spicy orange fragrance

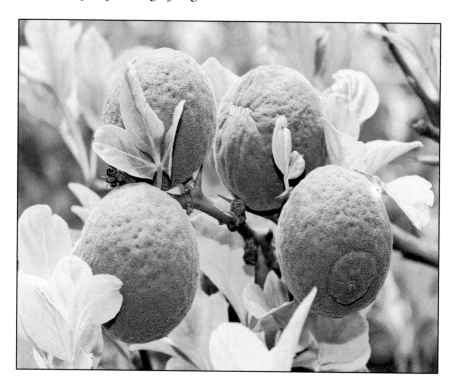

PHYSICAL

Bitter Orange has a strong faintly floral fragrance and is native to Asia and the Mediterranean and its essential oil is taken from the leaves of the orange tree, whereas Neroli is taken from its flower. This Orange plant is relaxing and prevents the body from constricting and tightening up. It reduces stomach pains that are induced from fear and increases energy and focus.

Warning do not administer to Children and pregnant or breastfeeding women.

EMOTIONAL

This is a very gentle oil and has a very quiet fragrance giving a sense of a calm and relaxed spirit. Its scent gives a hint of this oil's hidden personality, quiet but strong. Bitter Orange affects the nervous system by reducing stress and helping to cope during uncomfortable confrontations and difficult conversations and in situations like "fight or flight."

Bitter Orange is best inhaled when dabbed on to the wrist before dealing difficult and tense situations or breakup. This oil is a great anti-depressant and an anti-hysteria, its beautiful zesty odor can drag anyone out of any emotional pit no matter how deep they sank.

BIBLICAL

"Baal Hanan, son of Abhor died, and Hadar reigned in his stead. The name of his city was Pau; his wife's name was Mehetabel, daughter of Matred, the daughter of Me zahab." (Genesis 36:39)

"And you shall take for yourselves on the first day, the fruit of the Hadar tree, date palm fronds, a branch of a braided tree, and willows of the brook, and you shall rejoice before the Lord your God for a seven-day period." (Leviticus 23:40)

Bitter orange comes from a group of trees called Hadar, which in the bible is called a majestic tree. The bitter orange looks very similar to the Etrog which is the Citron Fruit that is one of the four species used in the Jewish Holiday of Sukkot. It has the same texture and scent, and many people get confused between them. Hadar can be interpreted in a general way, not limiting it to a specific species, the Sages say this strictly refers to the Etrog only. This identification of the "fruit of goodly trees" in the Torah with the Etrog was accepted as far as we know without reservation. God's gives specific instructions of the Hadar fruit, referring to all the citrus family.

Hadar was also a name of a king who reigned over Israel and was married to Mehetabel, daughter of Matred and the grand-daughter of Me-Zahab, her name literally meaning, "made out of gold," this probably means that he was rich, that gold was of no importance to him. The chieftains of Esau were called by the names of their provinces and after king Hadar died their kingdom ceased and the names of their generations are delineated. Eight kings reigned in Edom before a king reigned in Israel and are enumerated in the Book of Genesis, the eight kings were, Ish bosheth,

David, Solomon, Rehoboam, Abiam, Asa, Jehoshaphat, and Jehoram. Edom rebelled against the power of Judah and had no king, so they appointed a king over themselves, but he went with Jehoram the son of Ahab and with Jehoshaphat to war against the king of Moab, but he was not considered a real king, but a governor. Of the first seven of these kings, the bible writes they ruled, and then their death, when the bible mentions Hadar the eighth king, it only writes about his rule without mentioning his death, his death is only mentioned in Chronicles, but not in Genesis.

This is a tree whose wood has the same taste as its fruit, and they grow in the tree from one year to the next. These plants are a symbolic group of species needed to celebrate and rejoice for seven days. The citron was written about by King Solomon in the Song of Songs and the Romans used to call them Persian Apples.

Black Cumin

Latin Name, Nigella Sativa
Aroma, Sweet, nutty, and earthy

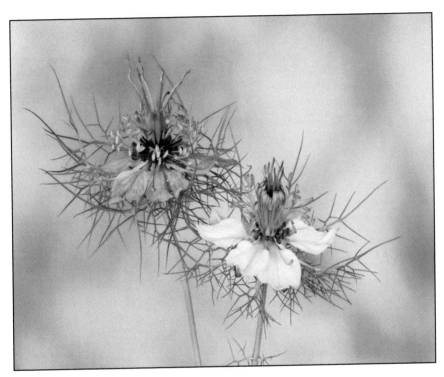

PHYSICAL

Black Cumin is a native of southern Europe, north Africa, and southwest Asia, this is a stunning plant with white, yellow, pink, pale blue, or pale purple flowers, with five to ten petals. Nigella seeds are self-sowing if the seed pods are left to mature. The seeds are used as a carminative and stimulant to ease bowel and indigestion problems. Black Cumin is administered to treat intestinal worms, nerve defects, reduce flatulence, and induce sweating. Its dried pods are inhaled to restore a lost sense of smell and is also used to repel some insects, like the way mothballs are applied.

Black cumin also known as black onion seed, or just nigella, they are used as a spice in Indian and Middle Eastern cuisines. The oil is extracted from the seed by cold compression and is an amazing antioxidant. Its anti-inflammatory abilities allow it to help arthritis sufferers, it lowers systolic and diastolic blood pressure. It can even reduce triglycerides and LDL and total cholesterol, while raising HDL cholesterol.

EMOTIONAL

Black Cumin has been proven to help in neurological and psychiatric problems as well as in pain control. It helps with epilepsy, Parkinson, anxiety, and drug dependence, and will aid improvement of learning and memory, sharpen alertness, elevate mood, and give a feeling of good health.

This oil stimulate energy and helps to recover from fatigue or hopelessness. It is an anti-depressant that supports the overcoming of anguish, grief, or heartache. Black Cumin helps to cope with life stresses and lows making it easier to rebound faster.

BIBLICAL

"Is it not so? When he smooths its surface, he scatters the black cumin and casts the cumin, and he places the prominent wheat, and the barley for a sign, and the spelt on its border."
(Isaiah 28:25)

"For not with a grooved implement is black cumin threshed, neither does a wagon wheel turn around on cumin, but black cumin is beaten with a staff and cumin with a rod."
(Isaiah 28:27)

"This too comes forth from the Lord of Hosts, He gave marvelous counsel, made great wisdom." *(Isaiah 28:29)*

Black cumin seeds have been mentioned in the Bible where Isaiah from the Old Testament reaps black cumin seeds and God compares this with the reaping of wheat. This too, like the custom of threshers of grain and those who flail black cumin and cumin, comes forth from God.

When the prophets admonish a man to bring him back to do good deeds, he does not admonish him forever because it is not productive and has no benefit. This is compared to sowing and plowing land, if we harrow our soil, we shall never be able to sow it, but soil that is free and open with plow shares is easier to work of the field. First, he makes wide furrows and later he makes small furrows. The plowman, as soon as he plows, smooths the surface of the soil and only after this he sows the land, the commentary explains that the way to sow black cumin is by "scattering it, and if he comes to sow cumin, he sows it by casting it Katzach which is a kind of food."

This is how God directs the prophets he sends to admonish a person, if the person he does not heed admonition, God shall penalize him with judgments of chastening in order that the effort of his admonition will help, like the one who smoothes the surface of the earth to sow, in order that the toil of his plowing that he plowed shall succeed. A wooden implement, made with grooves, and its name is "Morag," a threshing-board, and one cuts the straw with it to be straw fodder. The grooved tool is used to thresh the black cumin, for its seed making it easily extractable from within its straw.

The same system is used on regular cumin, they do not use the wheel of a wagon to thresh it, because the black cumin is easily beaten with a baton and the cumin with a cane. God compares the threshing of Black Cumin by using spiritual riddles and meanings through concrete and material forms. God says, by not harshly over threshing the seeds because they are very delicate, is like a person willing to accept reproof, so God will not be heavy with his decrees.

Black Pepper

Latin Name, Piper Nigrum
Aroma, Strong, hot and peppery

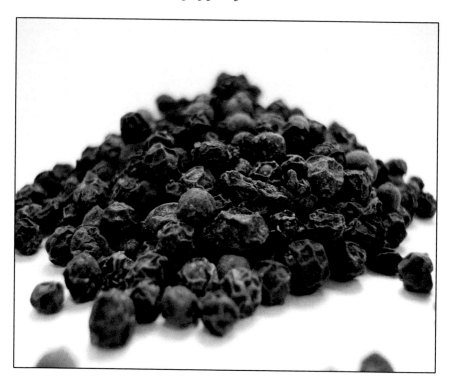

PHYSICAL

Black Pepper is a climbing plant that looks much like the Passiflora, passion fruit plant, and it has some fruit too called peppercorns. The fruits come in many colors, black, white, green, red, and pink, and are a native of tropical regions like the Middle East and Vietnam. They are used in many medicinal and beauty products and when dried, their essential oil can be extracted from the berries by crushing them. Black Pepper is an effective painkiller and reduces pain levels dramatically, it is great for inflammation especially when acute. It has anti-cancer properties and cleanses the system. It supports the immune system and circulatory system by excreting toxins efficiently. It also reduces hypertension and high blood pressure and improves blood circulation. Black Pepper helps the digestive system, fantastic for healing Helicobacter Pylori. It relaxes muscles spasms; stomach pains and works well against pathogens.

EMOTIONAL

Black pepper encourages fearlessness, providing strength and stamina with heightened endurance. It is motivational giving fortitude to venture into unknown places, this oil imbues faith and certainty in decisions and trusting one's own knowledge guiding every step of the way. Black pepper knows how to manipulate talents and ingenuity to create dreams to happen, it brings upon deep faith and certainty that protects and steers. With un-matched access to the Inner strength, this oil gives a powerful sense of spirit against adversity. With Black Pepper teaches how to listen and trust the inner voice and acquire inspiration from it.

BIBLICAL

"And they sat down to eat a meal, and they lifted their eyes and saw, and behold, a caravan of Ishmaelites was coming from Gilead, and their camels were carrying spices, balm, and lotus, going to take it down to Egypt. (Genesis 37:25)

"The charge of Eleazar the son of Aaron the kohen, oil for lighting, the incense of spices, the continual daily meal offering, and the anointing oil; the charge for the entire Mishkan and all that is in it, of the Holy and its furnishings." (Numbers 4:16)

"I have come to my garden, my sister, my bride; I have gathered my myrrh with my spice, I have eaten my sugar cane with my sugar, I have drunk my wine with my milk. Eat, friends; drink, yea, drink abundantly, beloved ones." (Song of Songs 5:1)

"I made myself gardens and orchards, and I planted in them all sorts of fruit trees." (Ecclesiastes 2:5)

"And Solomon reigned over all the kingdoms from the river to the land of the Philistines, and to the border of Egypt, they brought presents, and served Solomon all the days of his life." (I Kings 5:1)

"And three times in a year did Solomon offer up burnt-offerings and peace-offerings upon the altar he had built to the Lord, burning upon it incense upon the altar that was before the Lord, so he completed the service of the Temple." (I Kings 9:25)

Solomon recognized with his wisdom the veins of the earth which vein leads to Cush, and there he planted peppers; which one goes to a land of carob fruits, and there he planted carob trees. For all the veins of the lands all come to Zion, from where the world was founded, this is the meaning of, "all sorts of fruit trees." In biblical times the owner of many spices, was a rich man. Spices, herbs, balms, and wines were very much sought after and appreciated in those days.

"From Zion, the all-inclusive beauty."

People loved to come and hear the wisdom of Solomon, all kings of the world at that time had heard about his great wisdom. Hiram the king of Tyre sent his servants to Solomon, when he had heard that he had been anointed king in place of his father. Hiram was ever a lover of David, and they were great allies, Solomon sent word to Hiram, saying, since you knew my father, David then you know that he was not permitted to build the house of God because of the wars, which he was involved in. God put them under the soles of his feet, where the bible clearly states,

"You shall cross the Jordan and settle in the land the Lord, your God, is giving you as an inheritance, and He will give you rest from all your enemies surrounding you, and you will dwell securely."

When David conquered Jerusalem and crossed into Jordan to settle into the land the task was to be apportioned among the twelve tribes, every man was expected to recognize his portion and the territory of his tribe. After the conquering and the dividing of the land was completed, they obtained rest from the nations which God left around through whom to test Israel. The new generation that did not know about the miracles of the battles with Canaan and they did not witness the great acts of God, and began rebelling against God, and this happened only in the days of David.

Hiram supplied Solomon with cedar-trees, fir trees, and Tyrian constructors for the building of the Temple; in turn Solomon repaid him with wheat and olive oil. Solomon's and Hiram's builders were the Gebalites, who were a nation called Gebal who were skilled in the art of chiseling stones and building. Solomon hired them to hew them the rocks, and together they prepared the timber and the stones to build the house of God.

Cajaput

Latin Name, Melaleuca Leucadendra
Aroma, Strong, slightly sweet, Camphoraceous

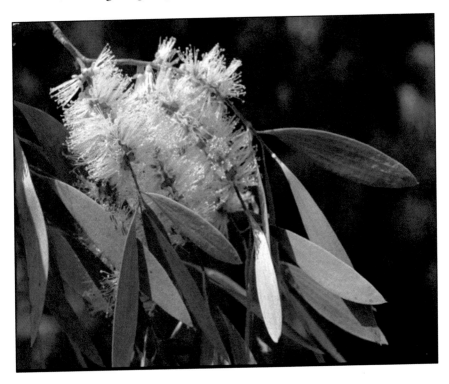

PHYSICAL

Cajaput oil is a wonderful essential oil that has been described as camphire, not to be confused with camphor. Its strong scents give a wonderful fragrant scent which wafts far forward and evaporates into the distance. Cajaput comes from the Eucalyptus, Tea Tree and Niaouli family raised in Australia. The Aborigines often used the cajaput tree bark for shields, canoes, roofing material and timber. It has a very sharp smell, all three of these oils contain anti-inflammatory properties. Coming from warm countries they learned to protect themselves from fungus wounds and skin damage. It is an anti-cancer for skin because of its dominant Cineol properties.

It melts away phlegm, eases respiratory infections of the bronchioles and even kills E-Coli. Cajaput kills infected bacterias caught from animals, impetigo that kids get from playing in the sand pit and psoriasis. Put a few drops into your aquarium to get rid of fungus. Cajaput is a painkiller for swollen joints anywhere in the body, from toxins that affect the shoulders and spinal problems.

EMOTIONAL

Cajaput oil stimulates the mind and promotes clear thinking, it relaxes, destresses, and relieves anxieties. Cajaput delivers the courage needed for introspection and helps identify dysfunctional behavior patterns in relationships. It stimulates cellular healing and bolsters the body to heal itself. Cajaput helps enhance self-esteem and enabling self-expression. It is believed to have mystical powers and has the power to protect against all kinds of evil powers.

BIBLICAL

A cluster of henna-flowers is my beloved to me, in the vineyards of Ein-Gedi." (Song of Songs 1:14)

"Your head upon you is like Carmel, and the braided locks of your head are like purple; the king is bound in the tresses." (Song of Songs 7:6)

"Myriads, like the plants of the field I have made you, and you have increased and grown, and you have come with perfect beauty, breasts fashioned, and your hair grown, but you were naked and bare."

"And I passed by you and saw you, and behold your time was the time of love, and I spread My skirt over you, and I covered your nakedness, and I swore to you and came into a covenant with you, says the Lord, and you were Mine." (Ezekiel 16:7-8)

Because of the levels of Cajaput's monoterpene alcohols, it is one of the ingredients that the Israelites needed to make Henna Powder and improve its skin stain characteristics. The word henna in Hebrew is kopher, this word is used several times in the Song of Songs, where it is known to be referred to as the henna plant. Camphire is Henna which originally grew in Egypt and India. Henna is regarded by Jews of Morocco and Yemen as a blessing, it is applied with complex patterns for luck as well as joy and beauty. It has become a popular tradition in modern Israel for Brides and their close family and friends to have beautiful designs painted on their hands and feet. In Judaism women's' beauty is very vital to the sanctity of marriage; a woman is expected to take care of herself and remain attractive to her husband. Beauty is an expression of perfection both inside and out, it is also related to the word for an eternity.

Henna branches are called a cluster of henna, a cluster in Hebrew means Eshkol, and is usually used to refer to a cluster of grapes. Here the word is intentionally used to refer to the henna's clustered flowers where the plant grows in a style of a cluster of grapes with small white and yellow odoriferous flowers. Ein Gedi is the name of a place in the south of Israel, where there is a legend that those vineyards in that place, would produce fruits four or five times a year. There runs a stream, which divides into many streams that sweetens the seas into which it mingles, many fish are swarming in those waters, very much alive and healthy. Fishermen would stand besides these streams all the way from Ein-Gedi to Ein-Eglaim, they spread their nets catching many kinds of fish from the great sea. On the banks of the streams from either side grew almost every kind of food bearing tree, their leaves never withered, and their fruits never stopped producing month after month ripe fruits. The legend was, "that its waters will emanate from the Sanctuary, and its fruit shall be for food and its leaves for a cure." This is symbolic of the many atonements and forgivenesses that God forgave the people of Israel for the many trials that they tried him when they wandered in the desert.

Calamus

Latin Name, Acorus Calamus
Aroma, Soft spicy, a little resembling cinnamon

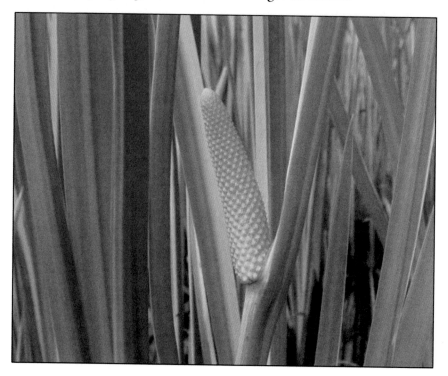

PHYSICAL

Calamus is an herbaceous flowering plant that has basal leaves that rise from a spreading rhizome, the leaves stand very straight and are flat and narrow, tapering into a long, acute point. The flower is a sweet flag that resembles an iris and has tiny green and yellowish flowers. It is native to India, Central Asia, China, and Japan and likes to live at the edges of small lakes, ponds and rivers, marshes, swamps, and wetlands. Calamus has been traded for thousands of years all over the Silk Road for its medicinal and healing qualities.

It was used to heal in treatments of inflammatory swellings and wounds, angina pectoris, severe sore throat, cough, arthritis, asthma, laryngitis, sinus congestion, sinus headaches, gastritis, gastric ulcers, colic pain, dyspepsia, diarrhea, anorexia, periodontal diseases, deafness, neuralgia, and shock.

Calamus has been banned from human use in 1968 by the United States Food and Drug Administration due to findings that the Indian Jammu version has a chemical called B-asarone, which is a cacogenic and develops tumors. The American Acorus Calamus does not contain this chemical and is safer to use.

EMOTIONAL

Calamus was used for anxiety, relieving panic attacks and clarifies perception and confusion. In Ayurvedic medicine it is used to help lucid mind and thoughts acting as a brain tonic promoting higher mental functions, much like Ritalin.

BIBLICAL

"Place fire into them and put incense upon them before the Lord tomorrow, and the man whom the Lord chooses he is the holy one; you have taken too much upon yourselves, sons of Levi."
(Numbers 16:7)

"Moses was exceedingly distressed, and he said to the Lord, "Do not accept their offering. I have not taken a donkey from a single one of them, and I have not harmed a single one of them."
(Numbers 16:15)

"Let each man take his censer and place incense upon it, and let each man present his censer before the Lord; there will thus be two hundred and fifty censers and let you and Aaron each take his censer." (Numbers 16:17)

"A fire came forth from the Lord and consumed the two hundred and fifty men who had offered up the incense." (Numbers 16:35)

"Spikenard and saffron, calamus and cinnamon, with all frankincense trees, myrrh and aloes, with all the chief spices."
(Song of Songs 4:14)

"Vedan and Javan gave spun silk into your treasure houses, iron wrought into ingots, cassia and calamus was in your stores."
(Ezekiel 27:19)

"Why do I need the frankincense that comes from Sheba, and the good cane from a distant country? Your burnt offerings are not acceptable, and your sacrifices are not pleasant to Me."
(Jeremiah 6:20)

The bible hints that Calamus is another version of "Cannabis" or Kaneh-Bosem as it is called in Hebrew, this plant was one of the thirteen oil essences used in the Ketoret, the incense for offerings to God. In the Bible it is referred to as sweet cane because of its sweet fragrance, pharmaceutical companies powder it down and use it for expensive perfumes.

Korach was the great grandson of Levi, and along with Dathan and Aviram, great grandsons of Reuben, contested the appointment of Aaron as high priest. Korach dissociated himself from the congregation in this persistent dispute. At the introduction of Korach, the bible omits that Korach is the direct descendant of Jacob, the reason being that Jacob prayed not to be mentioned in connection with this quarrel, his name is mentioned in connection with Korah, however, at the service of the Levites on the platform in the Temple, "the son of Korah, the son of Izhar, the son of Kohath, the son of Levi, the son of Israel." The reason Korah decided to quarrel with Moses was his resentment that Moses had appointed Elizaphan the son of Uzziel as chieftain over the sons of Kohath, who were Amram, Izhar, Hebron, and Uzziel.

Amram was the eldest, but his two younger sons received greatness, one became a king and other one a high priest. Korach expected that he was entitled to receive the second position since he was the son of Izhar, who is the second brother to Amram, but Moses appointed his youngest brother as chieftain. Korach assembled two hundred and fifty men, heads of Sanhedrin, most of them from the tribe of Reuben who were his neighbors. He dressed them with cloaks made entirely of blue wool and came and stood before Moses and asked him, "Does a cloak made entirely of blue wool require fringes "tzitzit" or is it exempt?" Moses replied that it does require fringes. Korach's men began laughing at Moses saying, "Is it possible that a cloak of another colored material, one string of blue wool exempts it from the obligation of techelet, and this one, which is made entirely of blue wool, should not exempt itself."

They accused Moses and Aaron, "you take by far too much greatness for yourselves." All of them had heard the words of the commandments at

Sinai straight from the mouth of the Almighty. The felt that since Moses have taken the role of kingship for himself, he should not have chosen the holy position of high Priest for his brother. Moses was devastated, this was their fourth rebellion, he became physically disheartened, and his hands were shaking, he did not know how much more he could take. Moses told Korach that God will tell him what to do in the morning, he told him since nighttime is a time of drunkenness and is improper to appear before God. His real intention was to delay the conversation with God in the hope that Korach might retract his opposition and hopefully draw close to him by then.

Korach refuses to reason with Moses, he tells his people that "among the different nations, there are various forms of worship, and they have many priests, and they do not gather in one temple. The Israelites, however, have only one God, one ark, one bible, one altar, and one high Priest and you two hundred and fifty men are all seeking holiness and I too would prefer that!" Korach continues, "here, take for yourselves the service most dear, it is the incense, more cherished than any other sacrifice, but it also contains deadly poisonous herbs, by which Nadab and Abihu were burnt, therefore be warned," Korach then challenges God and says, "and it will be the one whom the Lord chooses, he will be the holy one." Korach was insinuating that he himself was already in the state of holiness. It was obvious that he was the one who should have been chosen. Moses challenged them back, warning them that they had taken too much upon themselves.

> *"I am telling you this so that you should not be found guilty. For the one He chooses will survive, and the rest of you will perish."*

Their sins were risking their lives, but Korach was not astute enough to see his folly, his logic was deceiving him. He saw in a prophesy that Samuel will be his descendant and his greatness was said to be Moses and Aaron combined. He also saw twenty-four "seers" of Levites emanating from his grandsons, all prophesying through the divine spirit and Korach thought because of all these merits he will be spared. The thought, "Is it possible that all this greatness that is destined to emanate from me, and I should remain silent?" He erred in thinking whom God will choose, that it referred to him. Korach however, did not "see" properly, because his sons had repented and thus did not die at that time. Moses, however, foresaw this, he began to whisper to Korach, but he saw that he was adamant and would not budge. Moses thought, "before the rest of the tribe join him and thus perish with him, I will speak to all of them as well." He then began to speak to them,

> "Listen to me, sons of Levi, you and your entire company who are assembled here are against the Lord, because I acted as God's messenger, and his instruction was to give the kehunah to Aaron, so this rebellion is not against us but against God."

Moses was distressed that God was angry and he begged him not accept the incense that they will sacrifice before God and let the fire leave it and not consume it. The next morning the two-hundred and fifty men place their incense before God and then stood at the entrance of the Tent of Meeting with Moses and Aaron. With words of mockery Korach went around all that night long to all the tribes and attempting to entice them to rebel against Moses saying, "do you think I care only for myself? I care for all of you too, these people came and took all the high positions and the kingship for himself and the kehunah for his brother," until they were all enticed. Then God told Moses and Aaron, "Dissociate yourselves from this congregation, and I will consume them in an instant." Moses warned the people of Israel to also separate from Korach and his men, and they did, until it was only Korah, Dathan, Aviram and their families at the entrance of their tents with their wives, their children, and their infants.

God created a special punishment to kill them through a death by which no man had died until now. As soon as God finished speaking with them, the earth beneath them split opened its mouth and swallowed them and their houses, including all the men who were with Korah and all their property. They descended alive into the huge grave and the earth covered them up, and they were lost forever. All the other Israelites fled in pure terror screaming, "Lest the earth swallow us up too!" Suddenly a huge fire flared up and consumed the two hundred and fifty men who had offered up the incense with Korach. Now they understood how greatly they provoked God, the Rabbis say, this mouth had already created on earth from the time of creation for this unique punishment.

> "And the earth will open its mouth and swallow them up,"

Once Calamus was commonly grown as a garden plant, it is a plant that thrives in wet areas and was imported to Israel from India via spice traders. It was also called Lemon Grass or Ginger Grass because of its resemblance to Cinnamon, Maimonides confirms it identify as an Indian plant.

Caraway

Latin Name, Meridian Fennel
Aroma, Pungent anise like flavor

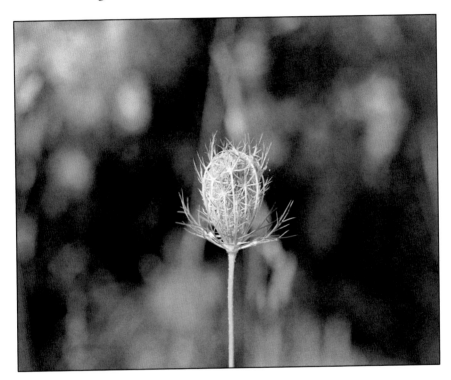

PHYSICAL

Caraway is native to Europe, Western Asia and North Africa, this plant is also a member of the carrot family and has white or pink flowers that grow in an umbrella shape. Also known as Kimmel Oil and comes from the Fennel and Cumin family. It has the same fragrance as fennel, anise, and licorice. Caraway is active with the Lymphatic System; it drains the body of excess mucus and improves mothers' milk.

Caraway eases PMS symptoms, it protects the uterus It combats cancerous cells such as breast cancer. Caraway fruit oil is also used as a fragrance in soaps, lotions, and perfumes. Caraway is also used as a breath freshener, and it has a long tradition of use in holistic medicine. It is an antihistamine and assists the digestive system, gall bladder and liver. It helps digestive issues and babies' gassy stomachs and should only be taken externally with a base oil, spread on stomach. Use as an herbal tea to sooth heartburn and to dispel worms.

EMOTIONAL

Increases circulation and improves conscious mind dispels feelings of sluggishness, paleness, stress, fatigue, and wane. It warms and stimulates gently and improves the mood. This plant has strong protective properties to maintain a deep inner balance. It is a great oil to use in a diffuser.

BIBLICAL

"Abram said, "Behold, you have given me no seed, and behold, one of my household will inherit me." (Genesis 15:3)

"He took him outside, and He said, "Please look heavenward and count the stars, if you are able to count them." And He said to him, "So will be your seed." (Genesis 15:5)

"He said to Abram, "You shall surely know that your seed will be strangers in a land that is not theirs, and they will enslave them and oppress them, for four hundred years." (Genesis 15:13)

"On that day, the Lord formed a covenant with Abram, saying, "To your seed I have given this land, from the river of Egypt until the great river, the Euphrates River." (Genesis 15:18)

"Is it not so? When he smooths its surface, he scatters the black cumin and casts the cumin, and he places the prominent wheat, and the barley for a sign, and the spelt on its border." (Isaiah 28:25)

"For not with a grooved implement is black cumin threshed, neither does a wagon wheel turn around on cumin, but black cumin is beaten with a staff and cumin with a rod." (Isaiah 28:27)

"This too comes forth from the Lord of Hosts, He gave marvelous counsel, made great wisdom." (Isaiah 28:29)

Caraway was a very common spice, known as a seed, mentioned in the bible, and known because of its similarity to black cumin. It is thought to be the product the passage is referring to in Isaiah, who was known to cultivate spices in the bible guided by God. He was instructed exactly how to thresh the black cumin and pepper to make it right. In modern times we use caraway in many dishes, salads, and rye bread for that unique flavor.

Abram said to God, "O Lord God, what will You give me, since I am going childless, and the steward of my household is Eliezer of Damascus?" Abraham points out to God that he is without an heir and his heart is broken about it, saying, "if only I had a son, my son would be appointed over my possessions." He has prayed to God many times, but to no avail, and he is afraid that his manservant Eliezer will inherit his possessions. God reassures him by saying, "this one will not inherit you, but the one who will spring from your innards he will inherit you." God took him outside of his tent to see the stars, the Midrash interprets this to mean, that God told him to check out of his astrology and showing him the signs of the zodiac where he was not destined to have a son. Indeed, Abram will have no son, but Abraham was destined to have a son, just like Sarai will not give birth, but Sarah will give birth and so God changed their destiny.

Even though Abraham believed God, he found the situation unbelievable, and asked God, "how will I know?" God answered him, "I am the Lord, who brought you forth from Ur of the Chaldees, to give you this land to inherit it." Abraham further asks God, "O Lord God, how will I know that I will inherit it?" God asked him to bring as a sacrifice three calves, three goats, three rams, a turtle dove and a young bird and Abraham divided each one into two parts. Abraham knew that God was forming a covenant with him to keep his promise and enable his sons to inherit the land. It was the custom in those times, that in order to form a covenant they had to divide the animals and pass the smoking furnace, which was a band of fire, between the two sections, this was the agent of the holy spirit of God, seen in the form of the fire.

Abraham divided up the animals but not the birds, because the animals represented to him all the countries of the world which will gradually perish, but the Israelites he likened to the young doves, as an allusion that Israel will exist forever. Suddenly all the birds of prey, said to be eagles, swooped down onto the carcasses and Abraham shewed them away. Because of this David the son of Jesse will be destined to destroy them, but they will not permit him from heaven to do so until the King Messiah arrives. From the time that Isaac was born until the Israelites' left Egypt

157

was four-hundred years, Isaac was sixty years old when Jacob was born, and Jacob went down to Egypt for one hundred and thirty years, totaling one-hundred and ninety years. The Israelites were slaves in Egypt for two-hundred and ten years, totaling four-hundred years.

Cardamom

Latin Name, Elettaria Cardamonum
Aroma, Fresh sweetish green, spicy

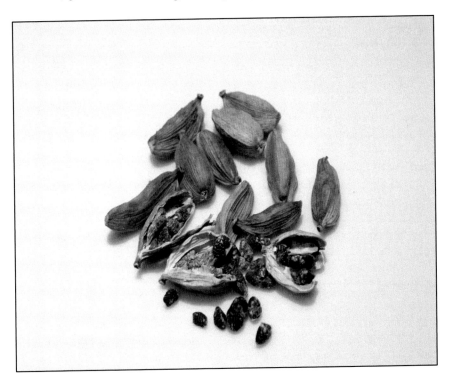

PHYSICAL

The oil comes from its green seeds, which must be kept in the freezer since it deteriorates quickly. Cardamom is used for the nervous system because of its relaxing properties, containing linalool like Lavender, making it a very rich relaxant. Cardamom is from the ginger family, and therefore it is great for the digestive system, especially for a flatulent stomach. Also used to relieve Fissura, hemorrhoids, nausea, and heartburn. Cardamom is also used for psoriasis, hemorrhoids and nervous headaches generated from stress, it is used to relieve wounds pains and nausea caused from chemotherapy.

In Arabic it is called "hel," and is drunk with black coffee as an enhancement with this amazing and unique flavor. Generally used in the coffee drunk after meals, because coffee constricts and produces stimulant acids which accelerate the system with adrenaline. These acids may cause high Blood Pressure and is best used in green coffee which is not roasted.

EMOTIONAL

This oil has the power to bring back memories of incarnation, giving wisdom to deal with responsibilities of this life. Cardamom encourages clarity, concentration and gives a feeling of very clear directions. It motivates moving forward with enthusiasm, confidence, and courage it's always a constant forward movement without looking back.

Cardamom opens the generosity of spirit, teaching graciousness and kind when dealing with others. Always the first to step forward and offer help and friendship to persons who needs it most, even if at first there was an aversion to them. It stimulates spiritual sensitivity and activates a deep and long buried magnanimous inner beauty allowing one to see with the heart.

BIBLICAL

"God said, "Let us make man in our image, after our likeness, and they shall rule over the fish of the sea and over the fowl of the heaven and over the animals and over all the earth and over all the creeping things that creep upon the earth." (Genesis 1:26)

"The traffickers of Sheba and Raamah they were your traffickers; with the best of all spices and with all precious stones and gold they gave your merchandise." (Ezekiel 27:22)

"And oil for lighting, and spices for the anointing oil and for the incense." (Exodus 35:8)

For centuries in the Middle East green cardamom powder was used as a spice for sweet dishes, as well as traditional flavoring in coffee and tea. Now a days Cardamom is used to a wide extent in savory dishes, but some Middle Eastern countries will still offer your coffee with cardamom. Since man was created in the likeness of the angels, because God knew they would envy man, so to prevent this situation, he consulted with the angels. Among the heavenly beings, there are some in God's likeness so there had to be some earthly beings in God's likeness too. If there are none in his likeness, then there would be envy among the all the creatures of Creation. Sometimes even God needs to consult with his heavenly household of angels to judge his earthly kings. God has a team of angels standing on the right as the defense, and his team of angels standing on the left are the prosecutors. The decree of the destructive angels of the left is taken into consideration as advice only by God, however the final word of the decree is always by the holy and merciful one.

Even though the angels did not assist God in the creation process, the scripture says that God consulted with his angel only to teach proper conduct and enhance the trait of humility. Every great person should consult with and receive advice from a lesser one. God created rules over the fish of subservience, if he merits, then he shall rule over the beasts and over the cattle. If he does not merit, he becomes subservient to them, and the beast will rule over him. Once God created man in his image, he created both male and female and commanded them,

> *"Be fruitful and multiply and fill the earth and subdue it, and rule over the fish of the sea and over the fowl of the sky and over all the beasts that tread upon the earth. I have given you every seed beasts of the earth."*

God equated cattle and the beasts to man regarding the food they were permitted to eat. He did not permit Adam and Eve to kill any creature to eat its flesh, but they were permitted to eat every green herb equal with the animals. When the sons of Noah came, however God permitted them to eat flesh, only because man's awareness had lowered and so in addition to the green herbs which he permitted to Adam and Eve, he added the permission to eat animals. At the completion of the creation, God stipulates that man was created on the condition that Israel accepts the Five Books of the Torah. The works of creation were all paused until the "sixth day," because the sixth day was the day God prepared himself for the giving of the Torah.

Carob

Latin Name, Ceratonia Siliqua
Aroma, Fresh sweetish musk, cocoa

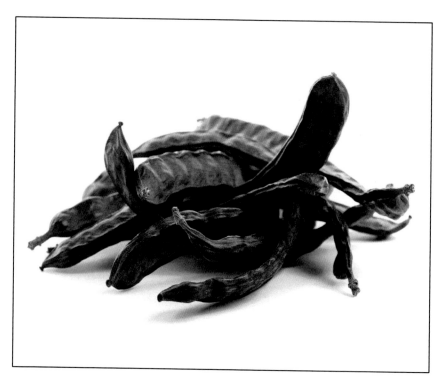

PHYSICAL

Carob trees are natives of the Mediterranean basin, the trees grow in abundance all over Israel to heights of six to ten meters because it thrives in dry climates and adapts very well to poor and salty soil. Its fruits are long pods that contain a sweet starchy pulp with a slightly chocolate type of flavor and is a member of the pea family. Most carob trees are dioecious, and some are hermaphroditic, so strictly male trees do not produce fruit. When the trees blossom in autumn, the flowers are small and numerous, spirally arranged along the inflorescence axis in catkin-like racemes borne on spurs from old wood and even on the trunk cauliflory; they are pollinated by both wind and insects. The male flowers smell like human semen, an odor that is caused in part by amines.

Carob seeds are processed to produce a gum used in the food industry as a thickener and its fruit contains important essential oils with antioxidant properties. In fact, it is the source for many products such as gum, sugar, and alcohol as well as for aromatic substances that are widely used in the perfume industries. Its oil contains hydrocarbons, fatty acids, sterols, carotenoids, waxes, tannins, coumarins, and flavonoids, and purification of its essential oils are processes that last for many years, the two most common extractions are, solvent and steam distillation. It is very often used as a chocolate substitute; the carbo is rich in fiber and low in fat. It may also be effective for weight loss because it helps to decrease the amount of ghrelin, the hunger hormone produced in the body.

Carobs does not contain oxalates which are the natural compounds found in many foods that bind to calcium, oxalates are generally eliminated in the stool, and bolstering more calcium excretion, and a diet containing high levels of oxalates can increase the chances of developing kidney stones,

EMOTIONAL

Carob is used as a chocolate substitute and unlike cocoa, carob contains no caffeine or theobromine. Both of Caffeine and Cocoa are stimulants, Caffeine affects the central nervous system and theobromine stimulates the cardiovascular and pulmonary systems. Acetone was extracted from fresh carob pods and were analyzed to contain tannins which acts as an antidepressant with both the action of adrenergic and the dopaminergic systems. Carob supports psychological and physical problems such as stress, depression, fatigue, and laziness. Carob is also rich with a wide variety of polyphenols as well as with a high antioxidant value and prevents stress-induced memory impairment and enhances learning and memory.

BIBLICAL

"He said: The LORD came from Sinai; He shone upon them from Seir; He appeared from Mount Paran, and approached from Ribeboth-kodesh, Lightning flashing at them from His right."
(Deuteronomy 33:2)

"I made myself gardens and orchards, and I planted in them all sorts of fruit trees." (Ecclesiastes 2:5)

"Among trees: the sumac, the carob, the nut, the almond, the grapevine, the pomegranate, the olive and the palm are subject to peah." (Mishnah Peah 1:5)

"The LORD will guide you always; He will slake your thirst in parched places and give strength to your bones. You shall be like a watered garden, like a spring whose waters do not fail."
(Isiah 58:11)

"They shall not build for others to dwell in, or plant for others to enjoy. For the days of My people shall be as long as the days of a tree, my chosen ones shall outlive the work of their hands."
(Isiah 65:22)

"They shall not toil to no purpose; They shall not bear children for terror, but they shall be a people blessed by the LORD, and their offspring shall remain with them." (Isiah 65:23)

In archeological studies, Carob was used by human beings since very ancient times, mainly by nations of the Mediterranean basin have such recorded uses. Ancient Egyptians were known to feed carob pods to their livestock, and it is also believed that they used carob gum as a form of glue in their mummification processes. The Aramaic word for carob is "kharubha," which is similar to the Hebrew word "harub." In Arabic kharrub, means "locust bean pod," and in English, it is also known as "St John's bread." Solomon had planted peppers in the past, which normally does not grow in Israel, then he experimented again and planted carob trees, he wished to take advantage of all the veins of all the lands that reach Zion. It is believed that it is from Zion that the world was founded,

"Out of Zion, the perfect beauty, where every kind of fruit tree is found, as the days of the tree that lives for a long time, as the Carob and similar trees."

The prophet Elijah appeared to Rabbi Shimon ben Yochai and his son Eleazar in the cave where they were in hiding from the Romans, there Elijah planted a carob tree and provided a well of spring water from which the two men ate and drank during the twelve years they spent in hiding, enabling them to escape prosecution by the Romans. Elijah visited them

164

twice daily and gave them lessons of the torah, one of the lessons Elijah taught them was how to make use of God's input into the physical parts of the universe. God had to "clothe Himself," to conceal his essence and to restrict the brightness and holiness he radiated, which would have been too overwhelming for the beneficiaries. The AriZal explains,

"All parts of the universe require that God's essence reduces its natural radiations, as all creatures in varying degrees are unable to withstand the brilliance of the emanations from God's essence unless they had first been screened to some extent."

Those who sow with tears will reap with song, he will go along weeping, carrying the valuable seeds; he will come back with song, carrying his sheaves. So, will Israel in exile sow charity in tears, and they will reap it when God pays their reward in the future. Ancestors sow seeds, with tears for their descendants, knowing that only their descendants will reap with joy the benefits of their work.

Rabbi Yohanan, also known as Choni the Circle maker, was wondering, "Is there someone who can fall asleep for seventy years in a dream?' One day, he was walking on the road and saw a certain man planting a carob tree.

Rabbi Yohanan asked him, *"How many years will it be until this tree will be laden with fruit?"*

The man answered him, *"it will take seventy years."*

Rabbi Yohanan asked him, *"is it obvious to you that you will live for another seventy years?"*

The man answered him, *"that man found the world with carob trees. In the same way as my fathers planted for me, I will also plant for my children."*

Rabbi Yohanan sat and ate his meal and soon fell asleep, a boulder encircled him, and he was not able to see around him, and he fell asleep for seventy years. When he awoke, he saw a certain man that was plucking the fruits of the carob tree.

Rabbi Yohanan asked him, *"are you the man who planted this tree?"*

The man answered him, *"I am the son of his son."*

Rabbi Yohanan said to him, *"now I understand from this that I fell asleep for seventy years."*

He saw that his donkey had given birth to several generations, and he went to his home, and he said to them, Is the son of Choni the Circle maker alive? They said to him, "his son is not, but the son of his son is."

Rabbi Yohanan announced to them, "I am Choni the Circle maker," and they did not believe him. So, he went to the study hall, and he heard the rabbis who were saying, "Our discussions are as clear as in the years of Choni the Circle maker.

He began coming to the study hall regularly and he would answer all the questions that the rabbis had. After some time, he thought he could reveal to the Rabbi and students his true identity, and Rabbi Yohanan said to them, "I am he, Choni the Circle Maker." They did not believe his story, and they did not give him the respect that was appropriate to a Rabbi of his caliber.

Rabbi Yohanan began to feel very upset about his situation, life as he knew it was gone, his peers and students were no longer alive, and he prayed to God for mercy and died. This is what is meant by the saying, "either companionship or death."

Carrot Seed

Latin Name, Daucus Carota
Aroma, Dry earthy

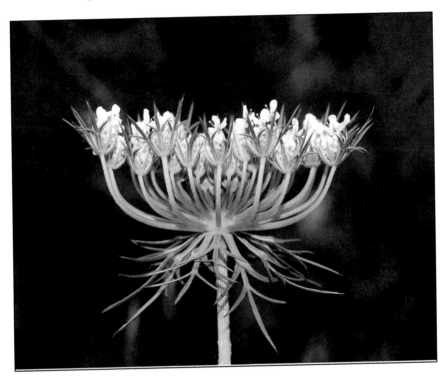

PHYSICAL

Carrot seed comes from Europe and southwest Asia whose names include wild carrot, bird's nest, bishop's lace, and Queen Anne's lace and resembles a royal crown. The oil is taken from the seeds, and contains Beta Carotene and Vitamin A. This means it is great for skin problems, especially acne, skin scars, stretch marks, dry skin, and eczema. Carrot Seed promotes cellular regeneration, skin nourishment, and reduces acne and wrinkles. The Vitamin A also helps liver problems such as hepatitis, cirrhosis, and mucus, this is a very expensive oil. As we know that Vitamin A is also used to improve eyesight and night vision.

EMOTIONAL

Carrot seed is helpful in uplifting emotions and reducing anxiety especially mood swings. This oil strengthens the spirit and eases that feeling of vulnerability allowing the feeling of encouragement and a sense of inner peace and security. It eases and relaxes busy minds that causes insomnia and soothes chronic emotional and enables the start of relaxation. Carrot seed oil stops those negative feelings of enslavement and obliterates the urge for negative actions.

Once people are released from their boundaries then they can begin to enjoy the fullness and totality of spirit so that the Carrot Seed can break through and teach appreciation of life.

BIBLICAL

"And it will cause thorns and thistles to grow for you, and you shall eat the herbs of the field." (Genesis 3:18)

For the land to which you are coming to possess is not like the land of Egypt, out of which you came, where you sowed your seed and which you watered by foot, like a vegetable garden." (Deuteronomy 11:10)

"And when the word burst forth, the Children of Israel increased the first of corn, wine, oil, honey, and all the increase of the field, and the tithes of everything they brought in abundance." (II Chronicles 31:5)

"And Ahab spoke to Naboth saying, "Give me your vineyard and I will have it for a vegetable garden since it is near my house, and I will give you instead of it a vineyard which is better than it, if it pleases you, I will give you money, it's worth." (I Kings 21:2)

We are taught to respect the earth and mixing plants seeds is not good for the land, this causes thorns and thistles to grow instead of vegetables. Carrots are native to Europe and southwestern Asia and are close relatives to parsley, cilantro, coriander, fennel, anise, dill, and cumin which are all grown for their leaves and seeds. While the Jews lived in the land of Egypt, they were required to bring water from the Nile by foot to water their plants, once in Israel, they learned that the Land of Israel absorbs water more easily from the rains of the heaven. The saying was "While you sleep in your bed," actually hints that there was no need to toil as hard in Israel as they did in Egypt to work the land, much like modern day "passive income."

King Ahab married to Jezebel desired Naboth's property which was adjoining to the palace land. Naboth explained to Ahab that his property was an inheritance from his parents, and he was forbidden to sell his land. Ahab sulked and went to bed crying and when his wife, Jezebel came home and found him lying face down on his bed, she asked him to explain.

"I will not give you the inheritance of my forefathers."

Jezebel did not understand how Ahab did not exercise his kingly power to simply confiscate Naboth's land. She told him to get out of bed and she would get the land for him, which she did by forging her husband's seal in a letter to the elders and officials of the city. She demanded that they proclaim a fast day immediately to atone "sins," and set up a false hearing against poor Naboth. She implanted two evil men in the witness box to testify against Naboth for blaspheme against God and king. Naboth was then removed and sentenced to death by stoning, once he was dead, Jezebel told Ahab to go and take possession of Naboth's vineyards. Some Sages say that the property of those executed by the king belong to the king, while others say that Ahab was the son of his Naboth's uncle, and he himself killed Naboth and his children and therefore inherited his property.

God was furious and ordered Elijah the prophet at that time to visit Ahab in Samaria, and he will find him in Naboth's vineyards where he has gone to take possession of it. God told Elijah to ask him straight, "have you murdered and also inherited?" God sent a message through Elijah telling Ahab, "In the place that the dogs have licked the blood of Naboth, shall the dogs lick your blood, and yours." Elijah told Ahab, "You sold yourself to anger your creator, and now you will sell yourselves there to your enemies." Elijah continued, "also concerning Jezebel, God spoke saying, 'The dogs will eat Jezebel in the valley of Jezreel," and all who die for Ahab will be devoured in the fields by the fowls of the sky.

God was so angry at Ahab that he said that there was no other king as evil as Ahab. The Scripture testifies that all those who worshipped calves out of fear of Ahab, because he would not allow them to go up to Jerusalem to return to the house of David. Ahab had forced them to worship Baal and the Asherah because Ahab had sold himself to idolatry, and this further added to the fury of God. Once Ahab heard these words, he immediately repented and tore his garments, he put a sackcloth over his flesh and he fasted, and he lay in the sackcloth and walked barefoot slowly. For this God had mercy on Ahab and did not bring disaster to his house in his days, but the decree that the dogs will lick his blood is impossible to come in the days of his son but will come upon him for sure.

Cassia

Latin Name, Cinnamomum Cassia
Aroma, Spicy, woody, and earthy

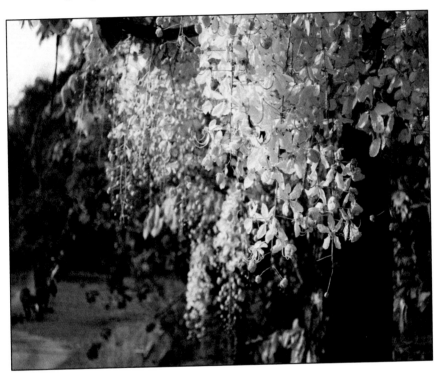

PHYSICAL

Cassia is also known as Chinese Cassia; it is an evergreen that originated in Southern China and East Asia. Not to be confused with Cinnamon, Cassia is often referred to as fake Cinnamon because has the same fragrance. Cassia does not have the same characteristics or properties that Cinnamon has. It is not as strong and can be used to heat without the intense constriction of Cinnamon. Cassia is a Camphoraceous oil and stimulates the blood system, lowers blood pressure. A great oil to use in a massage because of its ability to warm without affecting the heart.

EMOTIONAL

Cassia is all hugs; it listens and gives a great feeling, for those who keep their feelings locked inside, cassis extracts them out. This oil helps people who find it hard to voice their feelings and is perfect for heart-to-heart conversations. Cassia is used to help with deep emotional problems and melancholy. It is like reaching for the chocolates instead of asking for a hug. This oil helps prevent emotional eating and gives that loving feeling without needing the food. Its energy generates sensual warmth with masculine protective instincts.

BIBLICAL

"Myrrh and aloes and cassia are all your garments; more than ivory palaces, those that are Mine will cause you to rejoice."
(Psalm 45:9)

"Vedan and Javan gave spun silk into your treasure houses, iron wrought into ingots, cassia and calamus was in your stores."
(Ezekiel 27:19)

"Now the Lord blessed Job's end more than his beginning, and he had fourteen thousand flocks and six thousand camels and a thousand yoke of cattle and a thousand she-donkeys."

"And he had fourteen sons and three daughters."

"And he named the first Jemimah, the second Keziah, and the third Keren-Happuch."

"Nowhere in the land were women as beautiful as Job's daughters to be found, and their father gave them an inheritance among their brothers."

"Now Job lived thereafter one hundred and forty years, and he saw his sons and his sons' sons for four generations."

"Then Job died, being old and sated with days." (Job 42:12-17)

Cassia is one of the most difficult of the eleven spices to identify in the passages of Exodus. The word Cassia really translates as curtsey or bow. It comes from an aromatic bark of this fragrant tree, which is thought to be from the Cinnamomum. It was used as the fourth fragrance in the Ketoret, the holy incense blend of the temple of Jerusalem. Job was one of three royal advisors to Pharaoh when the Israelites were enslaved in Egypt. He was part of the team who assisted the king in deliberating over the plot to murder all male Israelite newborns. When Job understood the enormity of this proposal, Job was indifferent and did not have the courage to protest the decree, and this was the reason that his inaction later caused God to bring immense suffering upon his life. In just a single day, he loses all his children, many of his servants and livestock, and the remaining animals are captured and stolen. God had sent a destructive angel to test his faith, and indeed Job's reaction was of faith and humility. Job said,

"I came out of my mother's womb naked, and I will return there naked. God has given and God has taken, may the name of God be blessed."

The destructive angel wished to intensify Job's suffering by striking him with severe boils over his entire body, but Job refused to curse with his lips at his situation. The Talmud says that in his heart he may have cursed, but he still refused to actually say the curses out loud. He asked, "is it possible that we are willing to accept the good from God only without being willing to also accept the bad?" Finally, God openly admonishes Job directly, driving home to him all his inadequacies as a man, and his inherent inability to grasp the wisdom of God. God asks him, "where were you when I founded the earth? Speak up if you have understanding!" Job immediately recognizes his errors and begs God for forgiveness, and he prays for his companions, so God restores his fortune and increases it two-fold. Job's later years are defined by his phenomenal material success, until his passing.

Job had fourteen sons and three daughters and was very proud of his daughters, he named each girl according to her beauty. The first daughter he named Jemimah, because she was as white and bright as the sun. His second daughter he named her Keren-Happuch due to her large eyes, and his third daughter he named, Keziah because she had a beautiful natural fragrance, perfumed scent like the spice cassia. Job knew that nowhere in the land were there women as beautiful as his daughters, and Job was so advanced for his times; that he treated his daughters equal to his sons and left them their rightful share of his inheritance along with their brothers. He lived to the ripe old age of one-hundred and forty and managed to see four generations.

Cedarwood

Latin Name, Cedrus Libani
Aroma, Warm, sweet soft and woody

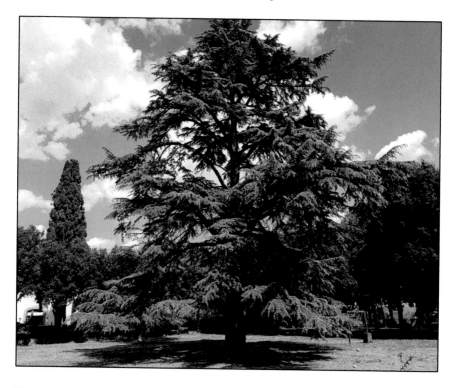

PHYSICAL

Cedarwood is indigenous to the Middle East and is a native of the Mediterranean basin, they grow in Israel in the Upper Galilee area and the Judean Desert. Its tree has needles, silver green leaves, pinecones, and they grow very tall, some up to forty meters with a massive trunk. Its oil is of a very heavy consistency and not very fluid but has a beautiful woody scent. It is a great oil that blends well with other oils, allowing them to be absorbed into the blood stream well. Cedarwood is an antiseptic, tonic and an anti-spasmodic and is good for young mothers, or young girls suffering from long painful periods. People with Epstein's Bar or tired and stressed who don't sleep well will benefit from this oil's quality. Cedar oil is a turpentine oil extracted from the wood, was used in ancient times as a preservative for parchments and garments. Use this oil for people who have a low immune system because of its regenerative qualities.

EMOTIONAL

This strong tree imbues a powerful feeling when it is inhaled. Cedarwood is good for empowering kids and adults, preventing fears of taking control and stops loving too much and being unable to forgive and encourages moving forward. It is also helpful clumsy people, unpopular kids and unfocused people who are not able to deal with life challenges, this is the oil. Cedarwood works via the spinal cord, giving courage and backbone, it does this by stimulating the hypothalamus and pineal gland, which are both associated with spiritual sight and development.

Cedarwood helps unite hope and reality and always driving forward till the end. For those who are afraid of everything, who are cowardly, this oil helps them get stronger. Cedarwood is an ancient spirit who has lived through many humankind existences, its superior soul stabilizes the earth and drives away negative influences and evil spirits.

Warning this oil is not to be used by nursing mothers because it constricts.

BIBLICAL

"And you shall say, So, said the Lord God, the great eagle with great wings and long pinions, full of feathers, who had diverse colors, came to the Lebanon and took the lofty top of the cedar." (Ezekiel 17:3)

"So says the Lord God, And I Myself will take from the lofty top of the cedar, and I will place it; I will crop off from the topmost of its young twigs a tender one, and I Myself will plant it upon a high and lofty mountain." (Ezekiel 17:22)

"In the mountain of the height of Israel I will plant it, and it will bear boughs and bring forth fruit and become a sturdy cedar, and under it shall dwell all birds of every feather; in the shade of the branches thereof shall they dwell." (Ezekiel 17:23)

"Behold Assyria was a cedar in Lebanon, with beautiful branches, shady woods, and of tall stature, and among the interwoven branches was its lofty top." (Ezekiel 31:3)

"Cedars did not dim it in the garden of God, junipers did not equal its boughs, and chestnut trees were not like its branches; no tree in the garden of God equaled it in its beauty."
(Ezekiel 31:8)

"It shall blossom and rejoice, even to rejoice and to sing; the glory of the Lebanon has been given to her, the beauty of the Carmel and the Sharon; they shall see the glory of the Lord, the beauty of our God." (Isaiah 35:2)

"The trees of the Lord are full of sap; the cedars of Lebanon, which he has planted" (Psalms 104:16)

The Lebanon Cedarwood Tree is called Erez in Hebrew and is mentioned several times in the bible always in an admirable context. This tree has many roles to play in the bible, one of which is to treat leprosy. The Kohen, who is the high priests uses the bark of the cedarwood tree to treat it, as ordered by Moses. In the bible it is always called the Cedars of God, it was one of the last visible evidence of the sweeping forests of Lebanon. In ancient times Lebanon was once a flourishing forest across its mountains. However, since then its timber was exploited by the many nations and civilization building their constructions for habitat, one of whom was King Solomon who also used plenty of cedarwood timber to build the Holy Temple in Jerusalem.

Prophecies in the bible are usually expressed in riddles and there is a riddle written where God compares Nebuchadnezzar to an eagle, and the kings of Judah are compared to the lofty tops of cedarwood trees. The eagle is described to have long pinions, which are their wide range wings and their bodies of diverse embroidered colors with beautiful ornate feathers. The lofty tops of the cedars are characterized to have all the foliage of the trees, God depicts them as Jehoiakim, one of the kings of Judah, and his large army of mighty men. The eagle flies above the trees and plucks at the top of the branches, whereby compromising and humbling Jehoiakim's legendary greatness and his monarchy. When the branches of the cedarwood trees are snapped and dropped upon the ground in a land of merchants, that is known as Babylon.

The second story goes, God took of the seed of the land, who is Zedekiah and his son, into a fertile field full of seeds located in Jerusalem the capital city of Israel. The seeds take root besides abundant waters and became deeply rooted besides these waters, giving the seed much greatness and dominion over his surroundings. The seed grows into a large mountain willow tree of many branches, spreading out with long overhanging lengths, and is a tree of low stature ordained to serve the king of Babylon. Its tendrils and branches are attracted to grow towards the king of Babylon, while underneath it is the king, a vine sprouting branches and growing many boughs and leaves. Now there was one specific eagle, who was the king of Egypt, he was gathering roots in anticipation of hunger, because a famine was expected to arrive in Egypt. The roots of this vine hungered and longed for the eagle; the Sages adduce that it is something similar to a leader's call of public gathering. The trees tendrils are sent forth towards him sending her emissaries to catch his attention, calling him to come to her, water her from the furrows of its planting, when the eagle in the riddle comes and waters the tendrils of the tree from the ditches, it has made for the beautiful tree.

The Hebrew prophet Isaiah mentions Lebanon cedarwood tree as an analogy to describe striving for merit and self-growth. He explicitly mentions the Cedarwood tree as a symbol of righteousness due to their conifer shape that points to the sky, which also signifies heaven. Cedarwood trees are often used as a symbol of immortality and spiritual elevation. Cedarwood trees are referred to in the bible with admiration at every mention because of their tall impressive and proud stature.

Chamomile

Latin Name, Anthemis Nobilis
Aroma, Sweet, fresh herbal and like an apple

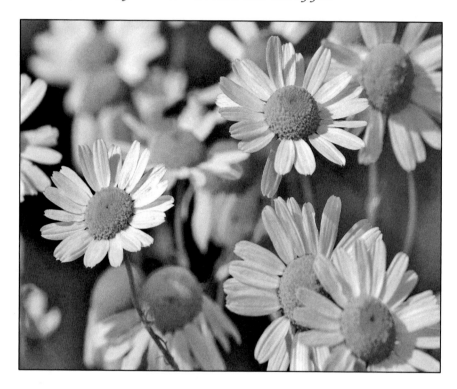

PHYSICAL

This Chamomile is found in dry fields and gardens and has a daisy like white flower. It is a native to Southern and Western Europe and the Middle East and is an herbaceous plant with strong fibrous roots. It is used in shampoo and conditioner and for rinses of natural blonde hair. Chamomile meaning "earth-apple" because of the apple-like aroma set forth from the plant. Chamomile blue refers to its chamazulene, which is a chemical compound with the molecular formula also found in wormwood and Yarrow. The chamazulene is the purified deep-blue essential oil is obtained using steam distillation, rather than from the plant itself.

Chamomile Roman essential oil is clear and contains ninety percent Esters and is waterier than other Chamomiles. This oil is great to use for crying babies with colic, it calms their stomach and relaxes them in general. Chamomile heals the painful cracked nipples that sometimes develop during breastfeeding. It reduces swellings a good oil to use if going through radiation treatments. This oil is a calmative, analgesic, an anti-spasmodic, an anti-inflammatory and a sleep aid. Even though this oil is very gentle, at the same time, it is very powerful and affects the nervous system. As an antiseptic and anti-spasmodic chamomile also combats fungus and parasites. As a sedative it is very relaxing and calming, it reduces stress and may cause sleepiness. It reduces hyperactivity and stress, takes away a bad mood and eases emotional problems. Since it affects the nervous system, it helps digestive and hepatic functions, it will sooth sore stomachs and irritable bowel syndrome. Chamomile German also solves skin and fungal problem and assists skin problems such as eczema and acne.

Warning do not administer to Pregnant Women because it can cause uterine contractions and miscarriage. Do not use this oil on a regular basis, too much use of more than a month can affect the thyroid causing it to absorb less Iodine, though babies can use for it for slightly longer.

EMOTIONAL

This chamomile encourages calm relaxation, a very still and gentle type of relaxation. It's so soothing that it gives out a deep feeling of serenity and if meditating, a sense of acute spiritual awareness is achieved with a unique experience of real Inner peace with an understanding and harmonizing unity. Chamomile is very soothing to the soul; its peacefulness resonates beyond the realms of auric light, it reaches way into the inner child, allowing access to the mysterious within and unites individual spirituality. Their petals motivate the expression of appreciation and gratitude for all the fragrances that this flower contributes to this world.

Chamomile encourages communication and understanding in a perceptive way. It's empathetic and patient manner awards the ability to be calming and soothing spiritually, chamomile petals open towards the sun and pulls in the solar energy, absorbing a deeper wisdom of the cosmos while at the same time maintains a down to earth characteristic due to its earthy fragrance helping to clarify the meaning of life. Meditation with this oil encourages the feeling of clarity to open to deeper meaning within.

BIBLICAL

"And the screen of the gate of the courtyard was the work of an embroiderer, made of blue, purple, and crimson wool, and twisted fine linen, twenty cubits long, and its height in the width was five cubits, corresponding to the hangings of the courtyard." (Exodus 38:18)

"Speak to the children of Israel and you shall say to them that they shall make for themselves fringes on the corners of their garments, throughout their generations, and they shall affix a thread of sky-blue wool on the fringe of each corner."
(Numbers 15:38)

"And two doors of olive-wood, and he carved upon them carvings of cherubim and palm trees and open flowers, and he overlaid them with gold; and spread the gold upon the cherubim, and upon the palm trees." (I Kings 6:32)

"A voice says, "Call!" and it says, "What shall I call?" "All flesh is grass, and all its kindness is like the blossom of the field."
(Isaiah 40:6)

"Speak to the children of Israel and you shall say to them that they shall make for themselves fringes on the corners of their garments, throughout their generations, and they shall affix a thread of sky-blue wool on the fringe of each corner."
(Numbers 15:38)

'There were spreads of white, fine cotton, and blue, embroidered with cords of linen and purple, on silver rods and marble columns; couches of gold and silver, on a pavement of green, white, shell, and onyx marble." (Esther 1:6)

Chamomile was well known to the Israelites, they used it for many medicinal purposes as well as for aesthetics. This oil is so special because the color of this oil changes from blue to yellow while in storage. The Holy temple of Jerusalem decorated the Cherubs using palm trees and many open flowers, overlaying everything. Chamomile was also known as one of the countless flowers of the field, just like Marigold, Hibiscus and Roses. Chamomile in Greek means "on the ground" and the commentary for these passages explains that God says, "What shall I call?" And the voice answers him "Call this, all flesh is grass" All those who are haughty their greatness shall be turned over and become like grass." Chamomile is a very modest plant that naturally grows close to the ground, even though it is a very beautiful plant it insists on being quiet and gentle, just like how we should aspire to be.

All flesh is grass, meaning a person's end is ultimately to die; therefore, if a person has a tendency towards kindness but doesn't do any kindnesses, it as though their blossom of the field that is cut off and dries, being they are unreliable and have no power to fulfill promises. If a person dies just like dried out grass, the blossom will wilt, and their promises are null. No one lives forever and actions are way more important than words, so it is these actions which are left behind in the end, it takes a lot more power and self-discipline to act on promises. A person whose heart moves him to generosity, is called "generous-hearted" in Hebrew it is called "Nadiv Lev," they were all the generous hearted people who decided to make offerings of gold, silver, or copper to God.

"Upon a lofty mountain ascend and herald, O herald of Zion, for the promise of the tidings emanates from the mouth of Him Who lives forever."

The term "techelet," which is a very specific shade of blue is mentioned throughout the bible many times. The high priest wore garments with blue designs embroidered on his tunic, there were also garments with which they used to cover the holy furnishings at the time they departed on their journeys. Tzitzit is a wool garment worn by men with four corners, corresponding to the four expressions of redemption that were promised by God in Egypt,

"I am the Lord,"

"I will take you out from under the burdens of the Egyptians, and I will save you from their labor,"

"I will take you to Me as a people, and I will be a God to you, and you will know that I am the Lord your God,"

"I will bring you to the land, concerning which I raised My hand to give to Abraham, to Isaac, and to Jacob which I will give it to you as a heritage,"

"I will redeem you with an outstretched arm and with great judgments,"

"I am the Lord."

Dyed light blue, the color of the sky which appears opposite the sun when there is a clear sky. Blue wool is dyed into that same light clear blue mentioned, using the blood of the chilazon, the color mix is to be made with very clear directions. The chilazon, the commentary says is a type of fish whose color is like the color of the sea and whose blood is black like ink. However, the Hebrew word Chilazon means a snail, so today it is not clear which creature it actually is. This specific fish in the bible was found in the Mediterranean Sea, and its blood was placed in a pot and blended with herbs, including chamomile. Another Midrash says it is also called "petil techelet," because of the bereavement the Egyptians suffered over the loss of their firstborns, the Aramaic translation techelet means bereavement. Moreover, the plague struck them at night, and the color of techelet is like the color of the sky, which blackens at dusk; the eight threads of the Tzitzit symbolize the eight days that the Israelites waited from when they left Egypt until they sang the song at the Red Sea.

The numerical value of the word Tzitzit is six hundred, ten + ninety + ten + ninety + four hundred = six hundred add to this the eight threads and five knots, there is a total of six hundred and thirteen. This coincides with the number of commandments in the Torah, the Midrash says, the heart and eyes are the spies for the body. They are its agents for actions, both good and bad, the eye sees, the heart desires, and the body acts. Today Jews wear these four cornered wool garments called Tzitzit every day and it is not colored with that unique blue dye. The Tzitzit still have specially knotted ritual fringes, or tassels on each of the four corners consisting of four strands which are knotted in a special formulation depending on which custom a person goes by.

Cinnamon

Latin Name, Sassafras Cinnamomum Zeylanicum
Aroma, Warm, spicy, sweet

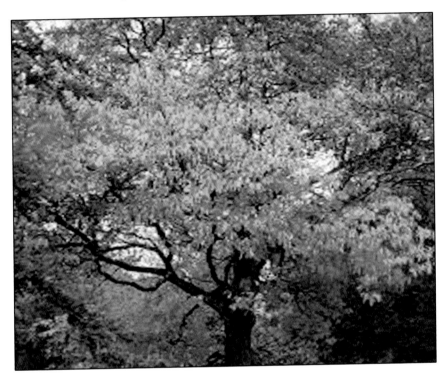

PHYSICAL

Cinnamon is obtained from the inner bark of the Cinnamomum Zeylanicum tree which has a berry fruit. It heals conditions such as bronchitis or diabetes and assists pancreas functions by transferring sugar out from the blood stream. The oil is extracted from the bark of the tree, which has a very different characteristic from the oil taken from the leaves. It is cut from the stems of the Cinnamon Tree and dries in curled rolls looking like sticks, which can then be made into oil or powder. Cinnamon is very active in killing bacteria, viruses, and infections such as streptococcus, its actions are very similar to those of black pepper. It is an analgesic, an anti-inflammatory, it heats and is also a stimulant thinning blood and causes sweating. It also contains Cyanamid Aldehyde and kills ants, bugs, and mice.

Warning do not administer to Pregnant Women, people suffering with High Blood Pressure or children under age 3.

EMOTIONAL

In humans it lowers stress, fears, and causes people to talk about their fears. Cinnamon elevates to the upper selves of the mind, it calms hysteria, relaxing both emotionally and physically. Cinnamon raises self-confidence and self-image and help the emotionally drained. It clears trapped emotions from a past trauma and it releases feelings of jealousy and insecurity.

BIBLICAL

"And you, take for yourself spices of the finest sort, of pure myrrh five hundred-shekel weights; of fragrant cinnamon half of it two hundred and fifty-shekel weights; of fragrant cane two hundred and fifty-shekel weights." (Exodus 30:23)

"Spikenard and saffron, calamus and cinnamon, with all frankincense trees, myrrh and aloes, with all the chief spices." (Songs of Songs 4:14)

"I fanned my couch with myrrh, aloes, and cinnamon." (Proverbs 7:17)

The bible makes specific mentions of this spice many times, the first we hear about it is when Moses is commanded to use both sweet cinnamon and cassia in the holy anointing oil. Cinnamon was an integral ingredient of the Ketoret, this incense is described in great detail in the bible and Talmud. It was the main spice used for offerings on the specialized incense altar at the time when the Tabernacle was in the First and Second Holy Temples of Jerusalem. Cinnamon was blended with Myrrh and Aloes that were used as a seductive perfume sprinkled on a lover's bed. In the beautiful Song of Songs, King Solomon describing the beauty of his beloved who has cinnamon scents on her garments which reminds him of Lebanon.

The bible often mentions that garments of kings and scholars which often smelled of myrrh, aloes, and cassia, hinting that these oils were expensive and not everyone had the luxury of having access to them. Some barks of Cinnamon trees have no scent and are smell just like ordinary wood, while there are other Cinnamon trees that have the rich aroma of a fragrant bouquet. In the bible God always found it necessary to specify and ensure that the incense should be made up of the good fragrant trees. Cinnamon trees grow in the land of Israel in abundance, and goats and gazelles love to reach up to the tops of these trees and eat from them.

It is written in the bible that when Abram was ninety-nine years old the time had arrived for his name to be changed to Abraham. It was also time for him to be circumcised as part his covenant with God, and that all male children born after him shall also be circumcised at the age of eight days. Abraham recognized God at the age of forty-eight but never got circumcised then, the Midrash says it was to discourage proselytes. Another missed opportunity for him to be circumcised would have been at the age of eighty-five, when God spoke with him between the pieces, "covenant between the splits," which means these were interval of events in which God revealed himself to Abraham. These were a series of covenants, and in one of the first of these events, God announced to Abraham that his descendants would inherit the Land of Israel. God wanted to ensure that Isaac would be the consequence of a holy source, therefore God did not convince him to be circumcised before, not even at the age of eighty-six, when Ishmael was born.

God said, "I will set up a cinnamon tree in the world: just as the cinnamon tree yields fruit as long as you manure and hoe around it, so [shall Abraham be] even when his blood runs sluggishly, and his passions and desires have ceased."
(Bereshit Rabbah 46)

Clary Sage

Latin Name, Salvia Sclerae
Aroma, Nutty, warm, light and musky

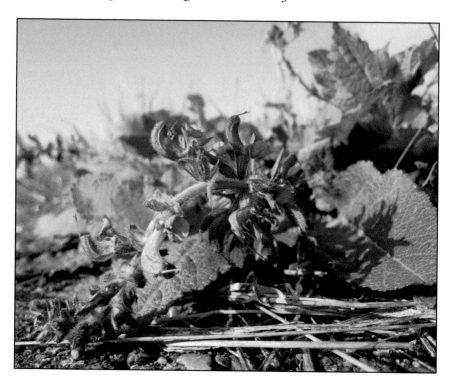

PHYSICAL

There are over three-hundred species of sage in the world, which is an herbaceous plant native to the Mediterranean and not all the Sage species are used for medical purposes. They specific strains are identified by their flowers, which all have mouths with lips. Their flower colors range from pale mauve to lilac or from white to pink. Clary Sage is a hormonal plant, with estrogen and in labor it can reduce birthing pains. It is an anti-inflammatory and can help acne and other hormonal skin issues. Because of its hormonal properties it may help reduce or heal cysts on the womb. It affects the nervous system and is a relaxant and may be used as a sedative to encourage sleep and calm nerves, Clary Sage also reduces convulsions, epileptic fits, and other nerve disorders.

Warning, this oil is not for kids!

EMOTIONAL

Clary Sage enhances hormonal and awareness intuitions focusing on keeping calm and confident as much as possible. Clary Sage exudes a sense of fulfilment in a devoted heart, developing satisfaction and pride in personal success. Clary Sage places problems into perspective, with convincing realization that problems are only what is made of them. This oil grounds and gives tranquility and a feeling of spiritual prosperity.

This is the true tree of abundance and prosperity, it has a very captivating and strong fragrance, uncovering time with a magnitude of possibilities to love and be who the person desired. Clary Sage will ensure that time is never judged in the same way ever again, enhancing the enjoyment of every moment and monetizing time masterfully. Use this oil when feeling the need to self-focus.

BIBLICAL

"Moses said to the children of Israel: "See, the Lord has called by name Bezalel, the son of Uri, the son of Hur, of the tribe of Judah." (Exodus 35:30)

"And He put into his heart the ability to teach, both him and Oholiab, the son of Ahisamach, of the tribe of Dan."
(Exodus 35:34)
"Bezalel made the ark of acacia wood, two and a half cubits long, a cubit and a half wide, and a cubit and a half high."
(Exodus 37:1)

"And he made the menorah of pure gold; of hammered work he made the menorah, its base and its stem, its goblets, its knobs, and its flowers were all one piece with it." (Exodus 37:17)

"And six branches coming out of its sides, three menorah branches from its one side and three menorah branches from its second side." (Exodus 37:18)

"Three decorated goblets on one branch, a knob and a flower, and three decorated goblets on one branch, a knob and a flower; so, for the six branches that come out of the menorah."
(Exodus 37:19)

"And on the stem of the menorah were four decorated goblets, its knobs and its flowers." (Exodus 37:20)

This plant grows all over Israel, being indigenous of the Mediterranean, the Menorah in the Holy Ark of the Temple of Jerusalem is intricately designed with a plant that completely describes Clary Sage. Since it was Bezalel, the son of Uri who totally devoted himself to the work of building the holy Temple of Jerusalem, more so than the other wise men of that time, he had the merit of being personally mentioned by name in the bible for his contribution to the work. Oholiab was also mentioned for his work on the holy Temple together with Bezalel, he the descendant of the tribe of Dan, which were considered to be from the lower ranking of the tribes. Dan was the son of the handmaiden Bilhah, Jacob's fourth wife and yet God compared Oholiab to Bezalel equally for their work of the Mishkan.

Bezalel was the descendant of the greatest of all the tribes, Judah, and his task was to fulfill what it is said in the bible, "and a prince was not recognized before a poor man." Oholiab was a widow's son, his mother was from Dan, and his father was from Naphtali, it was Rachel who said, "I twisted cords; I went through contortions until I was able to compare to my sister Leah." If Leah would boast that it was her descendant Bezalel, who will have the honor to build the Tabernacle, she would have to be informed that he will require one of the sons of Dan to help him. Rachels continues, "also, if Solomon, the descendant of my sister, will build the Temple, some of the sons of Dan and Naphtali will have to participate with him." God imbued them with wisdom of the heart, to do all sorts of work of a professional craftsman and master workers, such as embroiderers and weavers with blue, purple, and crimson wool, and linen.

Bezalel, the son of Uri was given the credit to have created all that the Lord had commanded of Moses. Bezalel's intuition for building the Temple coincided with what God told Moses on Mount Sinai, which was to first make the furnishings and afterwards the Mishkan. Then later Moses commanded Bezalel to do the opposite of what God had commanded him. Once Moses realized that he had made a mistake he admitted to Bezalel, "you were in the shadow of God," which is the translation of Bezalel's name. So, he first made the Mishkan, and afterwards he made the furnishings. Bezalel was also solely responsible for the formation of the menorah, God showed him with his own finger, because it was a complicated project and Bezalel had difficulty constructing it. It was made from one solid block of gold weighing a "talent," that need intricate hammering, Bezalel pounded it with a hammer, and cut it with a chisel to form the extend limbs as desired by God. It was not to be made limb by limb and then connected, from its base, which was hollow, to its flower above the legs, the menorah itself and everything attached to it was one large unit. The flower was the finest of all hammered work and the design of it was a flower God had revealed to Bezalel on Mount Sinai. Then God said, "now see and make, according to their pattern which you are shown on the mountain." Bezalel constructed the menorah physically, but the one who really made it was God himself.

Clove

Latin Name, Eugenia Caryophyllata
Aroma, Rich, warm, sweet, and spicy

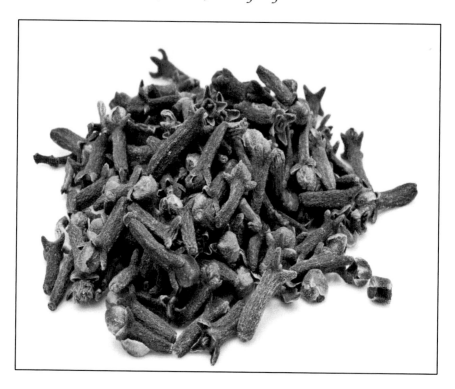

PHYSICAL

Clove is an evergreen plant and a native of Indonesia, India, Madagascar, and Pakistan. It was brought over to the Middle East by Arab traders that then made its way to Israel. It is an aromatic stimulant like Cinnamon and Nutmeg, both contain eugenol, which is a colorless to pale yellow aromatic oily liquid extracted from these plants to make essential oils. Clove is an anti-inflammatory and an analgesic, it is amazing as a first aid painkiller for dental emergencies and trauma, tooth aches and other mouth issues. Clove has many antimicrobial properties against fungi and bacteria. Clove helps inflammations, pains, blood flow and acts like Ben Gay, it stimulates the blood to bring healing cells to the wound area and it soothes pains. It is also an antiseptic and helps prevent the growth of disease that cause microorganisms and sterilizes your wound. Clove also help soothe and stop nausea and can be prepared as a tea.

EMOTIONAL

Clove encourages stimulation and regeneration of emotions, inspiring a trust to spring from within transporting the spirit into the innermost being bringing warmth to the soul. Clove is very action based, it is constantly moving and pushing forward, this oil makes things happen while not allowing anything to stand in its way.

BIBLICAL

"He breathed into his nostrils the soul of life." (Genesis 2:7)

"And the woman saw that the tree was good for food and that it was a delight to the eyes, and the tree was desirable to make one wise; so, she took of its fruit, and she ate, and she gave also to her husband with her, and he ate." (Genesis 3:6)

"And the Lord God made for Adam and for his wife shirts of skin, and He dressed them." (Genesis 3:21)

"And the Lord said to Moses, "Take for yourself aromatics, balsam sap, onycha and galbanum, aromatics and pure frankincense; they shall be of equal weight." (Exodus 30:34)

"And she gave the king one hundred and twenty talents of gold and very abundant spices and precious stones; there were never such spices as those that the queen of Sheba gave to King Solomon." (II Chronicles 9:9)

The Kabbalah teaches that smell is the connection between the physical and spiritual and a direct connection to the soul. The Talmud says, "Smell is that which the soul benefits from, and the body does not." When God created Adam out of the earth, he gave him life by breathing into him through his nostrils. Fragrance is the method used to ease the soul's pain, the Midrash says that when Adam and Eve sinned by eating from the Tree of Knowledge, they used all their senses except for their sense of smell for this sin. When the serpent approached Eve, she understood his words very well and they appealed to her, so she believed him. The snake saw that his words brought delight into her eyes, so he said to her, "and your eyes will be opened," meaning now you will know good and evil. Eve made sure that Adam and all the cattle and beasts to also eat the forbidden fruit. Eve now knew she was in trouble and did not know what the consequence of her actions would be, she was worried lest she die, and Adam will live, and God will bring another woman for him to marry.

Some legend says that God made for Adam and Eve shirts made of skin, which were as smooth as fingernails that fastened over their skin. Other sources say that they were made of a material that derives from skin. He may have used the fur of rabbits, which is soft and warm, and made them shirts out of that. Now that man has become mortal and had the ability to choose between good and evil, God could no longer allow them to reside in the garden of Eden. Unlike the cattle and the beasts, humans have unique privileges over all earthly beings, while God has his unique abilities among all the heavenly beings. God became suspicious that Adam and Eve may abuse their privileges of astuteness and awareness and mislead the animals into believing they were God. So, God sent the Angels of destruction to keep them out of the garden of Eden, they frightened and subdued Adam and Eve with sharp blades preventing them from re-entering ever again. If man would not have reached out to Tree of Life and eaten from it, he would have lived forever, then God would not have sent them out of the Garden of Eden.

Clove is considered in the bible as one of the worlds sweet scents and was implemented in almost all the bible's aromatic blends. Some commentaries say that the Queen of Sheba brought it to King Solomon as one of her many expensive gifts. It is used every week after the Shabbat in a ceremony that marks the symbolic end of Shabbat, and escorts us into the new week. The ritual involves lighting a special Havdalah candle that has several wicks, after blessing a cup of wine comes the smelling of sweet spices. In the commentaries clove is referred to as a root spice which in Hebrew is "Sh'chelet" which is described as smooth and shiny as fingernails "Ziporen" because of its shape.

Coriander

Latin Name, Coriandrum Sativum
Aroma, Sweet, warm, and spicy

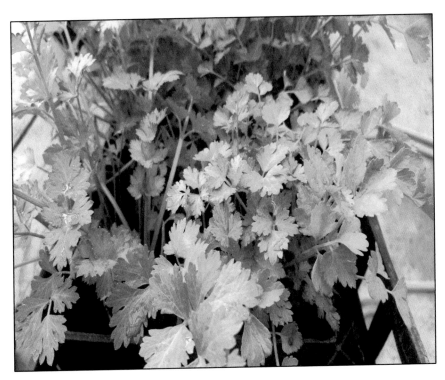

PHYSICAL

Coriander is also known as Chinese Parsley and grows wild in Israel. Fifteen dehydrated fruits known as coriander seeds were found in the Nahal Hemar Cave in the Judean Desert near the dead sea in Israel and this may be the oldest archaeological find of coriander. The oil is harvested from fruit of the plant, which are the seeds and not from the leaves. The seeds smell strong and taste sweet, their oil is like turpentine and evaporates. Coriander excretes phlegm by making coughing, reduces swellings and gassy stomachs, and because it is a diuretic it gets rid of excess bodily fluids.

Coriander seeds contains camphor and acts as a pain reliever, forcefully numbing the brain from feeling pain. It heats the stomach and the digestive tract, contracts rheumatic pain and excretes toxins. For people who are bedridden this oil helps relieve bed sores. This is an amazing oil, it can work in many different capacities, it contains flavonoids and carotenes. It is an anti-inflammatory, antioxidant, and an anti-cancer oil as well as an aphrodisiac, Ancient Egyptians used it in their love potions.

EMOTIONAL

Coriander gives that much needed peace, completely reduces fatigue by drastically lowering stress levels. Like a powerful drug it affects the neurological system and can incite a zombie feeling if too much is taken. This oil also gives courage in creativity and imagination helping focus for longer periods of time and enhances the memory.

BIBLICAL

"So, he said to them, that is what the Lord spoke, Tomorrow is a rest day, a holy Sabbath to the Lord. Bake whatever you wish to bake, and cook whatever you wish to cook, and all the rest leave over to keep until morning." (Exodus 16:23)

"So, they left it over until morning, as Moses had commanded, and it did not become putrid, and not a worm was in it." (Exodus 16:24)

"The house of Israel named it manna, and it was like coriander seed, it was white, and it tasted like a wafer with honey." (Exodus 16:31)

"Now the manna was like coriander seed, and its appearance was like the appearance of crystal." (Numbers 11:7)

"The people walked about and gathered it. Then they ground it in a mill or crushed it in a mortar, cooked it in a pot and made it into cakes. It had a taste like the taste of oil cake." (Numbers 11:8)

Manna was the "bread from heaven" which sustained the Israelites during their forty years of wandering through the desert, after their escape from Egypt and before arriving at Canaan. It described as, "a fine, flake-like things like the frost on the ground" and was said to arrive with the dew during the night. It was said to be like a coriander seed in size but white in color and like frost in the morning, it had to be collected before it was melted by the heat of the sun. It had the appearance of bdellium, which are semitransparent gum resin. The Israelites ground it and pounded it into cakes, which were then baked, resulting in something that tasted like cakes baked with oil. Raw manna tasted like wafers that had been made with honey and the Israelites were instructed to eat only the manna they had gathered for each day. Stored manna "bred worms and stank". The exception being that which was stored the day before the Sabbath, where they had to prepare twice the amount of manna gathered and this manna did not spoil overnight.

One time when the energy was low in the Sinai desert, and the people of Israel were looking to complain about everything, much to God's shock, it was evil to his ears. When God heard all their complaints and whining, mostly from the distinguished and prominent ones among them, his anger flared. God spread a large fire from him among them, consuming them, the Midrash says that when God is angry at the Israelites, he refers to them as "the people," but when he is pleased with them, he refers to them as "my people." The Israelites had no reason to complain, they were just looking for a pretext to grumble and lament about, they wanted God to hear their baseless complaints. "Woe is to us! How weary we have become on this journey! For three days we have not rested from the fatigue of walking." God flashed right back at them by saying, "I meant it for your own good that you should be able to enter the Land immediately." Later the people cried out to Moses to ask God for forgiveness and the fire died down and sank into the earth, had it spread along one of the sides of the camp, it would have gradually rolled along that entire side and caused more irreversible destruction.

Another bout of complaints started up about their strong cravings for meat and started a demonstration demanding to have a variety of food which included meat. They reminisced about the fish, cucumbers, watermelons, leeks, onions, and garlic that they were fed for free by their Egyptian masters. In fact, bricks were the currency the Egyptians used when bargaining for food with the Israelites. They conveniently forgot their workload that was laid upon them, had they remembered well, they would recall nothing was given to them free of charge, at that time they were just free from the burden of precepts. The manna changed into everything except the items the Israelites claimed they missed, and it is because they are harmful for nursing mothers. A nursing woman should not eat any garlic or onion, for the baby's sake, and was not because God did not love them or did not want them to eat those foods. The manna tasted very much like coriander seed and the Israelites said, "We have nothing but manna to look at," whereas God, inscribed in the bible, "the manna was like coriander seed," as if to say, "see, all you who inhabit the world, what my children are complaining about, the manna is excellent in so many ways!"

Cypress

Latin Name, Cupressus Sempervirens
Aroma, Woody, warm and spicy

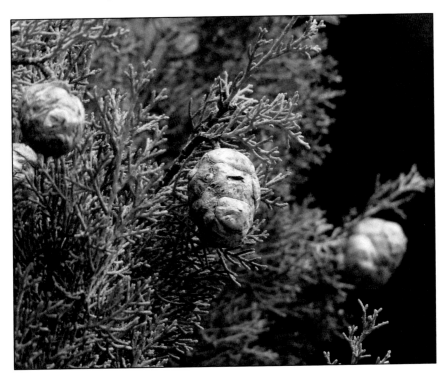

PHYSICAL

Cypress is native to the Mediterranean and some of its species are known to have lived for over a thousand years. It is an evergreen coniferous tree that can grow up to thirty meters with a completely upright trunk. This tree guards its own territory, it comes from the needle family and the essential oil is extracted from those needles. Cypress essential oil constricts blood cells and will stop bleeding from hemorrhoids, nosebleeds, and extra heavy bleeding from menstruation. It is a diuretic and will excrete excess body fluids such as profuse sweating or water retention. Cypress will also help if standing a lot at work and suffer from varicose veins. Cypress is great for acne and oily skin because of its cleansing astringent properties and helps with respiratory problems.

EMOTIONAL

This oil controls fear and is often associated with comforting and change. Cypress is in-between physical and spiritual and can assist in the passing over of a spirit. Cypress gives confidence, energetic protection, inner peace, and universal wisdom. It instills within the willpower to move on when purpose is lost. It has a particularly calming and soothing effect on irritable, angry, and stressed-out people.

BIBLICAL

"And God said to Noah, "The end of all flesh has come before Me, for the earth has become full of robbery because of them, and behold I am destroying them from the earth." (Genesis 6:13)

"Make for yourself an Ark of gopher wood; you shall make the ark with compartments, and you shall caulk it both inside and outside with pitch." (Genesis 6:14)

"And this is the size you shall make it, three hundred cubits the length of the ark, fifty cubits its breadth, and thirty cubits its height." (Genesis 6:15)

Noah's ark was made from Cypress Wood, Gopher wood in the Bible was actually known as Cypress, in Biblical and modern Hebrew the name for it is brosh. Gopher is a Babylonian word translated into Hebrew as qadros to mean cedar which in turn is also translated as brosh. There were many trees from Biblical times that had resinous wood, such as pine, cedar, fir, teak, sandalwood, ebony, wicker, juniper, acacia, and boxwood, all of which are mentioned in the Bible.

At the time of Noah, when the world was already quite populated, men and women mingled. Men would beautify and adorn women and entice them to enter the nuptial canopy, and noblemen would enter and have relations with her first. They would have relations also with married women, males and even animals. When coming from a position of authority, in today's world, it may be called rape, incest and pedophile. When God saw this behavior he said, "Let My spirit not quarrel forever concerning man, because he is also flesh, and his days shall be a hundred and twenty years." God did not wish to upset his spirit by complaining and quarrelling because of man, for a long time now God was having an internal argument with himself, whether to destroy or to have mercy on man. God thought even though man is only flesh, he nevertheless will not subordinate himself before me as is the nature of man. Until a hundred and twenty years I will delay my wrath towards them, and if they still do not repent, I will bring a flood upon them. This decree had already been issued twenty years before Noah begot children.

There were also many fallen angels living on earth among man who procreated with the daughters of man, they would bear children to these angels, called "mighty men," and they would rebel against God. There were some men of high repute, Irad, Mechujael, Methushael, also known as men of desolation, because they were destroyed. These good men were wiped out and uprooted from earth by the mighty men, and their absence made the world desolate. God saw that evil men were getting powerful on earth, they were getting away with their every imagination of evil, and God regretted that he created man upon the earth, this made his heart grieve. His thoughts to reconsider what to do with man, and he reached the decision to implement his plan of starting the flood.

"I will blot out man, whom I created, from upon the face of the earth, from man to cattle to creeping thing, to the fowl of the heavens, for I regret that I made them." (Genesis 6:7)

Only Noah found favor in the eyes of God, he had three sons, Shem, Ham, and Japheth. Since the world was full of corruption, full of immorality and idolatry, God informed Noah that he was going to destroy the earth, unlike when a pestilence comes upon the world and kills both good and bad alike. This time God wanted to create a disaster that would only annihilate only the bad and save the good, God directed Noah to start building an ark for himself and his family. In many ways God wanted to convey that relief and rescue was available to all the people of the earth, therefore he burdened Noah with such a specific and long arduous construction. God was hoping that the people of Noah's generation would see him occupying himself with the construction. Noah worked on the ark for one hundred twenty years and many people would ask him, "why do you need this?" Noah would say to them, "God has destined to bring a flood upon the world," in the hopes the people in the world would repent.

God then announced a clear warning that in only another seven days, he will make it rain upon the earth which will last for forty days and forty nights, the intention will be to blot out all beings he made, off the face of the earth. Noah was six-hundred years old at the start of the flood, and he too, was finding it hard to have faith and believe that the flood would happen. Noah did not enter the ark until the waters forced him to do so, the flood started to rain upon the earth slowly and gently at first. The Midrash says that God brought the rains down with mercy to give the people on earth yet another chance to repent and the floods would then have been rains of blessing instead. However, the people did not repent, and the rains became a flood. In fact, the people of his generation had been saying, "If we see him going into the ark, we will break it and kill him." So, God said, "I will bring him in before the eyes of all, and we will see whose word will prevail!" The rains rose off the earth, which was now submerged in water, above the peaks of all the mountains. The waters then became much more powerful, and the ark floated safely on the water and Noah and those with him in the ark survived.

Eucalyptus

Latin Name, Eucalyptus Camaldulensis
Aroma, Clean and pungent

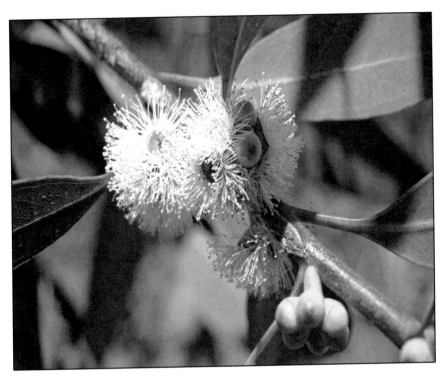

PHYSICAL

The eucalyptus tree is originally from Australia and is an adjustable tree that absorbs water; therefore, they were imported into Israel. Eucalyptus trees are known as gum trees because they exude Kino from their barks, this is an astringent tannin which is acid. It is an anti-bacterium and stimulates the internal walls of the bronchioles to excrete the mucus that is lodged from the nose and lungs. It is an oil for babies and children who have bronchitis, to help their respiratory system excrete phlegm and mucus.

This oil is good for people with cystic fibrosis when used in a humidifier or rubbed onto their backs. Eucalyptus is an antiseptic repellant, use it for low immune system and wounds. Eucalyptus helps the pancreas work better and is used to help people with diabetes. This is the oil to use for joint pain, great to massage with on sore muscle and joints. Mosquitos do not like this odor and it is used in a formula to prevent bites.

EMOTIONAL

Eucalyptus helps to deal with emotions in situations that need personal adjustment or change in a certain behavior pattern seen recurring over the years. Eucalyptus works great for groups at work or home for brainstorming, just try using this oil and see the results from it, it is a great essential when trying to develop a team. This oil builds team spirit, allowing ideas to formulate in developing a business with the right people on board. It focuses everyone to be on the same page when throwing out their ideas.

Eucalyptus helps emotional fatigue, or when feeling grey, alone, sad or fed up. It emotionally supports people who cry easily and is good for the middle child or people who may get insulted easily. Meditating with Eucalyptus oil helps see life from a different point of view. It gives a clear internal vision and wisdom, helping in becoming more assertive with more back bone. This is an amazing oil to use in a diffuser if feeling overloaded with emotions, this oil will help release them giving powerful and reliable confidence.

Warning, not to be used on children under the age of 3

BIBLICAL

"Fortunate is the man who has found wisdom and a man who gives forth discernment," (Proverbs 3:13)

"For its commerce is better than the commerce of silver, and its gain is better than fine gold;" (Proverbs 3:14)

"It is more precious than pearls, and all your desirable things cannot be compared to it." (Proverbs 3:15)

"Length of days is in its right hand; in its left hand are riches and honor." (Proverbs 3:16)

"It's ways are ways of pleasantness, and all its paths are peace." (Proverbs 3:17)

"It is a tree of life for those who grasp it, and those who draw near it are fortunate". (Proverbs 3:18)

Eucalyptus Trees are not mentioned in the bible and were originally imported into Israel from Australia in the later part of the ninetieth Century. These trees are indigenous of Australia and were never in this side of the hemisphere in biblical times. If you ask any Israeli what the most popular tree in Israel is, they will probably tell you the Eucalyptus tree, since it can be found planted all over Israel. Israel brought them over to solve our irrigation problems and dry up our swamps. When the state of Israel was being developed agriculturally, Israeli scientist and agriculturists studied technologies to develop it from a dry arid desert, into a major exporter of fresh produce in the world, despite the geography of the country.

Jewish immigration into Palestine, the name given to the land by the Romans, began in the late nineteenth century, once the Jews arrived, so did the Arabs from neighboring countries in search of work. When the Jews first arrived, the country was deserted and devoid of almost all life, there was nothing here. They immediately got to work clearing out the rocky fields and began constructing homes. They drained the swamplands and replanted all the forests spoken about it the bible. They became experts at irrigation and neutralized soil erosion and washed the salt out of the land. Jews who escaped or survived the holocaust joined in the creation and development of Israel and in 1948 and they reestablished the state of Israel.

One who learns and becomes wise this is real wisdom, it is only until a person has become so accustomed to his knowledge that he can easily express it with his mouth. As in any exchange, when a person wishes to exchange something for merchandise, each person takes that which they chose home. However, if a person says to his friend, "teach me your chapter, and I will teach you my chapter," then both chapters learned are securely established in each of them, and more valuable than fine gold. There is nothing equal to this value, and you cannot put a price on knowledge, those who take advantage of their ability to learn and engage in study, even just for their own sake, will live a life of assured riches and honor. For those who grasp knowledge and draws it near, should remember that God created the earth with wisdom. So, don't allow wisdom to be curved away from before your eyes, because is shall be "life for your soul," for this is the real tree of life.

A little after the establishment of the State of Israel, long boulevards of eucalyptus trees were planted along roads. This was done at the request of the then Prime Minister and Minister of Defense, David Ben-Gurion. The idea behind this was to make it difficult for our enemies to detect movement or to be able to see what is going on in our roads, the boulevards were called thereafter "Ben-Gurion Boulevards."

Fennel

Latin Name, Foeniculum Vulgare Dulce
Aroma, Warm, sweet, aniseed and pepper

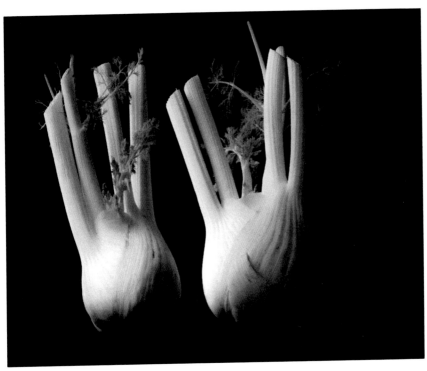

PHYSICAL

This plant is an awning that has a licorice fragrance and is a relative of the carrot family, it is indigenous to the shores of the Mediterranean. Fennel is highly aromatic and tastes similar to anise, dill and black cumin. It is a calmative, diuretic, as well as an antiseptic, an anti-spasmodic and is great for the digestive tract, helping to secrete digestive enzymes. Fennel is a relaxant, it lowers blood pressure, rids the body of mucus and balances humidity, it clears dry throats it helps humidify it to feel less dry. This oil encourages production of mother's milk and helps produce corticosteroids and cortisones making it a great anti-inflammatory.

EMOTIONAL

Fennel oil is so relaxing that it gives a certain unique feel of emotional quietness. It has a very subtle strength which clears and purifies people's auric field. Fennel encourages and enlivens, motivating clarity and preservation, reliability, and assertiveness.

BIBLICAL

"And God said, "Behold, I have given you every seed-bearing herb, which is upon the surface of the entire earth, and every tree that has seed bearing fruit; it will be yours for food."
(Genesis 1:29)

"And to all the beasts of the earth and to all the fowl of the heavens, and to everything that moves upon the earth, in which there is a living spirit, every green herb to eat," and it was so."
(Genesis 1:30)

"And the Lord said to Moses, "Take for yourself aromatics, balsam sap, onycha and galbanum, aromatics and pure frankincense; they shall be of equal weight." (Exodus 30:34)

"As Shamir, stronger than flint, I have set your forehead; fear them not, neither shall you be intimidated by them, for they are a rebellious house." (Ezekiel 3:9)

"And they made their heart as hard as a Shamir, in order not to listen to the Torah and to the words that the Lord of Hosts sent, through His spirit by the earlier prophets. And there was great anger from the Lord of Hosts." (Zechariah 7:12)

"And I will make it a desolation; it shall neither be pruned nor hoed, and the Shamir and desolation will come up over it; and I will command the clouds not to rain upon it." (Isaiah 5:6)

"The vineyard of the Lord of Hosts is the House of Israel, and the people of Judah are the plant of His joy; and He hoped for justice, and behold, there was injustice; for righteousness, and behold, an outcry." (Isaiah 5:7)

Fennel was used as a spice like dill in the bible, and in the Talmud, fennel is called "shumar." The Galileans did not consider it a spice, but it was regarded as such in Judah, fennel flower was known as katzah because it comes from the seed of the fennel flower. It was used as a spice on bread, and it is very likely that fennel was one of the seed-bearing herbs the bible often talks about. The Midrash states that any plant that is primarily used as animal fodder may only be consumed by humans for medicinal purposes, such as shumar. The result of mixed seeds combining fennel and parsley is also called rock-parsley.

Fennel is also called "Shamir," which in the bible is known as a legendary worm or stone created on the eve of the Sabbath and is said that it could cut any stone. Solomon was said to have built the Temple with this worm and the Midrash says this is probably the development of the original thorn or prickle used as a point for engraving as is written,

"The sin of Judah is written with a pen of iron, with a diamond point, engraved on the tablet of their heart and on the horns of your altars." (Jeremiah 17:1)

This is a spiritual meaning through concrete or material forms; as a figurative meaning, implying that a sin is deeply engraved into the world and time can and never be erased. The Midrash explains that the pen of iron had a diamond point, preserved by Jeremiah which he called "an iron wall," Another meaning of Shamir is preservable, conserved, preserved, capability or even fitness.

The vineyard of God is the House of Israel, the vineyard represents Adam, and the pride God has of his creation, just like a farmer would have of his vines growing in his grapevines. In the Garden of Eden, God planted the area around the tree of knowledge with the choicest vines, as the beginning of his formation was from the place of the altar. God built a tower and breathed into Adam's nostrils the spirit of life taken from the heavenly beings. The Midrash says that Adam was not immediately expelled from the garden of Eden, it only happened after he was rude to God. In fact, God was ready to give Adam another chance, he really did not want to throw him out of the Garden of Eden. In another source we find that God appointed guards to prevent Adam from eating from the Tree of Knowledge, and he fenced the tree inside ten layers canopies, clearing it completely from temptation.

God hewed a spring flowing with the fountain of wisdom hoping to produce grapes that Adam would be thankful about and praise God. Instead, it produced wild berries with putrid fruits because Adam had reviled and blasphemed God. What God decided to do to him, he did, he removed the hedge around the tree and expelled Adam from amidst his canopies. God cursed him that the fruits shall be eaten up and Adam's end will be to die and to be ruled over by wild beasts then he was expelled from the enclosure of Paradise, into where Adam and Eve were to live thereafter in desolation. The trees were neither to be pruned nor hoed so that they will learn from him their deeds, the Shamir and desolation ensued of because the temptation to perform corrupt deeds had ruled over him and his posterity.

Fir

Latin Name, Abies Alba
Aroma, Fruity, pine

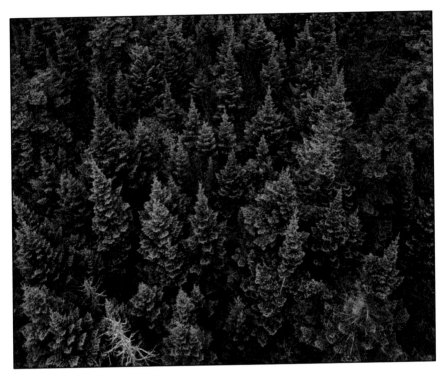

PHYSICAL

Fir is an evergreen coniferous tree that is closely related to Cedar Trees. Fir trees sometimes reach heights of eighty meters and are distinguished by their unique needle like leaves and very different type cones. Its oil is great for babies and pregnant women, but it should be applied onto clothes and not directly on the skin. Fir is an anti-depressant, and expectorant and an antiseptic oil and for adults can be used directly on the skin as a pain killer for joint and muscle pains. Patients suffering from arthritis can rub this oil directly onto their pain.

It is also used as a prevention for colds and flu's, it strengthens the immune system. This oil is also suitable for older people, they can use this oil even with their medications and steroids. Fir oil possesses a soft, sweetly resinous fragrance. Their clean, fresh aroma of silver fir exerts a powerful calming influence encouraging a restful sleep.

EMOTIONAL

The best thing about this oil is its ability to provide an uplifting and refreshing sensation. Fir essential oil promotes mental clarity and blends very well with many other oils. Fir assists lung complaints and sore bodies. An excellent oil that boosts energy throughout the body, soothing joints and muscles.

BIBLICAL

"And they shall come and all of them shall rest in the desolate valleys and in the clefts of the rocks and in all the thorn bushes and in all the shrines." (Isaiah 7:19)

"So says the Lord God: And I Myself will take from the lofty top of the cedar, and I will place it; I will crop off from the topmost of its young twigs a tender one, and I Myself will plant it upon a high and lofty mountain." (Isaiah 17:22)

"In the mountain of the height of Israel I will plant it, and it will bear boughs and bring forth fruit and become a sturdy cedar, and under it shall dwell all birds of every feather; in the shade of the branches thereof shall they dwell." (Isaiah 17:23)

"I will give in the desert cedars, acacia trees, myrtles, and pines; I will place in the wilderness boxtrees, firs, and cypresses together." (Isaiah 41:19)

"In order that they see and know and pay attention and understand together that the hand of the Lord did this and the Holy One of Israel created it." (Isaiah 41:20)

"The beams of our house are cedar, and the rafters are fir." (Song of Solomon 1:17)

All the trees mentioned in the passages of the bible that do not produce fruit were specifically designed by God to be used for building purposes only. Whenever God wishes to bless the Israelites, he says, "that in the place of thorn bushes, fir trees will come up." The commentaries explain that God gave cedars and acacia trees to live through many generations of civilizations in the desert. As powerful as humans are, most trees outlive humans by a long time and because of their centuries of presence in the land, God gave these trees the opportunity to develop great wisdom, goodness, and peace. The sad thing is that humans tend to take advantage of trees, abuse their abundance, we forgot to respect them and look at them in awe, and if God respects them shouldn't we.

When caught in the thicket of a tree that entangles, it is possible to become very much entangled in it. Many of the biblical wars would occur within thick forests, enemies would assume their opponents were camouflaging themselves in the trees and charge in to strike only to find themselves caught by the branches and thickets of the trees.

"Not like the shadow of a tree and not like a flying bird, which casts a shadow for days or years or casts a shadow for one hour, but like the shadow of the wings of a bee, which has wings but has no shadow." (I Chronicles 29:15)

Trees silently watch us through the generations and in their wisdom, they say nothing and don't judge. Many times, the reward for remaining silent receives a reward, the Midrash says, "and Aaron was silent," Aaron did not repeat that Moses told him he expected to be glorified and sanctified by God in front of all the people of Israel. For this Aaron merited that God's divine speech should be addressed especially to him, like when God spoke to Aaron and said, "drink neither wine nor strong drink." The Midrash says that when all the trees of the forest tremble, the sound of trees that do not produce fruit is heard louder than the trees that produce fruit trees.

Frankincense

Latin Name, Bosvellia Levona
Aroma, Warm, sweet, balsamic, and spicy

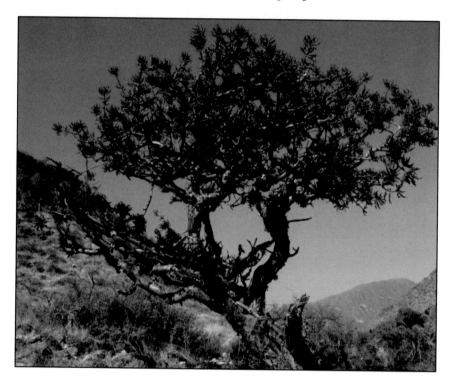

PHYSICAL

Frankincense is an aromatic resin used in incense and perfumes; these resins are taken from barks of trees that bleed resins. Frankincense has been in the Middle East area since biblical times and is written many times in the Bible. It is an anti-fungal balm which enables the tree to protect itself preventing anything to penetrate the tree and cause damage. Because of its connection to the sacral chakra, it helps with problems based on the lower part of your body. It eases constipation, hemorrhoids, and lower back pain.

Frankincense is also an anti-inflammatory and is a pain killer for intense and inflamed injuries. It calms and heals damaged skin from acne and acne scars.

Warning do not use this oil if you are pregnant or suffer from epilepsy.

EMOTIONAL

Connected to the sacrum chakra, Frankincense is good for grounding, especially in relationships. For those who suffer from low self-esteem, or even no self-esteem Frankincense restores confidence giving the confidence that allows the possibility to see different points of views and develop and understanding individuality. This is great for people who are dealing with sorrow, damaged emotions, this oil knows how to comfort. Frankincense helps deal with basal terrifying fears, like the fear of existence, survival and pain that doesn't seem to go away.

BIBLICAL

"And if a person brings a meal offering to the Lord, his offering shall be of fine flour. He shall pour oil over it and place frankincense upon it." (Leviticus 2:1)

"And he shall lift out of it in his fist, from the fine flour of the meal offering and from its oil and all the frankincense that is on the meal offering, and he shall cause its reminder to go up in smoke on the altar as a pleasing fragrance to the Lord." (Leviticus 6:8)

"And you shall place pure frankincense alongside each stack, and it shall be a reminder for the bread, a fire offering to the Lord." (Leviticus 24:7)

"And he had made him a large chamber, and in previous times they would put there the meal offering, the frankincense, and the vessels, and the tithe of the corn, the wine, and the oil, which were ordained for the Levites and the singers and the gate sentries, and the heave offering of the priests." (Nehemiah 13:5)

"And they shall come from the cities of Judah and from the environs of Jerusalem and from the land of Benjamin and from the lowland and from the mountain and from the Negev,

bringing burnt offerings and sacrifices and meal-offerings and frankincense, and those bringing thanksgiving offerings to the house of the Lord." (Jeremiah 17:26)

"Spikenard and saffron, calamus and cinnamon, with all frankincense trees, myrrh and aloes, with all the chief spices."
(Song of Songs 4:14)

Frankincense is named in the Bible by its Hebrew name, which is Levona, the root of which is the word white, "Laban." This oil was one of the main oils used in the Ketoret incense at the altar during biblical times in the Holy Temple of Jerusalem for meal offerings and incense offerings. The Ketoret was a blend of aromatic fragrant perfumes consisting of spices and gums to be burnt in worship of God at the Holy Temple. The exact blend of the sweet spices and of the aromatic condiments used in making the incense offering was a carefully guarded secret at the time of the Bible. The intense secret of the technique and exact proportions of the incense offering was to prevent its fraudulent replication to worship foreign gods.

The Bible teaches us that there is one law that applies to all offerings both for regular Israelites and for the Kohen, and that is that they all must use oil blends that contain frankincense, and the Kohen's meal-offerings must be burned entirely. Frankincense is known for its ability to produce Alpha Waves resulting in its unique ability for a spiritual connection to God. It is known as the Intuitive Antenna and a great tool for effective meditation and prayer. There are a total of eleven spices with which the bible suggests creating the incense and they must be pure. Only the important blends are prescribed specifically in the bible, otherwise other blends are left to the discretion of the pharmacist, but all blend varieties must generate a cloud of smoke.

Whatever varieties made, they all contributed to the sweet-smelling fragrances, the specifically name blends would only contribute to what was visible to the eye but could not be inhaled and no specification of quantities is mentioned in the bible. The bible did demand that the oils were blended synergically, all the spices should be equal to one another, God relied on the "handiwork of the perfumers." After everyone completed their incense, they were deposited in front of the Holy Ark so that their fragrance would elevate.

God told Moses verbally in great detail about "fragrances" and "incense," they are different names for different ingredients. There are three main ingredients that are connected to the anointing oil, they are resins that come from balsam tree trunks or unique plants. God instructed Moses for the anointing oil which is an incense, to use Myrrh, Frankincense and Cinnamon, which are also ingredients included in the Ketoret. The bible instructed Moses to take spices which the people were unfamiliar with but were also part of the mixture which made up the incense.

Galbanum

Latin Name, Ferula Gummosa
Aroma, Fresh earthy, musky and woody

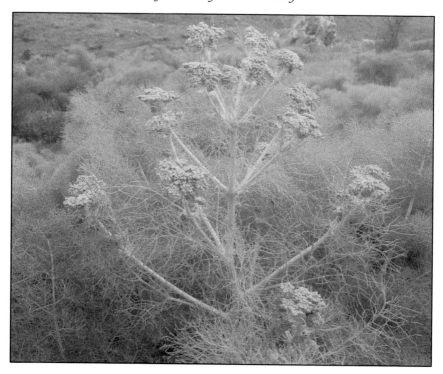

PHYSICAL

Galbanum is an aromatic gum resin from the celery, carrot and parsley family and is an herb species. Their taste is described as a disagreeable, bitter taste, a peculiar musky odor. Galbanum oil is an anti-arthritic, anti-rheumatic, anti-spasmodic, cicatrizing, circulatory, decongestant, detoxifier, emollient, insecticide, anti-parasitic, and vulnerary substance.

It reduces scars from wounds, boils, and scars from acne, pimples and rejuvenates your skin. Galbanum can reduce the signs of aging and wrinkles. This oil keeps parasites, fleas, mosquitoes, ticks, and bed bugs away, this does this for our pets too.

EMOTIONAL

Since Galbanum essential oil was an ingredient used in the Holy Anointing Oil at the Holy Temple of Jerusalem, it has regal and spiritual qualities. It teaches the important lesson to respect oneself, and to think kindly of others, this oil helps let go of past and residue issues that may have been lingering around too long. Galbanum changes the thought process and belief system teaching the embracement of new ideas, whether if a person is inclined towards religion or spirituality or not, Galbanum will guide. This oil is very calming and grounding, it gently shows possibilities of new directions while questioning to choose the divine paths and open hearts.

BIBLICAL

"And the Lord said to Moses, "Take for yourself aromatics, namely balsam sap, onycha and galbanum, aromatics and pure frankincense; they shall be of equal weight." (Exodus 30:34)

"And you shall make it into incense, a compound according to the art of the perfumer, well blended, pure, holy." (Exodus 30:35)

"And he shall take a panful of glowing coals scooped from the altar before the LORD, and two handfuls of finely ground aromatic incense, and bring this behind the curtain." (Leviticus 16:12)

"And he shall place the incense upon the fire, before the Lord, so that the cloud of the incense shall envelope the ark cover that is over the tablets of Testimony, so that he shall not die." (Leviticus 16:13)

"And he brought up offerings on the altar which he has made in Beth El on the fifteenth day of the eighth month, in the month that he had fabricated from his heart, and he made a festival for the children of Israel, and he went up to the altar to burn the incense." (I Kings 12:33)

The Bible says that Galbanum is a spice with a vile odor and the reason for this according to the Scripture, is that it was counted in amongst the ingredients of the ketoret, this is to teach that we should not look disapprovingly at transgressors. We must include them with us when we assemble for fasting or prayer, they must be counted with us. The Israelites incense burning was performed by the priests in the Tent of Convocation, this continued all throughout their journey in the Sinai Desert on their way to Israel. These incense offerings also continued throughout the beginning years of their settlement into the land, and they did so in the Temple, which was built by King Solomon in Jerusalem, and later in the Temple built by returning exiled Jews.

Offerings were delivered at the western side of the altar, just before the entrance into the Holy Temple. The incense had to be grounded finely. The Midrash explains that the incense was to be the finest quality as well as being grounded finely. On the eve of Yom Kippur any incense previously crushed would be re-crushed to an even finer consistency for use on this formidable day. The incense is placed on the fire before God, in a way so that the cloud would form from the incense to screen the cover over the Ark. Now king Solomon was a very strict king and heavily taxed the Israelites, his people, and when he died, they were hoping that his son Rehoboam who was to succeed him would be an easier going and lenient king.

After Rehoboam was crowned in Shechem, he took counsel with the elders who were his father's advisors, they recommended him to continue in his father's way and be kind to the people. Rehoboam did not like this advice, so he sought advice from the younger counsel of men, he asked them, "What do you advise that we reply to this people who have spoken to me saying, 'Lighten the burden which your father has placed upon us'?" The younger men also being Rehoboam's peers, having grown up with him, scoffed when they heard the request of the Israelites for leniency and recommended him to tell the Israelites, "My little finger is thicker than my father's loins, where my father did burden you with a heavy yoke, I shall add to your yoke; my father flogged you with whips, but I will flog you with scorpions." Jeroboam the son of Nebat heard of this while he was still living in Egypt, to where he himself had fled from king Solomon, he and all the people appealed to Rehoboam, but the king did not listen. The Israelites said,

"What share do we have in David? And no heritage in Jesse's son.
To your homes, O Israel! Now see your house, David,"
(I Kings 12:16)

218

When king Rehoboam sent Adoram his minister who oversaw tax collection to collect taxes, the people pelted him with stones and killed him, forcing the king to flee to Jerusalem. Israelites revolted against the House of David and when they heard that Jeroboam had returned, they declared him king over all Israel, only the tribe of Judah remained under the rulership of Rehoboam. When Rehoboam collected his men and tried to wage war with Jeroboam, he chose one hundred and eighty thousand warriors from the house of Judah and Benjamin. God immediately sent word to Shemaiah, the prophet at that time and demanded that he tell Rehoboam, "you shall not go up and you shall not war with your brothers, the children of Israel; return each man to his home for this thing has been brought about by Me." God declared Jeroboam king over Israel and the people were divided into two states, Judah and Samaria, giving Jeroboam a unique opportunity to become a great and God-fearing king.

Jeroboam's fear that the kingdom may be tempted to return to the original House of David got the better of him. The Israelites always took their three times a year pilgrimage to Jerusalem bringing offerings and sacrifices to God, here is where Jeroboam made a fatal mistake. He was afraid that the hearts of his people will return to Rehoboam the king of Judah, so he forbade the Israelites to go to Jerusalem to offer sacrifices to God. Instead, he built two temples, one in Beth El and the other he built in Dan. He told the people, "It is far for you to go up to Jerusalem; here are your gods, O Israel, that have brought you up from the land of Egypt." Jeroboam appointed his own priests who were not necessarily from the tribe of Levi, who are God's appointed priestly line. He replaced all the original festivals God had given to the Israelites with his own fabricated ones. Jeroboam ordered his people to bring up their offerings to his altars in Beth El only, they were to slaughter their calves there to the priests he had appointed in the high "holy" places he had created, and there the people went to burn incense.

God was furious and disappointed with Jeroboam, God summoned over a man of God to meet him at the alter in Beth El and he said,

"Altar, altar, so said the Lord, behold a son will be born to the house of David, Josiah will be his name, and upon you he will slaughter all the priests of the high places who offer sacrifices on you, and human bones will they burn upon you." (I Kings 13:2)

The prophet gave a sign on the day on which he prophesied, warning Jeroboam, the altar will split by itself, and the ashes will be spilled to the ground. The angry Jeroboam stretched out his hand from over the altar saying, "seize him!" As soon as he extended his arm, it stretched out and became stiff, so he was unable to bring his hand back to his body. God avenges the honor of a righteous man swiftly; being more important than avenging his own honor. Jeroboam's disdain for the righteous man God had chosen for this task, caused his punishment and not the fact that he was standing and offering sacrifices to pagan deities. It was only after Jeroboam pleaded with the prophet to beg God in his behalf, that his arm recovered to its original state.

God knew that Jeroboam was still in a state of rebellion and had every intention to continue burning sacrifices to his idols and tried to persuade the man of God to bribe him with delicacies and gifts. The prophet refused to either eat or drink at the king's palace because God had commanded him not eat bread nor drink water, during this mission. God further warned him to neither return by the same road he had arrived in Samaria. The prophet chose another route home, listening to God and not returning the way he had entered Beth El. There was an elderly prophet living in Beth El who followed the prophet from Judah, he found him resting under a terebinth tree. He asked him, "are you the Man of God who came from Judah?" to which he replied: "I am he." The old man offered him to come to his house to eat some bread and drink some water and still the prophet from Judah refused. So, the old man lies to him saying, "I too, am a prophet like you, and an angel spoke to me by the command of the Lord, saying, "bring him back to your house, and he shall eat bread and drink water." The prophet believed him and ate with him, while they were sitting at the table, the word of God came to the false prophet who had brought him back and warned him of what he had done, by offering food to the man of God he had forced God's holy spirit into the presence of baal. God told the prophet from Judah,

> *"Because you have rebelled against the word of the Lord, and you did not keep the commandments that the Lord your God commanded you. You shall not eat bread nor drink water and your corpse shall not come to the grave of your forefathers."*

After had eaten bread and he had drunk, the old man saddled the donkey for the prophet whom he had brought back. On his way home a lion killed the prophet of God, and his corpse was flung in the road, where both lion and the donkey stayed standing alongside his body. Passersby who saw the corpse with the lion came to tell the old prophet the strange sight they had just seen. When he arrived at the scene, he saw that the lion had not eaten the corpse and neither had it killed the donkey. The old prophet respectfully carried the corpse of the Man of God, onto his donkey and brought it back to his own city in Samaria to eulogize him and bury him. After he buried him, he told his children, "At my death you shall bury me in the grave wherein the Man of God is buried; next to his bones, place my bones." Even after this freaky incident Jeroboam did not return from his evil ways, the Midrash says that God grasped him by his garment and said to him, "repent and I and you and the son of Jesse will stroll in Paradise," where Jeroboam refused, and so God cut him off and destroyed him from the face of the earth.

Geranium

Latin Name, Pelargonium Graveolens
Aroma, Flowery rose, sweet and soft

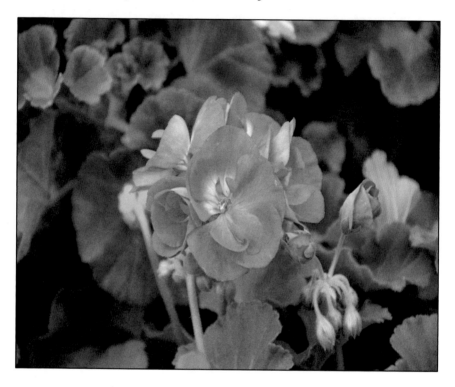

PHYSICAL

Geranium is a flowering plant known as cranesbill; they are found throughout the warmer countries of the world but are mainly found in the Mediterranean regions. Their flowers have five veined petals and are usually found in red, white, pink, purple or blue. This oil awakens the body and is great for extreme fatigue and stress reduction. This oil incites hyper activeness, combats viruses, fungus, strengthen the immune system against infections such as candida. This oil balances the hormone system and helps stabilize irregular periods and other vaginal problems. It is a diuretic, an antiseptic, and an anti-depressant with regenerative qualities. Geranium is also an anti-spasmodic and anti-infectious oil, a real multi-talented essential oil. Geranium lowers sugar levels and aids thyroid, adrenal, wrinkled skin, acne, and skin pigmentation. Use this oil as part of a cleanser to help generate elastin and antigravitation of the skin. Because this oil is great for skin, it is also great to use for scars and infectious wounds.

EMOTIONAL

Geranium supports the kidneys, which in holistic medicine is associated with fear. Fear is the main cause of most depressions, sufferers of exaggerated fear and loss of focus are usually administered Geranium, which is one of the main oils used as an antidepressant. Geranium helps in being less undecisive and giving confidence to make the right choices. Geranium gives the feeling of being cushioned and mothered, as well as an assurance of being taken care of. Geranium resonates with Mother Earth; it represents the feminine energy and reproduction.

BIBLICAL

"A voice says, "Call!" and it says, "What shall I call?" "All flesh is grass, and all its kindness is like the blossom of the field."
(Isaiah 40:6)

"The grass shall dry out, the blossom shall wilt, for a wind from the Lord has blown upon it; behold the people is grass.
(Isaiah 40:7)

"The grass shall dry out, the blossom shall wilt, but the word of our God shall last forever." (Isaiah 40:8)

"As for man his days are like grass; like a flower of the field, so does he sprout."

"For a wind passes over him and he is no longer here; and his place no longer recognizes him."

"But the Lord's kindness is from everlasting to everlasting upon those who fear Him, and His charity to sons of sons."
(Psalms 103:15-17)

Geraniums grow mostly in the eastern part of the Mediterranean region and are the most popular plant for gardens all over the world. Its oil is a popular choice to be used for meditation and awakening of the soul. Ancient Egyptians used Geranium as an effective treatment for cancerous tumors. There are an infinite number of beautiful flowering plants such as

Geranium, known in the bible as the plants of the field, God uses the analogy of flowers blossoming and then wilting to represent a life span many times in the bible. Just as people who became strong through their good deeds, will then be eligible to merit from the good deeds of their forefathers. The choice of being good or bad is just that, it is a choice, time passes by very quickly and the choices made during life determines the quality of life a person leads, the consequence of which then ripples down to future generations. This is the reality, the time will come when the flower wilts and dies and life is over, but deeds of a lifetime last forever. The commentaries explain many times that doing good deeds and kindnesses during our lives make us blossom and flower, however bad deeds make us wilt and dry spiritually.

People who adopt traits of haughtiness and exert bullying and superiority over smaller people than themselves, God judges them the harshest, by reminding them that their rulership is worthless, and shows them that also the princes and the kings are only human. After a person dies, his vanity is converted to become just dust, we all came from the dust, and we all will return to the dust. A person who understands this will put their heart to good, because all spirits both of children and adults ascends above to heaven and stands in judgment of God. However, the spirits of beasts descend below earth, without having to give any accounting of their lives. A man must rejoice in his good deeds and take value in the toil of his hands, he should rejoice and eat, but not exaggerate in his desires, like to covet riches, and accumulate what is not his. He should always be happy with his own portion and after he dies his children will have, and they too will learn to prosper with the riches that he earned and benefit from his example as a good role model.

Ginger

Latin Name, Zingiber officinale
Aroma, Hot, sweet, and sharp

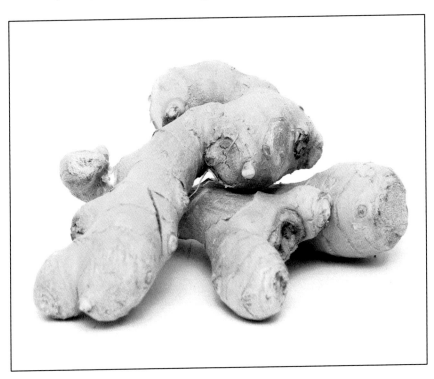

PHYSICAL

Ginger is an herbaceous plant and part of the Turmeric and Cardamom family and originated in the tropical rainforests from the Indian subcontinent to Southern Asia. It comes in clusters of white and pink flower buds that bloom into yellow flowers, whose rhizome, ginger root or ginger, is widely used as a spice and a folk medicine. Ginger is a pungent tasting aromatic plant of the genus of the Zingiber, the ginger family is known as amomum cardamomum. Ginger is one of the most well-known plants in the world and is used for both cooking, baking drinks and remedies. It was an Indian luxury spice that had great Jewish demand in biblical Israel.

Its oil is a strong anti-inflammatory and assists in joint pains works like glucosamine. Also rids the body of toxins and helps the body digest food after meals and lowers triglycerides. Take ginger to eliminate that feeling of having overeaten to ease the digestive system. This oil is an antiseptic, an analgesic, and an expectorant, it helps coughs and the respiratory system, though do not use this oil if there is fever. Use Ginger for car sickness, it prevents vomiting, and slice Ginger root into tea.

EMOTIONAL

Ginger is encouragement, warmth, and empathy, with its courage comes assurance and confidence, and with the confidence comes optimism and with the optimism comes liberation. This oil is a secret power to being one's own personal hero, it is the craved for knight in shining armor. Ginger saves the faint hearted and the weak, making them feel capable and strong. Ginger gives the confidence to take the road to a brighter future.

BIBLICAL

> "And you, take for yourself spices of the finest sort, of pure myrrh five hundred-shekel weights; of fragrant cinnamon half of it two hundred and fifty-shekel weights; of fragrant cane two hundred and fifty-shekel weights," (Exodus 30:23)

> "And a shoot shall spring forth from the stem of Jesse, and a twig shall sprout from his roots." (Isiah 11:1)

> "And it shall come to pass on that day, that the root of Jesse, which stands as a banner for peoples, to him shall the nations inquire, and his peace shall be with honor." (Isiah 11:10)

The prophet Isaiah prophesized that Jesse would be the ancestor of the kingly throne of David. The shoot is symbolic of the royal scepter, that springs forth from the stem of Jesse, is an expression of a sapling, basically his seed. He prophesized that the Israelites will be cast into exile from their land and their hope will be lost until the Messiah, a descendant from David, shall come and redeem them. This prophecy was said to console those exiled, and God's spirit will rest upon the Messiah an essence of wisdom and perception he will be the heroic savior of the Israelites. He shall be filled with the fear of God for the wisdom instilled into him so he will know and understand who is innocent and who is guilty. He will judge with the speech of his lips the innocent with mildness and tenderness, and in the same way he shall smite the sinful of the earth harshly. In the days of the Messiah, it is predicted that a wolf will be able to live with a lamb, a leopard shall lay around with a kid; a calf, a lion cub and a fattened ox shall play together, and a small child may accompany them. Furthermore, a cow and a bear shall graze together in a field, all animals will live in harmony, and a lion will eat straw just like cattle.

When a snake ages, it becomes deaf and is then called a "pathan," because it cannot be charmed, and it becomes an even more dangerous snake. The prophecy continues that an infant will play over the pit of an old snake and over the eyeball of an adder, the weaned child shall stretch forth his hand without any harm. There will no longer be any harm or destruction on all God's holy mount, because all the people of the land shall be full in knowledge of God, just as water covers the seabed. So, when the day comes that the root of Jesse shall announce his arrival, the people should support him and gather around him with respect. Then God will save the Israelites for the second time, just as he acquired them from Egypt, when their redemption was absolute, without subjugation, but the redemption preceding the building of the Second Temple and is not counted, since they were subjugated to Cyrus. This time God shall gather all the lost tribes of Israel, all the scattered people of Judah, God shall gather them from the four corners of the earth.

The tribe of Ephraim shall no longer envy the tribe of Judah, the Messiah is the son of David, and the Messiah is the son of Joseph, and they shall not envy each other anymore. Israel will fly and run of one accord against the Philistines who are in the west of Israel and conquer their land. The bible denotes complete unity, "they shall be shoulder to shoulder in their unity to smite the Philistines." It is said that God will dry up all the seven seas, "with the strength of His wind." From the Egyptian sea the exiles of Israel will pass through it from Egypt, and from the Euphrates River, for the exiles from Assyria to cross. From all the seven exiles God will lead the Israelites back to Israel walking on dry land, it shall be like a highway in the midst of the water.

Ginger was also used as part of the Ketoret incense in the Holy Temple of Jerusalem. In the Talmud it explains that Gingers in Aramaic is Zangvila and Zangvil in Hebrew. The Rabbis allowed dry ginger to be chewed on Yom Kippur, which is the Jewish Holiest Day of the year and a fast day.

"If one ate dried peppers or dry ginger, he is not liable, because they are not fit to eat. If he ate them while they were moist, when they are fit to be eaten, he is liable."

Grapefruit

Latin Name, Citrus Paradisi
Aroma, Warm, sweet, fresh, and citrus

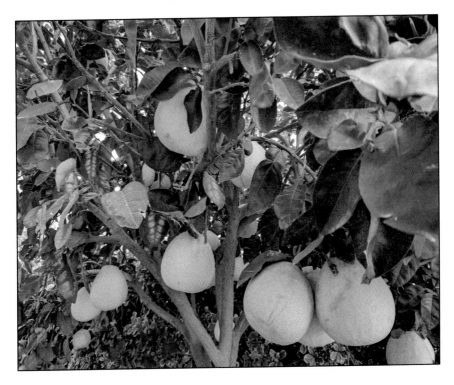

PHYSICAL

Grapefruit is a citrus fruit that is semi sweet and bitter at the same time and originated in Barbados. Apparently came about because it was an accidental mix between the regular sweet orange tree and the pomelo. It was thought to be the "Forbidden Fruit" from the Adam and Eve incident in the Bible, however it was misidentified. By the nineteenth century the grapefruit was spread all over the world, this hybrid accident was known as a shaddock fruit until it was named grapefruit because its fruits clusters like grapes. Like all the citruses Grapefruit contains Vitamin C and antioxidants. It lowers Cholesterol affect and its oil is extracted from the peels. Grapefruit affects the nervous system; each citrus fruit affects a different part of the nervous system. The limonene in this oil cures cancer and can be purchased in capsules, researchers have found that this citrus is very effective in healing breast cancer.

This oil has also been used to aid weight loss because it controls and balances your hunger pangs and gives the brain a sensation of satisfaction. It is good for skin; however, it is also phototoxic, and must refrain from going into the sun for two hours after use, it is better to use grapefruit oil at night. Also good for muscle pains and spasms, it is a blood thinner, lowers cholesterol and cleanses the lymph nodes.

Warning Grapefruit oil must NEVER be administered to people taking statins because it aggressively takes it apart in the liver.

EMOTIONAL

Grapefruit is good to cure a bad mood, this oil encourages joy, positivity, and confidence. It attunes the true inner self, alerting and stopping falling asleep at the job. It generates spontaneity and is a motivator energizing and uplifts the body and awakens the mind. Grapefruit awakens the spirit and forces one to face the world. It releases prayers from the inner heart with intent of being heard, forcing the connection with the angelic realm. This oil gives complete harmony so that the body and soul are completely in sync and hear each other.

BIBLICAL

"And the fugitive came, and he told Abram the Hebrew, and he was living in the plain of Mamre the Amorite, the brother of Eshkol and the brother of Aner, who were Abram's confederates." (Genesis 14:13)

"Exclusive of what the lads ate, and the share of the men who went with me; Aner, Eshkol, and Mamre they shall take their share." (Genesis 14:24)

"And he planted an eishel in Beer-Sheba, and he called there in the name of the Lord, the God of the world." (Genesis 21:33)

"They called that place the Valley of Eshkol because of the cluster Eshkol the children of Israel cut from there."
(Numbers 13:24)

"And they turned and went up to the mountain, and they came to the valley of Eshkol and spied it out." (Deuteronomy 1:24)

"I made myself gardens and orchards, and I planted in them all sorts of fruit trees." (Ecclesiastes 2:5)

This fruit tree was not mentioned in the bible, but its family was many times, even though the grapefruit only arrived in Israel in 1920 it was immediately recognized as a hadar fruit. Grapefruits belong to the Citrus family, and in Hebrew as I mentioned before it is called Hadar, it includes the entire citrus family, Citrus Medica, orange, grapefruit, lemon, pomelo, key lime and more. The Bible is so versatile, that it is possible to connect the grapefruit to the Bible and see its affects and its relevance even today.

King Solomon planted many orchards with groups of fruit trees according to their type. Abraham would offer fruits for his many guests at mealtimes, he planted an "eishel" which bore an abundance of fruit and he called it, "God of the whole world." After they would eat and drink, when they would thank Abraham, he would say to them, "Bless the One of Whose foods you have eaten," directing them to thank the real source of his hospitality. Grapefruit in Hebrew is Eshkolit, and Eshkol means a cluster, usually of grapes. In English Grapefruit was given its name because it grows in a Cluster. When the fruit arrived in Israel, Israeli farmers wanted to name this new fruit an Israeli version of "Grapefruit" and came up with "Eshkolit"

Og, was the king of Bashan who came from a family of Rephaim, meaning "ghostly spirit," he was so large that he had to have his beds custom made from iron so they could hold him. Og was from the generation of the flood and was the only one who managed to survive the flood. Og was one of the Nephilim, "mighty men," who were still on earth during the time of the flood. He was a giant and his feet were still on the ground while the earth was flooded, though some sources say that it was Noah who saved him. Og entered Mamre as a fugitive to inform Abraham of his nephew Lot's capture in battle in Sodom. Abraham immediately armed his three hundred and eighteen trained men of his household, Eliezer, Aner, Eshkol, and Mamre, and they pursued them until the land of Dan. It was at this point he became weak, for he saw into the future that his descendants were destined to erect a calf there, "and Jeroboam placed one in Beth-el, and the other he placed in Dan." Abraham decided to divide his army and he and his servants flung upon them at night, "he and his servants, smote them," fought the kings and Abraham saved Lot and all his possessions.

The Midrash says that Og informed Abraham about Lot because he knew that Abraham would go out to war and hopefully be killed. His altruistic motive was that wanted to take Sarah and to marry her. Og himself escaped from the battle, because Amraphel and his allies did not kill him, he lived for many years until Abraham's descendants finally killed him.

Helichrysum

Latin Name, Helichrysum Augustifolium
Aroma, Powerful, fruity, fresh

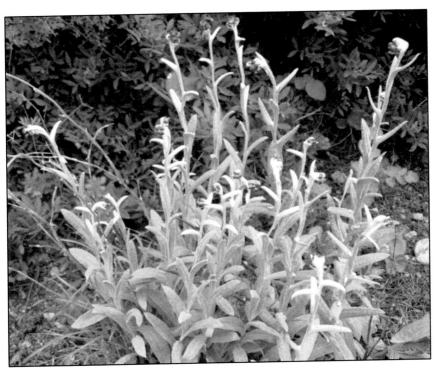

PHYSICAL

Helichrysum is a flowering plant also known as immortality, or everlasting flowers. It is a native of Africa, Madagascar, and some parts of Asia. It produces a yellow-reddish essential oil popular in fragrance for its unique scent, best described as a mixture of burnt sugar. Helichrysum is the biological broom, it gets rid of dead cells and cleans up the blood stream, as well as encouraging new cell to regenerate. This is the first oil to use after an operation and may be used directly on the wound.

It expels toxins, swellings and prevents thrombosis and bruising. This oil is great at fixing veins, cuts, wounds, and bruises. It is also used as an anti-parasite but because of its high cost, it is good to use geranium instead.

EMOTIONAL

Helichrysum encourages calmness and acceptance when one has lost touch with their spiritual self. This oil helps to achieve understanding and empathy for vulnerability when feeling it is time to expose one's true self. Helichrysum teaches patience and perseverance; it gives inner strength and awareness. To love truly involves acceptance of pain without compromise.

BIBLICAL

"And I will establish My covenant between Me and between you and between your seed after you throughout their generations as an everlasting covenant, to be to you for a God and to your seed after you." (Genesis 17:7)

"And I will give you and your seed after you the land of your sojourning, the entire land of Canaan for an everlasting possession, and I will be to them for a God." (Genesis 17:8)

"Those born in the house and those purchased for money shall be circumcised, and My covenant shall be in your flesh as an everlasting covenant." (Genesis 17:13)

"And God said, "Indeed, your wife Sarah will bear you a son, and you shall name him Isaac, and I will establish My covenant with him as an everlasting covenant for his seed after him." (Genesis 17:19)

"Do you not know-if you have not heard-an everlasting God is the Lord, the Creator of the ends of the earth; He neither tires nor wearies; there is no fathoming His understanding." (Isaiah 40:28)

"You, gates, lift your heads and be uplifted, you, everlasting portals, so that the King of Glory may enter." (Psalms 24:7)

"You, gates, lift your heads and lift up, you, everlasting portals, so that the King of Glory may enter." (Psalms 24:9)

"Before the mountains were born, and You brought forth the earth and the inhabited world, and from everlasting to everlasting. You are God." (Psalms 90:2)

"But the Lord's kindness is from everlasting to everlasting, and His charity to sons of sons." (Psalms 103:17)

"For he will never falter; for an everlasting memorial will the righteous man be." (Psalms 112:6)

Helichrysum, known as Red Everlasting and in Hebrew it is called, "Dam Hamakabim," which translated into English means "Blood of the Maccabees," and can be found growing all over the Upper Galilee, Central Israel, and the Judean Hills. Dam Hamakabim is a protected plant in Israel and the flower has become the icon of our Memorial Day for Israel's Fallen Soldiers and Victims of Terrorism. The name "Blood of the Maccabees" is derived from a legend saying that in every spot where the flower grows, a drop of blood had spilled on the earth. The Midrash says that one drop of blood that came out of the righteous man Micaiah, whose was struck and fatally wounded by his friend was enough of an atonement for all Israel. Blood of the Maccabees connects Israel's constant struggle for security today to the age-old struggle for our existence in Israel.

We continue to hope to see the day that all of Israel will be able to live in peace as we saw in the days of King Solomon. In the days of Solomon his son, when he comes to bring the Ark into the Holy of Holies and the gates cling to each other, Solomon recited twenty-four praises, but he was not answered until he said,

"Do not turn back the face of Your anointed; remember the kind deeds of David, Your servant." (II Chron. 6:42)

God made an everlasting covenant with Abraham and giving him the entire land of Canaan for everlasting possession. "I will be to you for a God, but if one dwells outside the Holy Land, it is as though he has no God," God tells Abraham, "As for me, behold my covenant is with you, and you must be careful to observe it." This observance entails that every male among you be circumcised. God says the covenant is between you and me, for all those living now, and for all those destined to be born, they must all be circumcised. God re-establishes his covenant with Isaac, because he was born holy, and was not the son of a mistress or a handmaiden, whereby Ishmael was and so could never have had the status that Isaac had. God says, "behold I have blessed him, and I will make him fruitful, and I will multiply him." Abraham loved Ishmael after all he was his son too and had him circumcised when he was already thirteen years old. On that very same day Abraham himself was circumcised when he was ninety-nine years old.

Hibiscus

Latin Name, Hibiscus Rosa-Sinesis
Aroma, Light, flowery, fresh

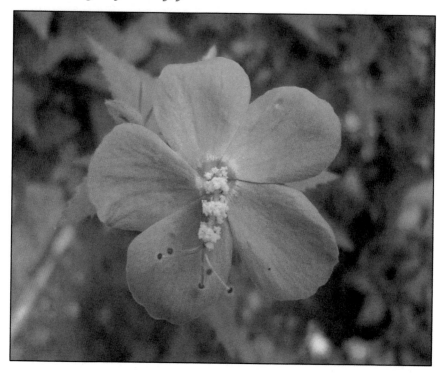

PHYSICAL

Hibiscus is an herbal plant as well as a woody shrub and grows in warm countries, such as Israel. Its flowers are large and trumpet like, with colors ranging from white, pink, red, orange, peach, yellow and purple. It is known in the Bible as the Rose of Sharon and admired for its many beautiful colors. They are used to make tea because of their sweet taste, vitamin C and antioxidants properties. Hibiscus tea extract is used also for weight management and lowering cholesterol. Use Hibiscus to help an upset stomach, for cancer prevention and liver disease. It also treats high blood pressure and is a diuretic to increase urination. It helps to combat bacterial infections, colds, flus, and skin infections.

EMOTIONAL

Hibiscus flower essence energizes the first and second chakras, releasing blockages in the lower back and spine. It gravitates to healing reproductive ailments and infertility problems, frigidity and feeling numb in life. Hibiscus soothes long-held scars from sexual trauma, its flower remedies assist in releasing pent up creative forces within the womb and sets it free to enjoy life again.

Warning do not administer to Pregnant Women or Nursing Mothers.

BIBLICAL

"I am a rose of Sharon, a rose of the valleys."

"As a rose among the thorns, so is my beloved among the daughters."

"As an apple tree among the trees of the forest, so is my beloved among the sons; in his shade I delighted and sat, and his fruit was sweet to my palate".

"He brought me to the banquet hall, and his attraction to me was symbolic of his love."

"Sustain me with flagons of wine, spread my bed with apples, for I am lovesick."

"His left hand was under my head, and his right hand would embrace me."

"I adjure you, O daughters of Jerusalem, by the gazelles or by the hinds of the field, that you neither awaken nor arouse the love while it is desirous."

"The sound of my beloved! Behold, he is coming, skipping over the mountains, jumping over the hills".

"My beloved resembles a gazelle or a fawn of the hinds; behold, he is standing behind our wall, looking from the windows, peering from the lattices."

"My beloved raised his voice and said to me, 'Arise, my beloved, my fair one, and come away. For behold, the winter has passed; the rain is over and gone."

"The blossoms have appeared in the land, the time of singing has arrived, and the voice of the turtledove is heard in our land."

"The fig tree has put forth its green figs, and the vines with their tiny grapes have given forth their fragrance; arise, my beloved, my fair one, and come away."

"My dove, in the clefts of the rock, in the coverture of the steps, show me your appearance, let me hear your voice, for your voice is pleasant and your appearance is comely."

"Seize for us the foxes, the little foxes, who destroy the vineyards, for our vineyards are with tiny grapes."

"My beloved is mine, and I am his, who grazes among the roses."

"Until the sun spreads, and the shadows flee, go around; liken yourself, my beloved, to a gazelle or to a fawn of the hinds, on distant mountains."

(Song of Songs 2:1-17)

This is the ultimate fantasy of King Solomon who adored women and could not get enough of them, he loved many foreign women especially the daughter of Pharaoh. He loved women of the Moabites, Ammonites, Edomites, Zidonians, and Hittites, however, the daughter of Pharaoh was beloved by him more than all of them. Of all the nations about which God had said to the Israelites, "you shall not mingle among them, and they shall not come among you, for certainly they will sway your heart after their deities," but Solomon did cleave to love to them all. Solomon had seven hundred royal wives and three hundred concubines, and his heart yearned still for more wives. When Solomon reached old age, he could no longer control his wives and they turned away from his heart and towards other gods, and this displeased God. When at first Solomon did nothing to stop them, this indicated that he was not completely devoted to God as his wives, just like his father David. Since Solomon did not protest against his wives as was expected of him, God blames him for their sins. Solomon then sends sacrifices to God for all his alien wives who had offered incense and slaughtered sacrifices to their foreign gods according to their deities. Twice God had approached Solomon regarding this issue, and he did not do as God as commanded to resolve this matter.

God said to Solomon, "For as this has been with you, and you have not observed My covenant and My statutes which I have commanded you, I will surely tear the kingdom from you, and I shall give it to your servant." God was telling him basically you knew that you were transgressing my precept. God rebuked Solomon for yet another matter, he built up a Milo, and with this building he enclosed into a breach to protect his wife, Pharaoh's daughter behind it. God said to Solomon,

"Your father made breaches in the wall for the pilgrims to enter, and you fenced it in, to create a labor force for Pharaoh's daughter, to station there her manservants and maidservants."

However, "I will not punish you in your days for the sake of David your father; but from the hands of your son, I shall tear it away. However, one tribe I shall grant to your son for the sake of David My servant, and for the sake of Jerusalem, the city which I have chosen." Jeroboam, the son of Nabat an Ephraimite, he was a mighty man of valor, was the man God chose to be king instead of Solomon's son. God will afflict David's descendants because of this comparable to the thirty-six years that Solomon was married to Pharaoh's daughter, he married her during the fourth year of his reign. The decree was promulgated on the kingdom of the house of David, and it was divided.

Ahijah, the Shilonite, the prophet, found Jeroboam on the way, and he was wearing a new garment, making sure the two of them were alone in the field. Ahijah grasped Jeroboam's new garment and tore it into twelve pieces, saying to him, "take for yourself ten pieces, for so has the Lord, the God of Israel, said, I shall tear the kingdom out of Solomon's hands, and I shall give you the ten tribes." But this decree was not to be for all times for in the days of the Messiah the kingdom will be restored to the kingdom of David, the rest of the events of Solomon and all that he did, and his wisdom are written in the book of the words of Solomon. The years which Solomon reigned in Jerusalem over all Israel were forty years. Then Solomon slept with his fathers and was buried in the city of David his father; and Rehoboam his son ruled in his place.

Hops

Latin Name, Humulus Lupulus
Aroma, Strong, pungent, herbaceous, and citrus

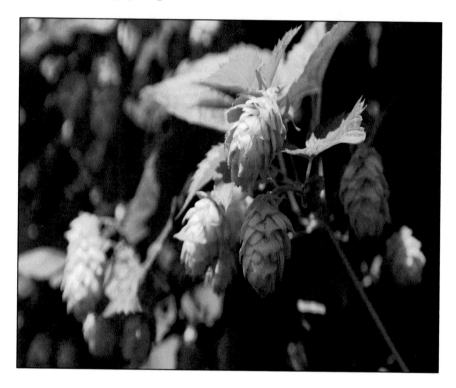

PHYSICAL

Hops is a plant with flowers shaped like cones and is a climbing plant that very much resembles a vine tree, it grows in Southern England and Western America. It is part of the Cannabis family and is mainly used to flavor and stabilize beer to give the bitter, zesty, or citric flavors. Its dried flowers are used to make medicine, as a sedative, antibacterial and anesthetic agent. Hops other features are, analgesics, appetite stimulant, and digestive stimulant and it increases the secretion of milk in lactating mothers. Hops is used for hormone replacement therapy and for relief of menstruation problems.

EMOTIONAL

Hops may be used in herbal medicine in a way like valerian, as a treatment for anxiety, restlessness, and insomnia. A pillow filled with hops is a popular folk remedy for sleeplessness, and animal research has backed up its sedative effect. Hops is used for people feeling unsettled, stubbornness or simply not wanting change. It helps to achieve changes in points of view, forces one to climb up and take control of their problems.

BIBLICAL

"So, the chief cupbearer related his dream to Joseph, and he said to him, "In my dream, behold, a vine is before me." (Genesis 40:9)

"And on the vine are three tendrils, and it seemed to be blossoming, and its buds came out; then its clusters ripened into grapes." (Genesis 40:10)

"For their vine is of the vine of Sodom, and of the field of Gomorrah; their grapes are grapes of Rosh, and they have bitter clusters." (Deuteronomy 32:32)

"Their wine is the bitterness of serpents, and the bitterness of the ruthless cobras." (Deuteronomy 32:33)

"Give strong drink to the one who is perishing and wine to those of bitter soul." (Proverbs 31:6)

"Let him drink and forget his poverty and let him remember his misery no more." (Proverbs 31:7)

"Wine mourns, the vine is humbled, all joyful hearted sigh." (Isaiah 24:7)

"In song they shall not drink wine; strong drink shall become bitter to those who drink it." (Isaiah 24:9)

"A cry for wine is in the streets; all joy is darkened; the joy of the land is exiled." (Isaiah 24:11)

"Ho! All who thirst, go to water, and whoever has no money, go, buy and eat, and go, buy without money and without a price, wine and milk." (Isaiah 55:1)

"So says the Lord of Hosts: They shall thoroughly glean like a vine the remnant of Israel; return your hand as a vintager over the branches." (Jeremiah 6:9)

Hops was a beer making agent, its oxidative reaction gives the bitter flavor to beer as well as flavoring it with its special hop aroma. It was discovered by the Israelites in biblical times and was adopted to make many varieties of alcoholic beverages, and very often was also used for medicinal purposes because of its many healing qualities. Alcohol is drunk for many reasons in life, for some as a comfort because they are suffering pain due to poverty or mourning. For others it is to celebrate either good or evil acts or for a bitter soul of envy. Alcohol is known to give pleasure for millions of reasons in a difficult world, and people who drink alcohol as an amenity for their conduct in this world, unfortunately leave with nothing. When enjoying alcohol regardless, for either happy occasions or sometimes sadder times, it heals and comforts the soul. After the vineyard has been gathered, and gleanings are left, and the poor come and glean them, so will they spoil and return and spoil.

Joseph had been brought down to Egypt, and Potiphar, Pharaoh's chamberlain, chief of the slaughterers, who was an Egyptian man, had purchased him from the Ishmaelites who had brought him down to Egypt. Potiphar took a strong liking to Joseph who served him respectfully, so he decided to appoint Joseph to manage over his house, giving him full control. Now Joseph was a very handsome man with a beautiful complexion, and soon Joseph found himself in the position of power. He began eating and drinking well and he enjoyed curling his hair, which made God unhappy,

"Your father is mourning, and you curl your hair! I will incite the bear against you."

Immediately afterwards, his master's wife lifted her eyes towards him, and she said, "Lie with me." Obviously, Joseph refused and said he had no intention of betraying his master, to which she replied, "in this house there is no one greater than I, and he has not withheld anything from me except you, insofar as you are his wife. Now how can I commit this great evil, and sin against God?" After many days that Joseph did not obey her and lie with her, and certainly would not have intercourse with her.

A special day of celebration had arrived, it was a day of rejoicing and a religious festival when the whole household went to the temple of their idols. She said, "I have no more fitting day to consort with Joseph than today. So, I am ill, and I cannot go." When Joseph came to the house that morning, he found that only Potiphar's wife was home. She grabbed at him by his garment, demanding that he lie with her, Joseph slipped out of his jacket leaving his garment in her hand and left the house. Seeing the empty garment in her hands humiliated and infuriated her, she began yelling, "look! He brought us a Hebrew man to mock us. He came to me to lie with me, but I screamed." She kept Joseph's garment as evidence for when her husband would come home later, accusing Joseph of abusing her.

When Potiphar his master heard his wife's accusing report of Joseph, "your slave did such things to me," that it flared his burning wrath. The Midrash says that she told him her lies about Joseph during intercourse and she demonstrated her meaning of "your slave did such things to me," meaning them to be acts of intimacy. So, Joseph's master threw him into prison, the same one where the king's prisoners were, and there he stayed. God protected Joseph during his stay in prison, by making him beautiful and charismatic so the warden would favor him. The warden entrusted all the new prisoners to Joseph and never inspected his possessions. After the event of Potiphar's wife slandering Joseph's righteous name, while he was in jail by the force of God, the cupbearer and the baker sinned against their master, the king of Egypt. A fly was found in his goblet and a pebble was found in his bread, God arranged it so, he wanted the King to turn his attention to the two chamberlains and not to Joseph and through them God would save him.

So, Pharaoh threw them also into the prison house where they all stayed a year in prison. One night both of them had dreams which were premonitions of their fates, and both were seeking interpretations of their dreams. That morning Joseph saw that Pharaoh's two chamberlains seemed very troubled, so, he asked them, "why are your faces sad today?" They told him their dreams and Joseph told him he could interpret them, so the chief cupbearer related his dream to Joseph, and concluded, "in my dream, behold, a vine is before me, on the vine are three tendrils, and it seemed to be blossoming, and its buds came out, then its clusters ripened into grapes. Pharaoh's cup was in my hand, and I took the grapes and squeezed them into Pharaoh's cup, and I placed the cup on Pharaoh's palm."

Joseph interpreted that the three tendrils commensurate three days, meaning in another three days, Pharaoh will confer with the officers, and restore you to your position, and you will place Pharaoh's cup into his hand, as you are accustomed to doing. Joseph asked him to please do him a favor and mention him to Pharaoh and get him out of this prison. Joseph told him was kidnapped from the land of the Hebrews, and he has no reason to be left in the dungeon. Now it was the chief baker's turn to have his dream interpreted and he saw that it went well for the cupbearer, so he proceeded, "in my dream, behold, there were three wicker baskets on my head, in the top basket were all kinds of Pharaoh's baking produce, and the birds were eating them from the basket atop my head." Joseph said again the three baskets represent three days, and he continued, in three days' time, Pharaoh will remove your head and hang you on gallows, where birds will eat the flesh off you.

The third day arrived, and it happened to be Pharaoh's birthday, and he made a large feast for all his servants, and he included the chief cupbearer and chief baker among his servants. He reinstated the cupbearer who then placed the cup on Pharaoh's palm, as for the chief baker, he was hanged as Joseph had predicted. However, cupbearer did not remember Joseph, and forgot about him for another two years.

Hyssop

Latin Name, Hyssopus Officinalis
Aroma, Sweet, rich, and floral

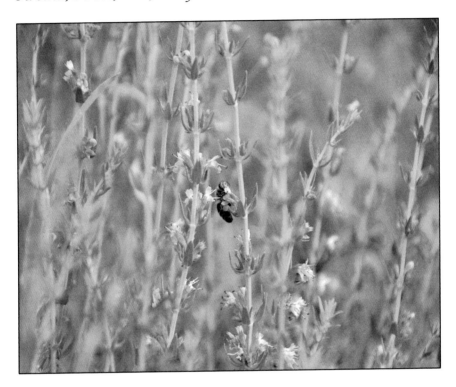

PHYSICAL

Hyssop is an herbaceous evergreen plant related to the mint family, it is a native of Southern Europe and the Middle East. It is a brightly colored shrub with woody stems with blue, pink, and sometimes white flowers. It has been used as an expectorant and an antiseptic for centuries in traditional medicine as a cough reliever and sooth sore throats. Its high concentrations of thujone and chemicals that stimulate the central nervous system.

This fresh herb is commonly used in cooking. Za'atar is a famous Middle Eastern herbal mix which has dried Hyssop leaves as one of the main ingredients

245

Warning Hyssop can cause seizures and even low doses, do not administer to children, Pregnant women and people suffering with epilepsy.

EMOTIONAL

Hyssop encourages awakening of the spirit, especially if it has been closed for a long time. It teaches acceptance and self-fulfillment. It gives encouragement to continue on in life while at the same time showing clarity. It brings balance and harmony, helping to establish spiritual and emotional connections. In the bible this oil was used in offerings to God to forgive sins, Hyssop gives the feeling of being cleansed and purified.

BIBLICAL

"And you shall take a bunch of hyssops and immerse it in the blood that is in the basin, and you shall extend to the lintel and to the two doorposts the blood that is in the basin, and you shall not go out, any man from the entrance of his house until morning." (Exodus 12:22)

"And God spoke to Moshe, saying, "This shall be the Torah of the leper in the day of his cleansing; He shall be brought to the Kohen." (Vayikra 14:1-2)

"And the Kohen shall go out of the camp; and the Kohen shall look, and behold, if the disease of leprosy is healed in the leper." (Vayikra 14:3)

"Then shall the Kohen command to take for him who is to be cleansed two birds alive and clean, and cedar wood, and scarlet, and hyssop." (Vayikra 14:4)

"And the Kohen shall command that one of the birds be killed in an earthen utensil over running water." (Vayikra 14:5)

"As for the living bird, he shall take it, and the cedar wood, and the scarlet, and the hyssop, and shall dip them and the living bird in the blood of the bird that was killed over the spring water." (Vayikra 14:6)

"The kohen shall take a piece of cedar wood, hyssop, and crimson wool, and cast them into the burning of the cow". (Numbers 19:6)

246

"A ritually clean person shall take the hyssop and dip it into the water and sprinkle it on the tent, on all the vessels, and on the people, who were in it, and on anyone who touched the bone, the slain person, the corpse, or the grave". (Numbers 19:18)

"Purify me with a hyssop, and I will become pure; wash me, and I will become whiter than snow." (Psalms 51:7)

The Hebrew name for Hyssop is Ezov and in the bible Ezov is described as a small plant that can be found on or near walls. Hyssop grows wild in Israel, in the Golan, Hermon, Galilee, Mediterranean coast and the Judean Mountains. It is considered a very holy herb used for divine wisdom and higher self and in Biblical times it was used for the purification of lepers. With specific instructions to make a formula which was then sprinkled over the "sinner," who was the leper or impure person to purify them. There are three different materials were mentioned in one sentence, cedar wood, hyssop, and crimson wool. These three types of very different objects correspond to the three thousand men who fell because of the sin of the golden calf.

A person afflicted with tzara'ath, leprosy, is brought for cleansing to the kohen who goes outside the camp to check if the lesion of tzara'ath has healed in the afflicted person. There were three types of camps, the first camp is for the Shechinah where the sanctuary is situated. The second camp was the Levite camp, and the third camp was the camp of the Israelites, where the ordinary Israelites encamped. The Kohen was sent during the time of his own uncleanness to cleanse the leper, he needed two live clean birds, a cedar stick, a strip of crimson wool, and hyssop. The Kohen ordered the slaughter of one bird into an earthenware vessel, over spring water, which was poured first at a quarter full into the bowl. Then the blood of the slaughtered bird was poured into the bowl. The next stage was to take the live bird, the cedar stick, the strip of crimson wool, and the hyssop, and dip them into the blood of the slaughtered bird and spring water. The cedar stick and the hyssop, however, were bound together with the strip of crimson wool, separately from the bird.

The Kohen then sprinkles the blood seven times upon the person being cleansed from tzara'ath, and then releases the live bird into the open field. The person being cleansed is then immerse with his garments into clean water, all his hair is shaved off, as is his beard, his eyebrows, and all other bodily hairs too, then he becomes clean. After which he may enter the camp, but he must remain outside his own tent for seven days, during this period he is prohibited to have marital relations with his wife. On the eighth day, he shall take two unblemished male lambs, one unblemished ewe lamb in its first year, three tenths of an ephah of fine flour mixed with olive oil as a meal offering plus one log of olive oil. Since a female animal is never brought as a burnt offering it is evident that this ewe lamb was to be sacrificed as the sin-offering. At the end the Kohen is to place some of the olive on the cartilage of his ear, and on his big toe.

The cedar is the highest of all trees, and the hyssop is the lowest of them all. This symbolizes that the one of high standing who acts haughtily, and sins should lower himself like a hyssop and a worm. Be careful from which position we talk to people, sometimes we are in a position to be above and be not so nice, until one day we fall to the lowest position and have to face others who are now high. Only after that will he then gain atonement. Worm translated into Hebrew means "Tola'at" and can also be translated as crimson.

Jasmine

Latin Name, Jasminum Officinale
Aroma, Sweet, rich, and floral

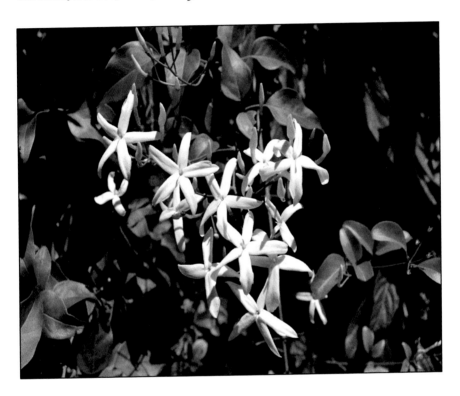

PHYSICAL

Jasmine is an evergreen shrub and is a climbing plant like vine, it has white or yellow flowers that have a divine fragrance, Jasmine fruits are berries that turn black when ripe. It grows in Morocco France, Egypt and India and has been used for many years as an aphrodisiac. Jasmine influences the central nervous system and cranial activity. It is an anti-depressant, and antiseptic, an anti-spasmodic and a sedative. For the worrying sort, this oil helps calm down, it also helps sleep if suffering from insomnia. It plays a huge role in female hormones; it heals damaged ovaries and quickens labor and helps in women's milk production. Jasmine also helps women suffering from post partem depression, and frigidity.

EMOTIONAL

This is an assertive oil, with a strong internal warmth that brings out the male side of a woman. It draws out feelings, abilities, and desires for success. Jasmine encourages uplifting optimism; it opens and stimulates one's sensitivity. Giving the beginning of a sense of harmony and profound awareness combined with inner inspiration and joy. Jasmine is great for an independent woman and strengthens the personalities of weaker men. It is a practical oil that solves problems and motivates one to be proactive.

BIBLICAL

"Now the man knew his wife Eve, and she conceived and bore Cain, and she said, "I have acquired a man with God,"
(Genesis 4:1)

"Reuben went in the days of the wheat harvest, and he found dudaim in the field and brought them to Leah, his mother, and Rachel said to Leah, "Now give me some of your son's dudaim."
(Genesis 30:14)

"And she said to her, "Is it a small matter that you have taken my husband, that you wish also to take my son's dudaim?" So, Rachel said, "Therefore, he shall sleep with you tonight as payment for your son's dudaim." (Genesis 30:15)

"When Jacob came from the field in the evening, and Leah came forth toward him, and she said, "You shall come to me, because I have hired you with my son's dudaim," and he slept with her on that night." (Genesis 30:16)

The dudaim are also called "love flowers" or mandrakes that are discovered mysteriously by Reuben, he finds the Jasmine in the field and brings them home for his mother. Rachel sees that he has them and asks for them, when Leah refused to relinquish her gift, Rachel offers her night with Jacob in exchange for the Jasmine and so Leah gave up all the dudaim to Rachel. Really classified as weeds and free for all to take, they are called jasmine in Arabic. The flowers have a divine aroma and was rumored to have the ability to make someone love you, and Reuben knowing that Jacob loved Rachel more, brought them for his mother Leah. When Rachel requested the flowers from Leah, she became very angry at Rachel and said, "Is it not enough that Jacob has established his dwelling with you, and is always with you?" Basically saying, now you also want my son's dudaim, is it not enough that Jacob loves you, and he spends most of his time with you. It was true Jacob's bed was permanently set up in Rachel's tent, but her problem was that she was barren, and she wished she would get pregnant, hoping that the dudaim would help. She was insanely jealous of her sister Leah who bore Jacob's sons and when she realized that Leah had no intention of giving her the dudaim, she traded her night with Jacob so she could have them. God did not approve of this deal and Rachel paid a high price for trading her night with Jacob, which was a belittling and disrespectful thing to do to a righteous man, "It was my night to be with him, but I give it to you in return for your son's Dudaim." and due to that fateful decision, she lost her merit of eternal burial alongside Jacob.

Reuben was only four years old when he found the Jasmines, and the bible says that he walked in the ways of the fathers of the world, meaning that he was a good little boy who was destined to rectify the sin of Adam. God praises Reuben's deeds, like every day their home is empty of food since they were still living in Laban's property. Laban was very stingy and did not care that Jacob's children only had a little bread with salt to eat. That day, Reuben was hungry, and being that there was nothing to eat at home, he went into the field to look for something to eat. Actually, the fields were an abundance of wheat, barley, grapes, figs, and pomegranates, but he had no right to eat any of them even if he craved them, because the field belonged to his grandfather Laban. Since the dudaim flowers were considered weeds that grow naturally, they may be taken by anyone. Reuben could not resist their tempting orange fruits with their beautiful fragrance. Reuben brought them to his mother Leah first and kept nothing for himself, he loved his mother very much and wanted her to enjoy them.

Reuben proved that his heart was pure as was his soul, unlike Adam and Eve in the Garden of Eden when Reuben picked the dudaim it was in the height of the wheat harvest, and he did not even for one moment attempt to steal any wheat or barley. The Midrash says this was the rectification of the first act of stealing in the world. Even though Adam and Eve were alone in the world where everything in the garden of Eden was theirs, except for the one tree that God withheld from them. But they could not resist their urge and took from the tree. As a punishment they descended from their previous greatness and never ascended again. Reuben was born twenty generations later rectified their sin; he was in a situation where nothing belonged to him except for the Jasmine. He saw the fruits, for him it was not even an option to try and taste them because he knew they were not his. Reuben's tribal flag depicts a picture of the dudaim, the fragrant scent of the Dudaim, was the Tree of Knowledge's amendment as this was the only sense that not involved in the sin of eating from the Tree of knowledge. When Reuben brought the dudaim to his mother Leah, she instinctively understood that it was the tree of Knowledge that transformed into the fruit of the Tree of Life. The virtue for Reuben bringing the Dudaim, jasmine flowers, which resulted in the birth of Issachar, who was from the good side of Cain the first born ever.

Issachar's birth was an allusion to Cain's rectification through him, both Eve and Leah were both on the same wavelength, which we know as Imma Ila'a, the supernal maternal aspect. Rachel and Leah were twins, just like Jacob and Esau. Leah was destined to marry Esau and Rachel was destined to marry Jacob. Leah found out Esau was evil and begged God to save her from him. God gave her to Jacob, and she married him before Rachel did. Both Rachel and Leah are direct descendants from Eve and are of a dual nature. Each one embodies a different aspect of her character; Leah owns the upper comprehension aspect. Rachel owns the lower sovereignty aspect and together they formed the complete typical feminine woman. The commentaries say that firstborn children take a double portion of the family inheritance because spiritually they participate in the conception of the following children. The commentaries continued to explain this passage which specifically refers to Reuben, Jacob's firstborn child who brought the dudaim which resulted in the birth of Issachar. The dudaim transferred force from Leah to Rachel and embodied a shift in the supernal realm, the blossoming of the Jasmine transferred the powers from the upper realm to the lower realm. Reuben who came from Cain rectified Cain's sin of killing his brother that stemmed from jealousy by causing Issachar to be born.

Juniper

Latin Name, Juniperus Drupacea
Aroma, Fresh, Fruity and Woody

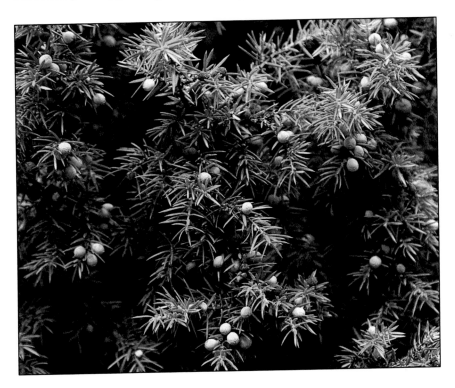

PHYSICAL

Juniper is a coniferous plant from the cypress family, it grows in Mount Hermon and Lebanon. Junipers are evergreens that grow at very high altitudes symbolizing strength and stature and can grow up to forty meters in height. Juniper berries are a spice used for flavoring "Gin" from the Gin & Tonic drink. Its leaves resemble cedarwood. It was brought to Israel because it grows in dry countries and absorbs water. Juniper does not need to be watered; it survives in all dry places.

Juniper emulsifies fats and assists the liver to digest it, one drop on your tongue before a heavy meal will help. It absorbs the water out of swellings, water retentions and fats. It is good to use in a deodorant, to absorb sweat. To make a deodorant, blend oil and water and add a few drops of juniper and watch it mix into a mayonnaise type mix. Good for blood vessels and capillaries, heals a sprained ankle much faster because of its ability to reduce the swelling. Can be used to prevent thrombosis and bruises. Juniper is an anti-inflammatory and helps balance muscle and arthritic pain. It heals inflammation from Gout, which is like a spur infection caught inside the muscle. It releases lactic acid pain, or pain from too much ripped muscles (DOMS), which is Delayed Onset Muscle Soreness. In this situation a lot of uric acid is released into your blood stream, showing high creatine levels in the Liver. Helps with bladder and urinary problems, lower back contractions at the end of the pregnancy.

EMOTIONAL

Dries up emotions, when crying a lot, it dries up bitter tears. For people stuck in a rut, Juniper cleans up the messy thoughts, it absorbs puddles and clears up the mind. It balances and helps regain homeostasis, it helps make important and calculated decisions. Juniper encourages inner vision, strength, vitality, and sincerity helping clear the path to the divine spirit, transmitting and facilitating prayers and enlightenment.

BIBLICAL

"Of junipers from Senir did they fashion you, all the planks; cedars from Lebanon they took to make a mast on you."
(Ezekiel 27:5)

"Cedars did not dim it in the garden of God, junipers did not equal its boughs, and chestnut trees were not like its branches; no tree in the garden of God equaled it in its beauty."
(Ezekiel 31:8)

"He went to the desert, a distance of one day's travel, and he came and sat under a juniper and requested that his soul die, He said, "Enough, now Lord take my soul as I am not better than my forefathers."
(I Kings 19:4)

"He lay and slept underneath one juniper and behold! an angel touched him and said to him, "Rise and eat." (I Kings 19:5)

"And the greater House he overlaid with juniper wood, and he overlaid it with fine gold, and he wrought upon it palm trees and chains." (II Chronicle 3:5)

"And Solomon made of the almog wood a path to the House of the Lord and to the king's palace, and harps and psalteries for the singers; none like them had been seen before in the land of Judah." (II Chronicles 9:11)

"Where birds nest; as for the stork the high junipers are its home." (Psalms 104:17)

"And he shall be like a lonely juniper tree in the wasteland and shall not see when good comes, but shall inhabit the parched places of the wilderness, a salty land that is uninhabitable." (Jeremiah 17:6)

"For he shall be like a tree planted by the water, and by a rivulet spreads its roots, and will not see when heat comes, and its leaves shall be green, and in the year of drought will not be anxious, neither shall it cease from bearing fruit." (Jeremiah 17:8)

Juniper in Hebrew is Arar and comes from the word childless and some even translate it as laid to waste. The Arar tree in the forest is deserted and alone, they mainly growing in Aroer which is an area in Samaria allotted to Reuben and is on the bank of the river Arnon. However even though Juniper contains a thorny exterior it conceals a beautiful secret, which is a tender edible heart. Once the heart is exposed to water, this nurtures the whole tree including its roots, which grow deep. Junipers grow tall in places where rivers flow around its base, and able to be seen by all the other trees around it. Its full height is taller than all the trees of the field, its boughs are multiplied, and when there is an abundance of water its branches grow long. They are beautiful trees generating pride due to their great height, where even Cedars cannot dim its elegance in the garden of God, they do not equal its boughs, and chestnut trees were not like its branches; no tree in the garden of God is equaled to the Juniper's grace. Juniper trees are natural survivors, it lives in the desert where there is no civilization.

When Jezebel sent a messenger to Elijah threatening that her gods would continue to operate unless he met with her at this time tomorrow saying, "I will make your life like the life of one of them." He got up and travelled to Be'er Sheba to escape her and save his life, there in the desert Elijah begged God to let him die already, claiming his life was long enough. He lay under a Juniper tree and slept when an angel woke him up and convinced him to eat and drink to give him strength on his journey to hide from Jezebel. After he ate, he gained enough strength for forty days and forty nights while he was up the mountain of Horeb. He found a cave where he was able to live in, it was in a cleft of rock exactly where Moses stood and spoke to God, then God appeared to him and asked him why he was there. Elijah tells God that his people has forsaken his covenant with him, they tore down his alter and killed God's prophets, telling God he is alone and afraid for his life.

God told Elijah to go and face him in the mountain, then God passed through the mountain and split it, via a sending camp of angels causing a strong wind and sending angels creating an earthquake and shattering the whole mountain to the ground. After the earthquake a camp of angels created a fire and after the fire there was a sound of a voice quietly praising the prophets of the nations. Elijah heard the voice and hid his face in his cape, he stood at the entrance of the cave and again God asked him why he was there, and again Elijah replied,

"I have been zealous for the Lord, the God of Hosts, for the Children of Israel have forsaken Your covenant, they have torn down Your altars, and they have killed Your prophets by the sword, and I alone remain, and they seek my soul to take it."
(I Kings 19:14)

God then tells him to continue his journey to Damascus and anoint Hazael to be king of Aram, anoint Jehu as king over Israel and to anoint Elisha as prophet to replace him. The Midrash says that God told Elijah, "I do not want your prophecy since you plead for the prosecution of my children." God said that those who escape the sword of Hazael, Jehu will kill, and those who escape the sword of Jehu, Elisha will kill, "I will leave over in Israel seven thousand, all the knees that did not kneel to the Baal and every mouth that did not kiss him."

Labdanum

Latin Name, Cistus Ladanifer
Aroma, Rich, musky, balsamic herb

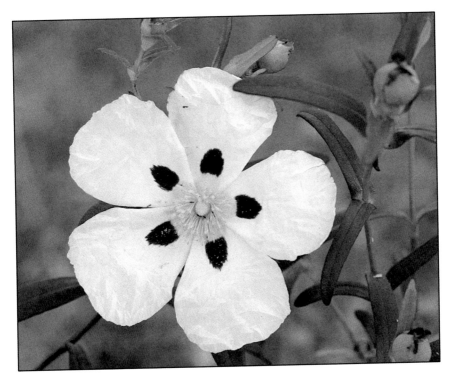

PHYSICAL

Labdanum is a sticky brown resin with a sweet and spicy fragrance, it is obtained from the shrubs of the Cistus Ladanifer which is a native to western Mediterranean regions. It is an evergreen shrub with a five-petal white flower and a beautiful maroon spot at the base of each petal. The whole plant gets covered with this sticky and fragrant resin, in ancient times labdanum was acquired by combing the beards and thighs of goats and sheep that used to graze on labdanum shrubs. This resin is oozed out in teardrop shapes and ages into a black solid onyx, thus called onycha.

It has very similar properties to lavender and is used for both perfumes and medicines. It knows how to help relieve bronchitis and difficulties in breathing, it heals colds, flus, and relieves respiratory tract infections much like an antibiotic. Also called Rock Rose because its roots depend on rocks by for anchoring to be able to grow producing flowers annually. The petals are in the shape of fingernails, and another reason to be called onycha which means nail.

EMOTIONAL

Cistus is used for trauma, shock and immediate trauma like during a war or a terror attack. This is the same plant used in Bach Flower Treatments "Rock Rose" where it is used to treat people suffering from shock, hysteria, or frozen shock. This oil deals with lack of ability or feelings of bad karma, use a few drops on the crown of the head. It is also used for nightmare for kids or babies birth trauma, just place a few drops on heels.

BIBLICAL

"And the Lord said to Moses, "Take for yourself aromatics, namely balsam sap, onycha Cistus and galbanum, aromatics and pure frankincense; they shall be of equal weight." (Exodus 30:34)

"And you shall make it into incense, a compound according to the art of the perfumer, well blended, pure, holy." (Exodus 30:35)

"And you shall crush some of it very finely, and you shall set some of it before the testimony in the Tent of Meeting, where I will arrange meetings with you; it shall be to you a holy of holies." (Exodus 30:36)

"And the incense that you make, you shall not make for yourselves according to its formula; it shall be holy to you for the Lord."
(Exodus 30:37)

This is the mysterious onycha ingredient in the holy incense Ketoret referred to in the bible. The exact instructions on how to make the Ketoret incense are in the passages of the Bible, their exact quantities and weights were kept secret for many hundreds of years. The Kohen was instructed by God to use only the best quality ingredients and is instructed how to blend and crush them and then how to offer it to God. Onycha is a root of a spice described as smooth and shiny as fingernails. The four ingredients, balsam sap, onycha, galbanum and pure frankincense are a blend mentioned explicitly, where God says shall be of equal parts, a weight for a weight, the weight of each was seventy units. They should be compounded thoroughly into an incense according to the art of the perfumer, they should be mixed as a sailor propels and oar to turn over the water, or as a person who beats eggs with a spoon. The ingredients must be pure so they can be holy, and these incense blends must not be made for personal use ever.

At the time of Jacob and his sons there was great famine in the land of Israel, when they finished all their stored grain, Jacob told his sons to return to Egypt and buy more food. Judah warned their father that they could not go back to Egypt without taking their youngest brother Benjamin. Joseph had not yet revealed to his brothers that he recognized them saying, "you shall not see my face if your brother is not with you." Jacob asked Judah why he told him that he had another brother, the brothers explained to Jacob, we were compelled to answer. The man asked if our father was still alive and asked if we had another brother. They said, "could we have known that he would say, bring your brother down?"

Judah told Jacob they had no choice, that he should send Benjamin with them to Egypt saying, "we will all come back alive." Judah personally guaranteed Benjamin's safety, he told Jacob, "If I do not bring him to you and stand him up before you, I will have sinned against you forever." Judah knew that they would not die of hunger, as for Benjamin, he was not sure whether he will be seized or not. However, it was certain that they would all die of hunger if they did not go to Egypt to buy food, so they had to go whether they liked it or not. Judah said in all this time they were dallying, they could have gone already twice and back, Jacob tells Judah to take a gift basket of a choice of products for the "man," they should take balm, honey, wax, lotus, pistachios, and almonds. He also told them to take double the amount of money with them and return the money that was somehow returned in error and take your brother.

Jacob said, hopefully this man will have compassion and will release you and your brothers, since he was an already bereaved man. Jacob was thinking "enough!" of his troubles since he had not enjoyed tranquility since his youth. He endured the troubles of Laban, who tricked him and pursued him with the intention of killing him. He had troubles with his brother Esau, who also wanted to kill him, then there were the troubles of Rachel, who died in childbirth. He also remembered the trouble of

Dinah who was violated and kidnapped by Shechem and the trouble of Joseph's disappearance. Now the trouble of Simeon who is being detained by the ruler of Egypt, and the trouble of Benjamin whom he demands that Jacob sends to him.

The brothers took the gifts and money and set out with Benjamin and soon stood before Joseph, when Joseph saw Benjamin again, he told the overseer of his house, "Bring the men into the house and gave orders to slaughter an animal and to prepare it, for the men will eat with me at lunch." When the brothers were brought into Joseph's house, they felt afraid, they thought this may be about the returned money. It was not customary for anyone who came to purchase grain to lodge in Joseph's personal home, people booked rooms in the city's inns. They feared that this was done to fabricate false accusations and put them into prison, and they told Joseph, "On account of the money that came back in our sacks at first, we are brought, to roll upon us and to fall upon us and to take us as slaves and our donkeys as well." They told Joseph about the returned money, which they only noticed once they got home saying, "we do not know who put our money into our sacks."

Joseph told the brothers not to worry, it was to their merit that they brought back the money and he brought Simeon out to them. Once again, they entered Joseph's house because the first time the brothers pushed him Joseph outside to speak to him at the entrance of his house, it was only after he said to them, "peace to you," that they followed him into the house. In the afternoon the brothers brought to Joseph the gift basket and bowed down to him to the ground, when Joseph once again inquired after their father asking if he was still alive. They assured him that Jacob was alive and well, and again bowed down to him to the ground. Joseph suddenly looked up and saw Benjamin, his brother, the son of his own mother, and he asked, "Is this your little brother, whom you told me about?" when Joseph saw his brother, he felt deep emotions for him and wanted to weep and he left the room to weep in private.

Joseph asked Benjamin, "do you have you another brother from your own mother?" to which Benjamin replied, "I had a brother, but I do not know where he is." Joseph asked, "have you any sons?" to which Benjamin told him that he had ten sons. Joseph asked what their names were, to which he told him, he then asked him, "what is the significance of each of these names?" Benjamin replied,

"All of them are connected to my brother and the troubles that befell him. My first son was named Bela because my brother seemed to have been swallowed up among the nations. My second son was named Becher because my brother was my mother's firstborn. My third son was named Ashbel because God put my brother into captivity. My fourth son was named Gera because my brother is a stranger in a lodging place. My fifth son was named Naaman because my brother was very pleasant to look upon. My sixth and seventh sons were named Ehi and Rosh because he was my brother, and he was my superior. My eighth son was named Muppim because my brother learned from my father's mouth. My ninth son was named Huppim because my brother did not see my wedding, and neither did I see his wedding. My tenth son was named Ard because my brother descended among the nations."

This immediately stirred Joseph's mercy causing him to weep in his room, once he composed himself, he came out of the room and dinner was served. They had to eat separately because it was against the law for an Egyptian to eat with a Hebrew, the brothers sat by order of age around the table. Joseph knocked his goblet with each brother announcing their names, with the sons of each mother sitting in order also. When Joseph reached Benjamin, he said, "This one has no mother, and I have no mother. Let him sit beside me." Joseph gave Benjamin a portion that was five times the size of the portions he gave to the other brothers, they all drank and became intoxicated with Joseph. The brothers had not drunk wine since the day they had sold him, but on that day they drank.

Lavender

Latin Name, Lavendula Augustifolia
Aroma, Fresh herbal and floral

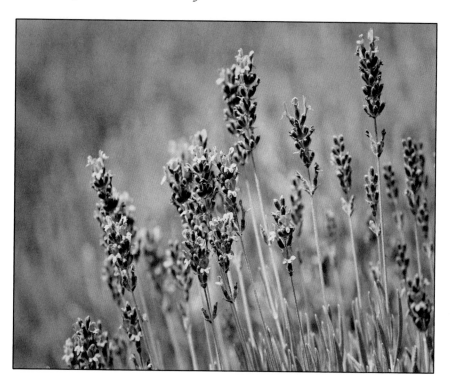

PHYSICAL

Lavender is a silverish green bush which can grow up to a meter in height, it has blue, purple-colored flowers and grows mainly in France. Lavender causes relaxation actions and puts you to sleep. Medical Lavender also known as English Lavender; it is a friendly oil capable of amazing things. It has many wonderful characteristics with a beautiful aroma. It is an anesthetizer and is a great help if you suffer from migraines and headaches. Excellent choice of oil for asthma sufferers, its influence on the nervous system as a relaxant and respiratory system helps coughs and allergies. Lavender is best known for its effect on the heart, and its ability to calm palpitations. This oil was used in the old days for these situations, best to always have Lavender at home. Inhale as soon as the palpitations starts and spread it directly on skin around the heart area. It is very often used in formulas to heal wounds, with its many healing properties. It is also used to treat scars and injuries, assuring a speedier recovery.

Lavender delays the onset of an inflammation and encourages the immune system to act, by delaying the release of histamines from the mast cells. These are the cells our immune system recruits to delay allergic reactions that release histamine and serotonin. Lavender increases the rate of chrome cell development to cause a reverse action to the release of histamine. This oil has a good effect on other essential oils when blended, because it reduces possible toxicity of other oils. It is a safe oil, it can be used directly onto the skin, on pregnant women and on babies.

EMOTIONAL

The word Lavender derives from the word Lavera, which means to wash. The Romans used Lavender in their baths and were the ones to bring Lavender to England. Till today it is a very popular plant in England. Lavender is sprinkled on sheets to give a very pleasant scent and a relaxing feeling. Lavender quietens and reduces stress, fears, and panic attacks. People who do not like the scent of Lavender is said to be a person who finds it hard to accept love, holistic therapists see this as an indication of emotional problems. Lavender gives the warmth needed and it protects like a mother in times of deep sadness, lavender lifts the heavy weight of sorrow, it wipes away the dark clouds and depression. When feeling despair or worried or have that trouble deep inside the spirit, or crying inside, lavender takes you right out of your troubles and dries up your tears. This is the most pliable of all the essential oils, it adapts itself and makes itself useful wherever needed. Replacement oils for people who really don't like lavender are mandarin and cinnamon.

BIBLICAL

"And He said, "Please take your son, your only one, whom you love, yea, Isaac, and go away to the land of Moriah and bring him up there for a burnt offering on one of the mountains, of which I will tell you." (Genesis 22:2)

"And the Lord said to Moses, "Take for yourself aromatics, balsam sap, onycha and galbanum, aromatics and pure frankincense; they shall be of equal weight." (Exodus 30:34)

263

"While the king was still at his table, my spikenard gave forth its fragrance." (Song of Songs 1:12)

Lavender was called nardus, spikenard or just nard in the Bible, spikenard, it is described to be shaped like a sort of cluster. It was one of the herbs used in the Ketoret for the purification ingredients in the time of the first Temple of Jerusalem, and nard is mentioned in the Song of Solomon as an expression of love as part of his love song.

God wants to test Abraham's faith, and he calls him one day, "Abraham, here I am." The Midrash says that it was really Satan accusing Abraham, and antagonized God that of all the feasts he prepares, he did not sacrifice even one bull or one ram to God. Then God says,

"He does everything only for his son Isaac, yet, if I were to say to him, sacrifice Isaac before me he would not withhold him."

God instructs Abraham with a "please" to bring his beloved son, the one he loves, when Abraham answered saying, "I love them both," God wanted to be very clear and said, "the only son of his mother, Isaac." He was to bring him to Moriah and bring him up there for a burnt offering on one of the mountains. The Midrash says the please was an expression of a request, but what God is actually saying to him, "I beg of you, pass this test for me, so that people will not say that the first one's tests had no substance." Mount Moriah was the choice of many holy sacrifices, it was also known as the "land of service," because there are many incenses growing naturally on this mountain, such as oregano, spikenard, and myrrh. In the future Mount Moriah is to be the choice to build the house of God.

The next morning Abraham arose early and saddled up his donkey, he took with him Isaac as well as Ishmael and Eliezer as escorts, because as a person of such great esteem, it was not permitted for him to go out on the road without two men, so that if one must relieve himself, the second one will remain with him. Abraham split up wood in preparation for the burnt offering and they set out to Moriah. On their third day of travelling, they saw Moriah at a distance, he paused for a while to think about what he was doing. Abraham did not want people to say that God confused and bewildered him suddenly and that his mind had become deranged. He wanted people to understand that it was of his own choice, the time he took to "think it over," was that people would understand that he also could had decided to not do it.

Abraham told Ishmael and Eliezer "Stay here with the donkey, and I and the lad will go yonder, and we will prostrate ourselves and return to you." He wanted privacy to see the place God had promised to him and right then and there Abraham prophesied without realizing it, that they will both return. Abraham took the wood piled it up and set Isaac on top of it and they both continued to the mountain. Isaac looked at all the items they took for the sacrifice and asked his father, "I am here, we have the wood, but where is the lamb for the burnt offering?" Abraham tells him that God will worry about the lamb once they get there, and if there will be no lamb, my son will be for a burnt offering, although Isaac understood that he was going to be slaughtered, he still went willingly with his father, both walking as one heart.

When they arrived at the exact location that God had selected, Abraham built the altar, arranged the wood, bound Isaac with his hands and his feet behind him where his ankles turned white. Abraham then placed Isaac on the altar on top of the wood, Abraham made up an incense blend using myrrh, spikenard, and other spices he found. He then reached out for the knife to slaughter his son, when suddenly angel of God called out to him from heaven and said, "Abraham! Abraham!" Abraham answered, "here I am." The angel then said,

"Do not stretch forth your hand to the lad, nor do the slightest thing to him, for now I know that you are a God-fearing man, and you did not withhold your son, your only one, from Me."
(Genesis 22:12)

Abraham asked the angel, "have I come here in vain? I will inflict a wound on him and extract a little blood." So, the angel told him to not do the slightest blemish on him, causing Abraham to be completely confused. At first God said that Isaac will be called his seed, then God retracted and said told him to take his son to be sacrificed, and now God is saying, "do not stretch forth your hand to the lad." God told Abraham he would never abuse his covenant with him,

"I did not say to you, slaughter him, but bring him up, you have brought him up; now take him down."

God said now he knows never to listen to Satan ever again, then Abraham looked up and saw a ram, and it was caught in a tree by its horns, so Abraham took the ram and offered it up as a burnt offering instead of his son.

Lemon Balm

Latin Name, Melissa officinalis
Aroma, Citrus, gentle and fresh

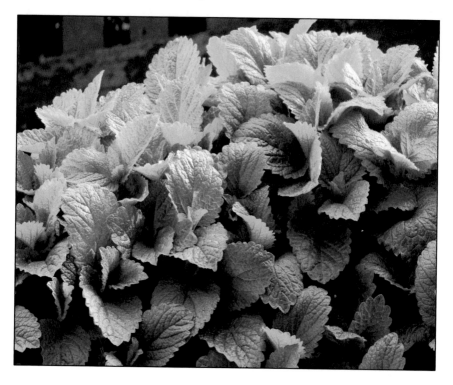

PHYSICAL

This is a Lemon Balm tree known as Melissa which comes from the mint family and is native of the Mediterranean Basin. During the summer season its small white flowers blossom and are full of nectar. It is these white flowers that attract bees, and this is also the reason this plant is called Melissa which means honeybee in Greek. Lemon Balm was used as a treatment of disorders of the gastrointestinal tract, nervous system, liver, and bile. It is an antioxidant and is very active against viral and fungal infections as well as herpes simplex and the flu.

It is also used as a sleep aid and digestive aid and for cognitive abilities, such as ADHD where it is considered a Ritalin alternative. This oil is used to help people suffering from Alzheimer's and dementia because of its abilities to rebuild brain cells. Appy to scorpion or animal bites for its antibacterial properties, this plant was grown in John Gerard's Garden, an English botanist with a large herbal garden in London.

EMOTIONAL

Lemon Balm is a relaxant and is used to lower Blood Pressure and calm people down. It acts much like dopamine because of its ability to reduce hysteria and anxieties for young girls, as well as relaxing fears from panic attacks and stress. Lemon Balm is widely used for its ability to bring acceptance, logic, and comprehension to one experiencing emotional shock from incomprehensible situations. When left with anger, fear, and grief from a deep loss this oil restores balance to resolute emotions. Lemon Balm gets into the depth of the psyche and drags one out of the rut. This oil uplifts spirit and assists to move forward and leave suffering behind. Lemon Balm is very calming and uplifting and brings joy into every cell of the being. Lemon balm has long been known as an herb that balances feelings, emotions and helps resolve moodiness and melancholia.

It acts revives and revitalizes the spirit bringing out the inner truth of Love. Melissa unblocks any overbearing heavy emotions, using its magical powers to bring success, peace, and purification. Lemon Balm works on an extremely high energetic frequency with the third eye chakra, great for meditations. Use it to release fears and negative emotions and acquire a quietened aura. Melissa, in Greek Mythology was a nymph who discovered honey from bees, it is believed this oil received its name from her. As one of the nurses of Zeus, rather than feeding the baby milk, Melissa fed him honey.

BIBLICAL

"And they sat down to eat a meal, and they lifted their eyes and saw, and behold, a caravan of Ishmaelites was coming from Gilead, and their camels were carrying spices, balm, and lotus, going to take it down to Egypt." (Genesis 37:25)

"Is there no balm in Gilead? Is there no physician there? Why then, has the health of the daughter of my people not been restored?" (Jeremiah 8:22)

"Judea and the land of Israel-they are your peddlers; with wheat of Minnith, balsam trees, honey, oil, and balm, they gave your necessities." (Ezekiel 27:17)

Lemon Balm is a native of this region and has been in Israel for centuries. Even though is not mentioned in the Bible, it was known and was used by the Israelites for medicinal purposes as well as a perfume. Balsam trees are generally called "pannag," and were then found in Jericho, and it was because of their fragrant scents, the city was called Jericho, in Hebrew the root word of Jericho "Re'ach" means scent after their reputed aroma in the city. The powers of these balms emanate healing throughout the whole world, and nothing is more beautiful than fragrance. In biblical times, being a wealthy person did not only refer to money, but it also referred to owning many oils, balms, and spices.

Jacob lived in Canaan in his father's property, one day when Joseph was seventeen years old and being a shepherd, together with his brothers guarding the flocks. Joseph was still a lad and was hanging out with the sons of Bilhah and Zilpah, his father's third and fourth wives. Joseph was frequently with the sons of Bilhah, because his other brothers despised him even though he acted friendly towards them. That day Joseph tattle tailed evil stories about the boys to their father, as always, any evil actions he saw his brothers, the sons of Leah do, he would tell his father. First, they ate limbs from living animals, second, they demeaned the sons of the handmaids by calling them slaves, third they were suspected of illicit sexual relationships and for these three tales Joseph was punished.

For the first report that his brothers ate the limbs of living animals, when they sold him, they slaughtered a kid and dipped his multi-colored coat in its blood and did not eat it alive. For the second report that he told Jacob about them calling their brothers slaves, Joseph himself was sold as a slave. For the third report concerning the illicit sexual relationships that he gossiped about them, Joseph himself had to deal with a scandal with his master's wife. The Midrash says that Joseph was an immature boy, always fixing his hair and touching up his eyes so that he would appear handsome. Joseph's features resembled Jacob's, and whatever happened to Jacob happened to Joseph, Jacob was hated, and so was Joseph. Jacob's brother Esau sought to kill him, as did Joseph's brothers seek to kill him,

268

Jacob loved Joseph more than all his sons, because he was a son of his old age; and he made him a fine woolen coat of green and blue wool. It was hard to miss, and the brothers noticed that their father loved Joseph more than all of them, so they hated him, and they could not speak to him in a civilized manner. To their credit, that they did not say one thing with their mouth and think differently in their hearts. To make matters worse Joseph had a dream which he told his brothers about which just caused their hatred for him to grow even more. Joseph said,

> "Listen now to this dream, which I have dreamed, behold, we were binding sheaves in the midst of the field, and behold, my sheaf arose and also stood upright, and behold, your sheaves encircled it and prostrated themselves to my sheaf."
> (Genesis 37:6-7)

Joseph's sheaves would remain standing erect in place, while the brothers' sheaves would bow down to him, the brothers were furious and said to Joseph, "now you think you reign over us, or you will govern over us?" The brothers continued their hatred of Joseph on account of his dreams and on account of his words telling evil tales about them to their father. Then soon Joseph dreamed another dream, "behold, I have dreamed another dream, and behold, the sun, the moon, and eleven stars were prostrating themselves to me." When he told his father about his dreams in the presence of his brothers, even his father got angry at him and rebuked him saying, "what is this dream that you have dreamed? Will we come I, your mother, and your brothers to prostrate ourselves to you to the ground?" Jacob did not realize that Joseph was referring to Bilhah, who had raised him as though she was his real mother. The last thing that Jacob intended was to make his other sons jealous of Joseph, so he asked them to forget the whole matter, even though he knew that there is no dream without meaningless components.

Jacob wanted to send Joseph to his brothers who went to pasture their father's flocks in Shechem, and Joseph wanted to fulfill his father's command even though he knew that his brothers hated him. Jacob told him, "Go now and see to your brothers' welfare and the welfare of the flocks and bring me back word." Jacob sent him to travel from the valley of Hebron until he would arrive in Shechem. Hebron is where his great-grandfather Abraham was buried, and Shechem is where the tribes had sinned and where Dinah was violated. Shechem was also where the kingdom of the house of David was divided, Joseph was found lost in a field until a man, said to be the angel Gabriel, asked him what he was looking for. He asked him if he had seen his brothers, he told Joseph that they had traveled away from this area, and he overheard them say they were going to Dothan. Joseph travelled there and found his brothers. When his brothers saw him arriving, they were not happy and plotted to kill him saying, "behold, that dreamer is coming."

They conspired a plan to kill him and throw him into one of the pits and will tell their father that he was devoured by a wild beast and see what happens to his dreams then, because, since they will kill him, his dreams will come to naught. Reuben heard their plans and protected Joseph and said, "let us not deal him a deadly blow," he did not allow them to shed his blood, but he did allow them to place him in the pit. Reuben's plan was to come back and save him later on from their hands and return him to his father. Later, God would testify for Reuben that his intention was to save Joseph and come back to take him out of the pit. He said, "I am the firstborn and the eldest of them all. The sin will be attributed only to me." The brothers stripped Joseph of his shirt and of the fine woolen coat which he was wearing, which his father had given to him, Joseph always got more than the other brothers. They found an empty pit that had no water in it, this indicating that there would be snakes and scorpions thriving in the dry pit.

Later the boys sat down to eat their meal, while they were eating, they looked up and saw a caravan of Ishmaelites arriving from Gilead, and their camels were carrying spices, balm, and lotus, obvious to the brothers they were on their way down to Egypt. Judah also protected Joseph and convinced the brothers not to kill him but to sell him to the Ishmaelites, "we shall not harm him, let us remember he is our brother and our flesh," and his brothers listened. Just then a caravan of Midianite merchants passed by, they saw Joseph in the pit, and they lifted Joseph out of the pit. The brothers sold Joseph to the Midianites for twenty silver pieces, and the Midianites sold Joseph to the Ishmaelites who brought him with them to Egypt. The Midrash says it was the brothers that pulled Joseph out of the pit, to sell him and in fact, he was sold many times over. Usually, Arab merchants would transport only petroleum and tar, which had a foul odor, this time God arranged it so they were transporting only sweet-smelling spices so Joseph would not suffer during this trip. The last sale was when the Midianites sold him to the Egyptian Potiphar, Pharaoh's chamberlain, and chief of the slaughterers of the king's animals.

Reuben who was not with his brothers at the time of the sale of Joseph, he had gone to help Jacob with something and only returned later. When he arrived at the pit and saw that Joseph was not there, Reuben ripped his garments as a sign of mourning. Reuben ran to his brothers screaming the boy is gone and how will he ever be able to flee from their father's pain. The brothers slaughtered a kid because its blood is very similar to human blood, they took Joseph's coat and dipped it into the kid's blood. They brought he bloodied coat home to their father, claiming they found it in a field, Jacob who recognized it as Joseph's coat, was convinced that a wild beast has devoured him; Joseph was most likely to have been torn up by these animals. God never revealed the truth about Joseph's fate to anyone because the brothers excommunicated and cursed anyone who would reveal it, including God. Only Isaac, however, knew that Joseph was alive, but he never revealed the truth either, because he knew that even God did not wish to reveal the truth to Jacob and Isaac wept over Jacob's distress.

Jacob tore his garments as is the custom, he put sackcloth on his loins, and he mourned for his son many days. Jacob mourned for twenty-two years, from the time Joseph left, until Jacob went down to Egypt. Joseph was seventeen years old when he was taken and was thirty years old when he stood before Pharaoh. There were the seven years of plenty, then the two years of the famine when Jacob came to Egypt adding up to twenty-two years. Jacob did not fulfill this honor for his own father and mother, he too left them for twenty-two years. There was the twenty years that he was in Laban's house, and two years that he was on the road when he returned from Laban's house, one and a half years in Succoth and six months in Beth-el. This is exactly what he meant when he said to Laban,

"This is twenty years for me in your house" (Genesis 31:41)

Jacob was taking responsibility for his actions and admitting that he deserved to get back for what he did. He ultimately made his own parents suffer for twenty years by neglecting to correspond with them. All Jacob's sons and daughters tried to console him, but he refused to be consoled, and he said, "because I will descend on account of my son as a mourner to the grave," and he wept for him. The Midrash says that Jacob never accepted any consolation because he always believed that Joseph was alive and never dead, as it is decreed in the bible, that a dead person should be forgotten from the heart, but not a living person.

Lemon

Latin Name, Citrus Limon
Aroma, Light, fresh, and citrus

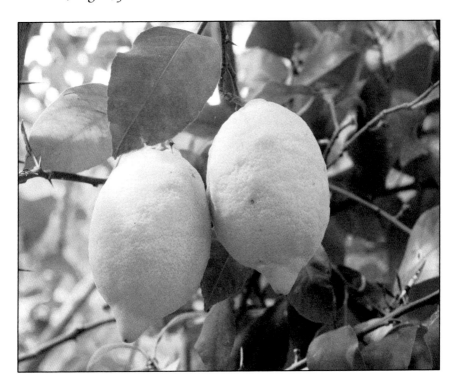

PHYSICAL

Lemon belongs to the famous citrus family and is a great antioxidant, great for sore throats and bronchitis. Lemon also heals wounds of the skin and is also used to lighten skin and help with pigmentation from the sun. Lemon oil is very phototoxic, so it must not be used if you plan to go out into the sun. However, it loses its photosynthesis when it is blended in a synergy mix. When mixed in equal amounts of essential oils, the lemon oil is no longer phototoxic.

Lemon is mainly used for its juice in cooking and baking all around the world. Its oil has many benefits too, it is a rich source of vitamin C, has numerous phytochemicals, including polyphenols, terpenes, and tannins.

Therefore, they have a very strong and recognizable fragrance. It also has anti-inflammatory characteristics and protects the blood cells from contracting serious illnesses. Lemon has been associated with a ten percent reduction in odds of developing breast cancer.

EMOTIONAL

Awakens and helps to stay alert to focus and learn, lemon oil is great for kids who suffer from ADHD. Lemon uplifts everything and helps to focus on the right things. It brings one back to basics of appreciation of life, love and all the good that is already had. Great oil for meditation, Lemon oil enables to meditate deeper and ultimately allowing to ask and open to receive what is needed.

BIBLICAL

"And you shall take for yourselves on the first day, the fruit of the Hadar tree, date palm fronds, a branch of a braided tree, and willows of the brook, and you shall rejoice before the Lord your God for a seven-day period." (Leviticus 23:40)

"And a letter to Asaph, the guardian of the king's orchard, that he gives me wood to make beams for the gates of the castle that belongs to the Temple and for the wall of the city and for the house to which I shall go, and the king gave me according to the good hand of my God upon me." (Nehemiah 2:8)

"May there be an abundance of grain in the land, on the mountain peaks; may its fruit rustle like Lebanon, and they will blossom forth from the city like the grass of the earth." (Psalms 72:16)

Hadar is the Hebrew word for all Citrus Trees, its other translation is beautiful, which literally means "fruit of a beautiful tree." Lemon is one of the citrus fruit's family members, just like oranges, lemons, grapefruit, pomelo, limes, and the citron. In Hebrew it's the "Etrog," citrus trees are mentioned many times in the Bible, and the first fruits of the season are picked and brought to Jerusalem in celebration of festivals. There are many laws regarding the fruits of trees, they must not be picked for the first three years of the tree's life. The fruits of the fourth year take on a very holy status and must be taken to Jerusalem to be eaten. It is a great curse for a person who planted a tree but does not merit to live and redeem it in the fourth year to eat its fruits. Sometimes it happens that a man plants a tree even though he knows he will not be alive when it grows to its full stature, this is one of the vanities that were given to creatures, they toil and someone else takes the fruits. It is important to rejoice in the appreciation of eating, drinking, and clean clothing.

David writes a special prayer blessing his son Solomon and his prophecy of the future messianic era, where people will live in abundance and their wealth will be expanded, there will be much goodwill placating people. They will feel appeased and happy because they know that God will give them plenty in the world to come. There will be a utopian peace for the people in those days, the mountains will bear a special peace when they produce fruit, people will not be jealous of his neighbor because each man will invite his friend to shelter under his vines, fruit trees or fig trees. The hills will bear peace for the people of Israel through their own righteousness that they will perform, where through them peace will flourish and last forever. King Solomon will always be remembered forever for his riches as well as his wisdom, and through all the days of the sun his name will be magnified. He will always be known as the ultimate ruler, people will always say, may you be wise and rich like Solomon. Blessed is God who performs wonders alone through his son Solomon and glorious is God's name forever, may his glory forever fill the entire earth, amen and amen, this is the end of the prayers of David the son of Jesse.

Lemongrass

Latin Name, Cymbopogon Citratus
Aroma, Citrus, fresh and straw like

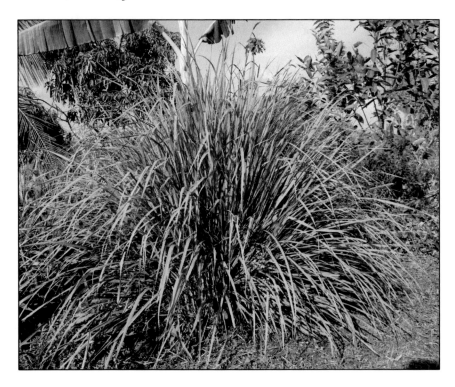

PHYSICAL

Grows in Sri Lanka and Madagascar, this oil is a cleanser and is great in the gardens and for animals. It grows rapidly in the garden and needs lots of water. Dogs love to dig up this plant and eat its roots. It contains many anti-cancerous properties and dogs know this instinctively, they understand and know what is good for them, it also kills animal lice and ticks. Lemongrass can identify dangerous cells, trap them, and export them out of the body via the liver. It is an antioxidant and is good for the skin and fungus infections.

Lemongrass is a killer of bacterias and was one of the main ingredients used in formulas to kill the Swine Flu bacteria. It is also an anti-inflammatory, it relaxes, relieves stress, depletes lactic acid in a massage and reduces high blood pressure. Lemongrass tackles acne and absorbs water like Juniper.

Warning, this oil is not for pregnant women or people suffering from glaucoma.

EMOTIONAL

Lemongrass encourages and uplifts with its powerful fragrance it does not apologize about its existence. It helps to get rid of regrets and shame with its complete straight forwardness. Even with its strong scent it is gentle and reminds us of who we are and strive to be.

If one is finding it hard to forgive, use this oil to help to release the anger and resentment. It is only beneficial to the health when one really forgives and "forget". This oil gives clarity and balance, helps make wise choices that come truly from within. This oil makes dreams come true with these small daily made choices, steering life in the right direction wished to arrive at.

BIBLICAL

"And I will give grass in your field for your livestock, and you will eat and be sated." (Deuteronomy 11:15)

"Vedan and Javan gave spun silk into your treasure houses, iron wrought into ingots, cassia and calamus was in your stores." (Ezekiel 27:19)

"Request rain from the Lord at the time of the latter rain; the Lord makes rain-clouds, and He shall give them rain; for each person, grass in the field." (Zechariah 10:1)

"For so said the Lord concerning the house of the king of Judah; You are as Gilead to me, O head of Lebanon, that I will surely make you a desert, cities not inhabited." (Jeremiah 22:6)

It is thought that the fifth ingredient in the anointing oil formula, also known as "Kaneh-Bosem" is Calamus, which is thought to be Lemongrass. The Bible says that it was an aromatic cane or grass, which was imported from a distant land by way of the spice route, and that a related plant grows naturally in Israel.

God told Jeremiah to give the king of Judah who was at the time sitting on the throne of David, and all the people who he reigns over, a message, which was a strong warning to listen to the Lord. He said, "Perform justice and charity, and rescue the robbed from the hand of the robber, and to a stranger, an orphan, and a widow do no wrong, do no violence, and shed no innocent blood in this place." The reward for doing as God says, he and his people will ride in chariots with horses. However, if he does not listen to the word of God, his house will become a destruction and be uninhabitable, and "even if you are as dear to me as the Temple, which is high on the mountain peaks of Gilead, I swear that I will make you a desert." Gilead being the mountain where the Temple was and from which balms and healing emanates to the whole world.

The warning continues, where God says he will send to the kingdom of Judah destroyers, each one with his weapons who will destroy his best cedars and burn them up, and all future generations will know and talk about what God did to his city. Simply because they renounced the covenant of God and worshipped idols. It will be forbidden to weep for their dead, such as, Jehoiachin and Zedekiah, whose carcasses were to be cast to the heat by day and to the cold at night, and whoever does bemoan them will be expelled from their home and never to return. Shallum the son of Josiah was now king of Judah, he was the fourth son of Josiah his father, the first son being Johanan, the second Jehoiakim, the third Zedekiah and the fourth Shallum. He also he shall not return to the kingdom, he was exiled from the land and died there, God despises a person who builds a house and lives without righteousness. God specifically points out that Jehoiakim, was a wicked man.

"I will build myself a wide house with spacious upper chambers, and he cuts out windows for himself, and it is ceilinged with cedar and painted with vermilion." (Jeremiah 22:14)

God had told Jehoiakim, Josiah your father, who demeaned himself with humility, did he not eat and drink and enjoy pleasure all the days of his life. Stealing money from the poor and the needy, crushing and oppressing them and they will not lament over his death. God tells the people they should cry the gates of the Temple Mount, which were made from the terebinths of Bashan, that they never listened to God at times of peace and instead had to wait to be punished and wish they were never born. God Inscribes, "this man childless, a man who will not prosper in his days, for no man of his seed shall prosper, sitting on the throne of David or ruling anymore in Judah."

278

God always forgives his people, "I will purify them of all their iniquity that they sinned against Me, and I will forgive all their iniquities that they sinned against Me and that they rebelled against Me. it shall be to Me for a name of joy, for praise and for glory to all the nations of the earth who will hear all the good that I do for them and fear and tremble because of all the good and because of all the peace that I do for it."

Litsea Cubeba

Latin Name, Citrus Medica
Aroma, Citrus, lemon, and lemongrass

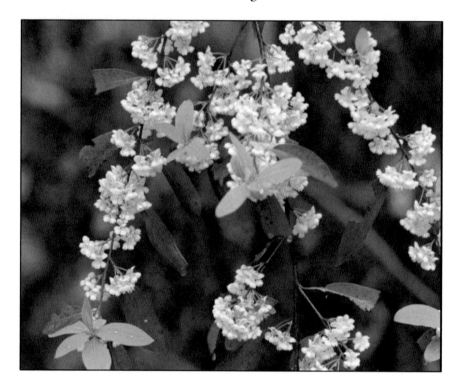

PHYSICAL

This tree is from China, it has dark orange flowers and is part of the citrus family which makes it phototoxic. It has a regenerating, energizing and refreshing aroma from its lemony fragrance, the essential oil extracted from the pepper-like berries of this evergreen shrub. Litsea Cubeba contains Linalool and can help kill cancer cells and when used in a diffuser it will dislodge phlegm. This plant is a mover of stagnated fluids and releases toxins, it is an anti-bacterium and helps skin irritations, acne, and other skin infections, including spots that have been there for a long time.

Litsea Cubeba is a relaxant and affects the neurological system, it lowers Blood Pressure and adjusts the heart rate and keeps the heart energetic and making breathing easier. It is an antibacterial and has antiviral properties which make it effective against common infections like colds and coughs.

EMOTIONAL

Litsea Cubeba's citrus lime fragrance is uplifting, refreshing with the unique ability to let go of worries and deep fears. It does this by excreting and cleansing the built-up toxins from the body that accumulated from fears. Intense fear happens when in a frozen state, like a "punch in the stomach," and left feeling unable to move and cope. Litsea Cubeba helps to clear all that, it pulls one out of hard to handle situations and releases pent-up anger that is hard to let go of.

Litsea Cubeba prevents taking things too seriously and shows how to learn to relax and be happy, being more assertive without being offensive, helping to find easier ways to obtain solutions. This oil is very soothing and reduces fury and aggression, use this oil to meditate, find ways to grow and achieve goals. It cleanses a room of bad energy and injects it with positive rejuvenating energy. A great oil to use when moving into a new house to start completely afresh.

This oil gives a sense of belonging when unsure of your role on this earth. It reduces feelings of rejection and separation and helps to realize that one is not alone. Either for an extreme extrovert or an extreme introvert, learn to be somewhere in between with this oil. Litsea Cubeba is the spirit of rejuvenation and eternal youth and brings only happiness and joy. It is the solar plexus chakra, which is responsible for mental and intellectual wellbeing,

BIBLICAL

"And the Lord God caused to sprout from the ground every tree pleasant to see and good to eat, and the Tree of Life in the midst of the garden, and the Tree of Knowledge of good and evil." (Genesis 2:9)

"And the woman saw that the tree was good for food and that it was a delight to the eyes, and the tree was desirable to make one wise; so, she took of its fruit, and she ate, and she gave also to her husband with her, and he ate." (Genesis 3:6)

"And you shall take for yourselves on the first day, the fruit of the hadar tree, date palm fronds, a branch of a braided tree, and willows of the brook, and you shall rejoice before the Lord your God for a seven-day period." (Leviticus 23:40)

"It shall blossom and rejoice, even to rejoice and to sing; the glory of the Lebanon has been given to her, the beauty of the Carmel and the Sharon; they shall see the glory of the Lord, the beauty of our God." (Isiah 35:2)

The Etrog is known as the Citron, which is the holiest fruit used in the Jewish holiday Sukkot, and in the bible the phrase "peri eitz hadar" refers to the Etrog as the most intended fruit in the citrus family. In the bible the Etrog has been cultivated for the Holy Land extensively, and many archeological legacies were found from during the period of the Second Temple era. There are mosaics featuring the Etrog found in the Maon Synagogue, the Beth Alpha Synagogue, the Hamat Tiberias Synagogue and more. All these sites display details of religious symbols and designs of the Shofar and the Menorah, as well as on the numerous Bar Kokhba coins.

God told Moses to inform the Israelites that he appointed holy days with specific designated times of the year for festivals where all of Israel will adhere to them. They should even proclaim the leap years for Israelites living outside the city to be able to ascend to Jerusalem for these festivals, giving them to the chance arrive in time and not lose hope and be encouraged to make their pilgrimage. Passover was appointed to be on the fourteenth day of the first month of Nissan, when a sacrifice should be offered to God in the afternoon. Starting on the fifteenth of the month they should eat only unleavened bread for a seven-day period, no work or labor is permitted during this time. Fire offerings should be brought to God for all seven days, Once the Israelites come into the Land which God is giving them, and they reap its harvest, you shall bring to the kohen a certain unit of measure, which was a tenth of an ephah, a bushel, at the beginning of their reaping to the Kohen.

On the first day of the seventh month will be Rosh Hashanah, which is the new year, and as an awakening to God the Israelites enlightenment will be evoked through the spiritual sounds of the shofar. Again, there shall be no work or labor and a fire offering shall be offered to God. Then on the tenth day of the seventh month shall be the day of atonement, Yom Kippur, where all Israelite atones, and for those who repent, does not atone for those who do not repent. Again, there shall be no work or labor and a fire offering shall be offered to God. Yom Kippur is the most serious day of the Jewish Calendar, where the punishment for not keeping this day is mentioned in many places in Scriptures where God says explicitly, "I will destroy," meaning destruction by premature death and not just be exiled. Yom Kippur is to be sanctified by wearing clean garments, prayer and not eating any food or drink for that day.

On fifteenth day of the seventh month is the seven-day festival of Sukkoth, for which each of the seven days a fire offering is to be offered to God and work and labor is forbidden. From the very first day take the fruit of the hadar tree, a date palm frond, a branch of a braided tree, which is a myrtle, and willows of the brook, and you shall use them in a ceremony to rejoice before God. The Israelites shall live in booths, known today as the Sukkah, and reside in it for seven whole days. So that all future generations should know that God took the Israelites out of the land of Egypt, and they lived in booths where the clouds of glory enclosed in the desert, forming a protective shelter for them against wild beasts and enemies. The Etrog tree was the notorious "Tree of Knowledge" in the Garden of Eden that Adam and Eve had eaten from.

Mandarin

Latin Name, Citrus Reticulata, C. Nobilis
Aroma, Sweet, light with combination of floral, fruity citrus

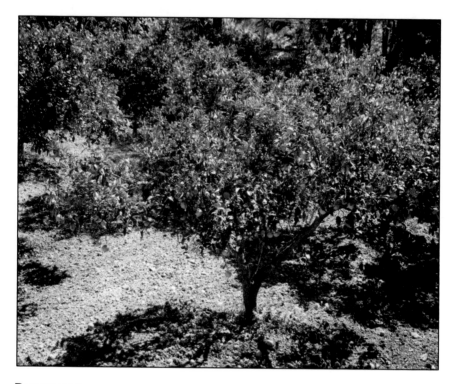

PHYSICAL

Mandarin or tangerine is a smaller version of the orange tree and is another member of the citrus family. The mandarin, the citron and the pomelo are the ancestors of the citrus trees. Its fruits are also smaller than the orange fruit and its peel is thinner. The version of this mandarin tree is a native of the Mediterranean region is called C. Nobilis. In Chinese medicine the dried peel of the fruit is used in the regulation of qi, and used to treat abdominal distension, to enhance digestion, and to reduce phlegm.

Mandarins are high in vitamins A and C and its oil is made from the peel of the fruit; it is antiseptic but very phototoxic. Mandarin is good for the metabolism and is an anti-inflammatory and a calmative and an anti-spasmodic.

EMOTIONAL

It is a great oil for children, especially those who were abused. Mandarin helps them gain self-confidence to play with other kids. Mandarin hugs and comforts as well as open your mind to show possibilities. This oil is great for Autistic kids and helps them be more open too. Mandarin gives a sensation of freedom; sweet taste is connected to sweet love. It is emotionally accepting and awakens neurotransmitters.

When meditating using mandarin, it allows for opening up and talking about things that were deep set inside. It also brings out creativity, Mandarin has such a gentle and sweet aroma that this is how it affects the spirit. Mandarin is a young oil, but it still attracts older people because of its ability to make one feel connected, loved, and hugged. Always lovely to smell this oil when wanting to feel elevated into other realms, also a great oil for meditation and in a diffuser.

BIBLICAL

"And the servant took out silver articles and golden articles and garments, and he gave them to Rebecca, and he gave delicacies to her brother and to her mother." (Genesis 24:53)

"When you come to the Land and you plant any food tree, you shall surely block its fruit from use; it shall be blocked from you from use for three years, not to be eaten." (Leviticus 19:23)

"Blessed will be the fruit of your womb, the fruit of your soil, the fruit of your livestock, the offspring of your cattle, and the flocks of your sheep." (Deuteronomy 28:4)

"And with the sweetness of the produce of the sun, and with the sweetness of the moon's yield," (Deuteronomy 33:14)

"And with the crops of early mountains, and with the sweetness of perennial hills," (Deuteronomy 33:15)

King Solomon in his wisdom planted all sorts of fruit trees all over Israel because he understood the veins of the earth and where they were located, and all the veins of the lands come to Zion. "From Zion, the all-inclusive beauty," God waters the mountains from his upper chambers and from the fruit of his works, the earth is sated. This refers to trees planted in the field, as opposed to the orchard, that do not bear fruit, but are destined to bear fruit in the future. The Sages explained that King Solomon planted many sweet fruits in the Temple grounds, which were gold, and as soon as non-believers entered the Temple, they withered. It is interesting to see that the ancient commentaries say, the taste of the tree tastes the same as its fruit. We can confirm that from their essential oils which also taste and smell the same as their fruit. The waters which lie in the depth of the earth ascend and moisten the land from below. Both Moses and Jacob blessed each tribe with very resembling blessings, Jacob blessing for Joseph,

> *"The God of your father, and He will help you, and with the Almighty, and He will bless you with the blessings of the heavens above, the blessings of the deep, lying below, the blessings of father and mother." (Genesis 49:25)*

That is to say that the ones who beget the children and the ones who bear the children will be blessed. The males will impregnate with a drop of semen that is fit for conception, and the females will not lose what is in their womb and miscarry their fetuses. With the sweetness of the fruits from the sun, because Joseph's land was exposed to much sun, which sweetened its fruit. The moon's yield is for some fruits that are ripened by the moon, such as cucumbers and gourds, also referring to fruits which the earth expels produce naturally every month. Joseph's land produced crops of early mountains and were blessed with the fruits that are first to ripen, because the height of the mountains advanced the ripening of their fruits.

Marigold

Latin Name, Tagetes Erecta
Aroma, Bitter scent

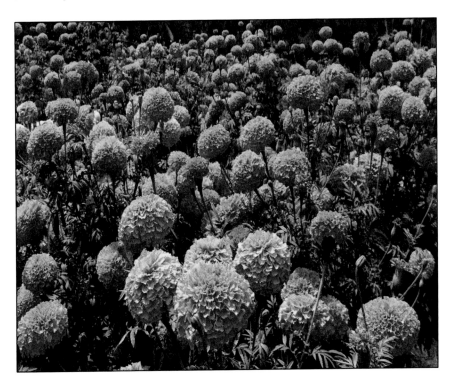

PHYSICAL

Marigold is an herbaceous plant from the sunflower family. They blossom with beautiful golden, orange, yellow, and white colored flower heads. They like to grow in wetlands, swamps and meadows and protects itself with its pungent odor to keep pests away. Marigold is used to heal large open wounds though it gets old very quickly and then gets brown and sticky. This oil is an anti-bacterium and heals wounds such as scrapes, cuts, burns and bites. Marigold is great for itchy skin, nappy or diaper rashes and other skin irritations.

It is also an anti-fungus helping with candida, fungus on toes and warts. It repels bugs and mosquitos and is a great plant to have in a garden to keep bugs away. Marigold is an antioxidant and helps prevent cardiovascular disease, strokes, and cancer. It has powerful flavonoids that can help to prevent diseases, with many other healing properties too. Its leaves are used to make tea to ease inflammatory bowel symptoms, helps with gastritis, acid reflux and ulcers.

Warning, Marigold essential is phototoxic and sensitive to the sun.

EMOTIONAL

Emotional trauma effects the body in the long term, this oil helps speed up the process and release the bad energy ingrained into the body. Let go of harsh self-judgement and self-blaming for long past situations that has no longer the power to change. This little flower symbolizes passion and creativity because it faces the sun, thus is said to have psychic powers with the ability to resurrect.

Marigold is connected to the third chakra, which is the solar plexus and is responsible for mental and intellectual wellbeing. It is all about being brave and combatting that inner self-doubt and facing problems. The orange gold color brings out a personal power for self-transformation and bringing out the hero within. It opens at sunrise and closes at sunset; this plant has prophetic powers and awareness.

BIBLICAL

"So long as the earth exists, seedtime and harvest, cold and heat, summer and winter, and day and night shall not cease." (Genesis 8:22)

"Desert and wasteland shall rejoice over them, and the plain shall rejoice and shall blossom like a rose." (Isiah 35:1)

"It shall blossom and rejoice, even to rejoice and to sing; the glory of the Lebanon has been given to her, the beauty of the Carmel and the Sharon; they shall see the glory of the Lord, the beauty of our God." (Isiah 35:2)

"He made them ride upon the high places of the earth, that they would eat the produce of the field. He let them suck honey from a rock, and oil from the mighty part of the crag."

(Deuteronomy 32:13)

Marigold is indigenous of the Mediterranean and although was not mentioned in the Bible by name, it was known as the "Flower of the Field." Since God destroyed the world once with the flood and saved only Noah and his family, he now makes a faithful promise to the Israelites that day and night shall not cease. God was so eager to save Noah so that the wicked of the generation should not kill him, that he made a promise to Noah, all the fruits he stores on board the ark, would not rot or become putrid. God made an order that the men sleep separately from the women that they should not engage in marital relations during their time in the ark. During the period of the flood the planets, the sun and the moon did not function, and days were indistinguishable from nights. After the flood God made a vow to never make another flood and in the future all the solar system shall never again cease to perform their tasks according to their natural course.

Jerusalem, called a wasteland, and Zion was called a desert, it was an arid, desolate land, a place full of howling jackals and ostriches, and God provided Israel with all their needs in the desert. Israel has many tall mountains with many flowers and fruits trees, and Israel being geographically higher than most countries, their fruits were quicker to bud and ripen than the fruits of other countries and olive trees grew from within the strongest part of the mountainous rock. Marigold has a unique and intimate rhythmical connection with the functions of the universe, because of its evenly designed petals and symmetry transmitting both harmony and order.

Myrrh

Latin Name, Commiphora Myrrha
Aroma, Warm, musty, and earthy

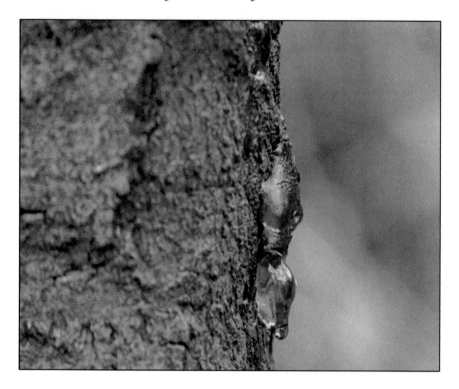

PHYSICAL

Myrrh is a natural gum or resin extracted from several small, thorny trees, its resin has been used throughout history as a perfume, incense, and medicine. A tree's wound penetrates through the bark and into the sapwood, this is the tree's resin, Myrrh gum, like frankincense, is such a resin. When people harvest myrrh, they wound the trees repeatedly to bleed them of the gum. Myrrh gum is waxy and coagulates quickly. After the harvest, the gum becomes hard and glossy. The gum is yellowish and may be either clear or opaque. It is an anti-inflammatory and is used for all bodily fluids and mucus, from having a sore throat right to hemorrhoids. It is an antiseptic and is used to soothe and heal mouth sores and cleanse teeth. Myrrh is an anti-fungal, and a remedy for indigestion, ulcers, colds, coughs, asthma, and lung congestions.

EMOTIONAL

Myrrh encourages fortitude and courage to heal wounds that are deep inside the soul. This unique type of fragrance enables one to let go of the need to battle and seek peace and calmness. This oil helps to open all possibilities, smashing out all limitations and allowing the mind to believe in its ability to achieve and succeed.

BIBLICAL

"And you, take for yourself spices of the finest sort, of pure myrrh five hundred-shekel weights; of fragrant cinnamon half of it two hundred- and fifty-shekel weights; of fragrant cane two hundred and fifty-shekel weights." (Exodus 30:23)

"And of cassia five hundred-shekel weights according to the holy shekel, and one hin of olive oil." (Exodus 30:24)

"You shall make this into an oil of holy anointment, a perfumed compound according to the art of a perfumer; it shall be an oil of holy anointment." (Exodus 30:25)

"Who is this coming up from the desert, like columns of smoke, perfumed with myrrh and frankincense, of all the powder of the peddler?" (Song of Songs 3:6)

"And let the king appoint commissioners to all the provinces of his kingdom and let them gather every young maiden of comely appearance to Shushan the capital, to the house of the women, to the custody of Hege, the king's chamberlain, the keeper of the women, and let their ointments be given them." (Esther 2:3)

In the Hebrew Bible, Myrrh is complimented as a rare perfume with intoxicating qualities in several places in the Old Testament Bible. Ishmaelite traders to whom Jacob's sons sold Joseph, their brother, sold Myrrh to the Israelites, which was one of the crucial ingredients of the Ketoret, the consecrated incense used in the First and Second Temples in Jerusalem. Myrrh is also listed as an ingredient in the holy anointing oil used to anoint the tabernacle, high priests, and kings. The Original Anointing Oil "Oil of Messiah" was first prescribed for the High Priest of the Temple, who was instructed to smear anointing Oil on himself before he blessed the children of Israel.

"Clouds of heaven returned, and went to the garden of Eden, and took from thence choice aromatics, and oil of olives for the light, and pure balsam for the anointing oil, and for the sweet incense. Beat some of it into powder and put some before the Pact in the Tent of Meeting, where I will meet with you; it shall be most holy to you. Next take choice spices: five hundred weights of solidified myrrh, half as much two hundred and fifty of fragrant cinnamon, two hundred and fifty of aromatic cane"

Aaron would make incense of spices go up in smoke on the alter every morning when he sets the lamps in order. He did this by cleaning the cups of the menorah from the residue ashes of the wicks that had burned the previous night. He would do this every morning and then rekindling them for the next day, once again make the incense rise in smoke so there was continual incense for God. Once a year Aaron would atone for the sins of the whole generation, using the horn of a bull and the blood of a kid. He would atone for ritual contamination regarding the sanctuary and all its holy things, this was on the holiest day of the year, Yom Kippur where the altar was sanctified for these things only, and for no other service.

The atonement used to take into consideration the total of every Israelite and give it to God in trade for their sins. They were counted not by count them by the head, but each person gave a half-shekel, and the Kohen would count the shekels so they will know the number. Keeping any plague away from them, because they believed the evil eye has power over numbered things, and pestilence will be allowed to enter their midst, as they did in David's time. From the age of twenty, everyone went through this counting process and gave offerings to God, all the silver from the atonements were taken into the tent of meeting and so God will remember to atone their souls.

God told Moses, "You shall make a washstand of copper and its base of copper for washing, and you shall place it between the Tent of Meeting and the altar, and you shall put water therein, so Aaron and his sons shall wash their hands and feet from it." The Midrash says the kohen would wash his hands and feet simultaneously, he would do this by laying his right hand on his right foot and his left hand on his left foot and wash them together. Before they enter the Tent of Meeting, they washed themselves with water so that they will not die. Whenever they approached the altar to serve, it was to make a fire offering to rise in smoke to God, and this became a perpetual statute, for the Kohen and his descendants, for their generations to come.

Then God told Moses to, *"take for yourself spices of the finest sort: of pure myrrh five-hundred-shekel weights; of fragrant cinnamon half of it two hundred- and fifty-shekel weights; of fragrant cane two hundred- and fifty-shekel weights, and of cassia five-hundred-shekel weights according to the holy shekel, and one hin of olive oil. You shall make this into an oil of holy anointment, a perfumed compound according to the art of a perfumer; it shall be an oil of holy anointment. Then you shall anoint with it the Tent of Meeting and the Ark of Testimony, and you shall sanctify them so that they become a holy of holies; whatever touches them shall become holy."*

Eleven ingredients were revealed to Moses when he was at Sinai. They were balsam sap, onycha, galbanum, frankincense, myrrh, cassia, saffron, oat, costus, aromatic bark, and cinnamon, that totals eleven. The oil of myrrh was used by Queen Esther in a purification ritual for the preparation of being King Ahasuerus's new queen. This cleansing process took twelve months, six months with oil of myrrh, and six months with sweet odors, which purified the women. In Biblical times this oil was used for anointing kings and prophets, now we use the oil to symbolize a priestly, regal, and higher self within ourselves, allowing us to connect and identify with God.

Myrtle/Hadass

Latin Name, Myristica fragrans
Aroma, Sweet, camphorous and herbal

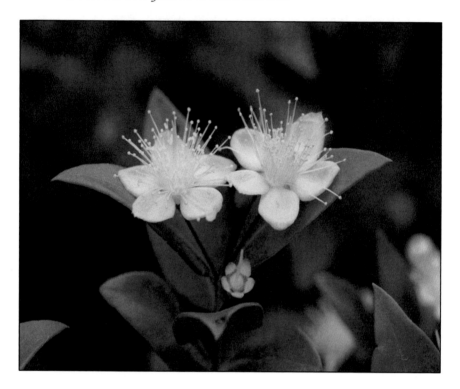

PHYSICAL

Myrtle is a flowering plant that is native to the Mediterranean region and is a smallish evergreen shrub with small star like flowers with five petals that are usually white. Its fruit is a round berry with several seeds inside it, which the birds love to eat. Myrtle has high levels of salicylic acid; a compound related to aspirin and is used for nonsteroidal anti-inflammatory drugs NSAID. This plant is great to reduce pain, decrease fever and prevent blood clots.

It's essential oil contains oxides like eucalyptus and is better for kids because it is gentle on their respiratory system. Myrtle excretes mucus, parasites and even acts as an auto immune and kills cancer cells. Myrle helps with allergies because it acts as an antihistamine. It does not burn the skin and can be used directly on skin for dermatitis or stomach pains.

EMOTIONAL

Its leaves are very green and very small, its flowers are also very small and white. But yet this tree is associated with royalty and confidence. Myrtle is considered capable and able, seen as very strong, "strong as a king." This oil does not damage DNA cells, it awakens the hypothalamus, and used for meditation. Use this oil if feeling sad and lonely to raise confidence and feel stronger. Hadass is great for kids to help them focus, much like Ritalin. This oil helps kids get their homework done.

BIBLICAL

"I saw tonight and behold! A man was riding on a red horse, and he was standing among the myrtles that were in the pool, and after him were red, black, and white horses." (Zechariah 1:8)

"And they answered the angel of the Lord who was standing among the myrtles, and they said, "We have walked about on the earth and behold! All the earth sits still and is at rest." (Zechariah 1:11)

"And that they should announce and proclaim in all their cities and in Jerusalem, saying, "Go out to the mountain and bring olive leaves and leaves of oil trees, myrtle leaves, date palm leaves, and leaves of plaited trees, to make booths, as it is written." (Nehemiah 8:15)

"Instead of the thorn shall come up the fir tree, and instead of the brier shall come up the myrtle tree" (Isaiah 55:13)

"They were your traffickers with adornments, with wraps of blue cloth and embroidery, and with treasures kept in chests, tied with ropes, enclosed in myrtle wood-in them was your merchandise." (Ezekiel 27:24)

"If you dream about myrtle, your property will prosper, and, if you don't have property, you will inherit property" (Berachot 57:1)

Myrtle means Hadass in Hebrew, it is one of the four species used in the Jewish holiday of Sukkot. Hadass is also Queen Esther's Hebrew name, which was compared to her good qualities. Myrtle is considered regal and a symbol of all good and beautiful, it symbolizes success and the eternity of life. Nettles are species of thorns usually compared to the wicked who will be destroyed, and the Myrtle is the portrayal of ultimate righteousness who will take their rightful rule. God says, there is a distinction and a difference, advantages, and superiority in his ways more than man's ways and in his thoughts more than man's thoughts, just as the heavens are higher than the earth; man is always intent upon rebelling against him, whereas God is always intent upon bringing man back.

Haran, Canneh, and Eden, were the traffickers of Sheba with the best of all spices and with all precious stones and gold. They would bring into Israel adornments, jewelry, and wraps of embroidered blue cloth. They would have all sorts of treasures kept in chests. The chests were covered with leather and decorated for beauty with a variety of nails forming rows and pictures, and they are called "kamatriah" in Aramaic and "bromim" in Hebrew and were tied and bound with linen ropes for beauty. The chests were placed inside other chests of myrtle wood, they would first open the outer chests and disclose the smaller chests within them. There were many ornaments inside those chests ready for merchandising. The Midrash says the outer chests were usually made of cedar wood, bromim, the chests were tied with ropes and placed in chests of myrtle, which is a species of cedar.

Zechariah, son of Berechiah, son of Iddo the prophet, saying, he had a prophecy which was extremely enigmatic, because it contained visions resembling a dream that required interpretation. In the eighth month before the commencement of the work resuming the construction of the Temple, which was on the twenty-fourth day of the ninth month. God was furious with your fathers who were in the generation of the destruction of the Temple, because they provoked him greatly. On the twenty-fourth day of the eleventh month, the month of Shevat in the second year of Darius' rule, God came to Zechariah the son of Berechiah, the son of Iddo the prophet, saying, that he saw tonight, a man was riding on a red horse, and was standing among the myrtles in a pool, and behind him were red, black, and white horses. The man was an angel, the red horse symbolizing the sword and with blood, the horses behind him confirming that he was prepared for the mission of God. The fact that there were among them many colors and sorts of horses, were meant as praise for God among myrtle trees of Babylon.

The angel who was speaking to him said, "I will show you what these are." The angel was riding the red horse, and the man standing among the myrtles replied and said, "These are the ones whom the Lord has sent to walk to and fro on the earth." Then they answered the angel, God who was standing among the myrtles, and they said, "We have walked to and fro on the earth and behold! All the earth sits still and is at rest." The angel spoke again, "O Lord of Hosts! How long will You not have mercy on Jerusalem and upon the cities of Judah, upon whom You are wroth for seventy years already?" God answered the angel who was speaking to me, saying good words and the prophet heard what God answered the angel, but from what the angel said to him, "Proclaim, saying, 'I am jealous for Jerusalem, and for Zion!" I know that He answered him good words. God says, "I have returned to Jerusalem with mercy; my house shall be built there, and a plumb line shall be stretched out over Jerusalem."

Myrtles are both the symbol and scent of the Garden of Eden. They have a beautiful fragrance but do not have a pleasant taste. This represents those who have good deeds to their credit despite that they do not have knowledge of the Torah.

Neroli

Latin Name, Citrus Aurantium
Aroma, Radiant, sweet, and floral

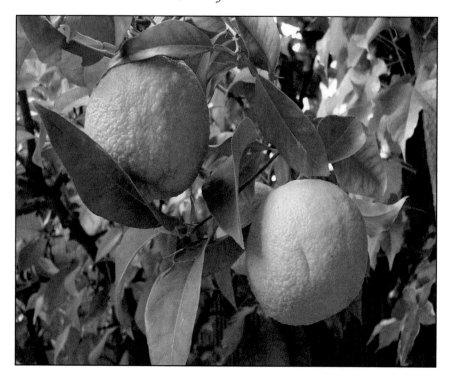

PHYSICAL

Neroli is an essential oil produced from the flower blossoms of the bitter orange tree. These Orange blossoms have beautiful fresh flowers that are used on the same day they are picked. The tree must be over three years old in order to use the flowers and usually a whole orange tree contains approximately six kilograms of flowers, this will make one kilogram of essential oil which is not phototoxic.

Neroli works on the brain stem, for comas, fainting, brain trauma and cell renewal. Use this oil directly on skin during childbirth. It helps skin wrinkles, for stretch marks allowing skin tissues to resume their shape after stretching from pregnancy.

EMOTIONAL

It affects the central nervous system and relaxes, relieves stress reminding of wide-open spaces. Neroli gives one a happy and joyful feeling and is great for teenagers to put their issues into proportion. Neroli lightens sorrows, comforts, and gives the sensation of complete joy. Helps to understand oneself and recognize how one has affected others and may have hurt them. It reflects and throws light on these situations and heals the rift and wounds caused.

Neroli fragrance enhances the feeling of being in love with its sweet excitement of a romantic encounter. This oil is very liberating, when inhaled one will feel an inner peace and feel guided into a better life. Neroli helps unite the subconscious mind with the conscious mind and exposes negative thoughts. This unison of both minds heightens awareness of the present and dissolves blockages. This releases a flood of positive energy to come streaming into one's higher selves allowing them to tap into their manifesting powers. Neroli helps enable to achieve the deepest and highest aspirations and desires. Neroli burns away negative thoughts, feelings, and habits. Meditate using this oil in a diffuser or just simply inhale, Neroli will uplift the spirit and bring one back to a peaceful state of mind.

BIBLICAL

"The choicest of the first fruits of your soil you shall bring to the house of the Lord, your God. You shall not cook a kid in its mother's milk." (Exodus 23:19)

"I will turn towards you, and I will make you fruitful and increase you, and I will set up My covenant with you." (Leviticus 26:9)

"The staff of the man whom I will choose will blossom, and I will calm down turning away from Myself the complaints of the children of Israel which they are complaining against you." (Numbers 17:20)

"And they took some of the fruit of the land in their hands and brought it down to us, brought us back word, and said, "The land the Lord, our God, is giving us is good." (Deuteronomy 1:25)

The orange blossom tree is a native of the Middle East and grew in most people's gardens in biblical times. The tree is very aromatic and was used to make citrus honey and orange blossom water. After Judah's daughter in law was twice widowed by the death of his two elder sons, Judah said to his daughter in law Tamar, "Remain as a widow in your father's house until my son Shelah grows up." Even though he promised to send for her when his third son was older, he was afraid lest he too will die, like his brothers. So, Tamar went, and she remained in her father's house and Judah had no intention of marrying her to Shelah. A woman who lost two husbands was considered to be bad luck and most people would be too superstitious to marry her. A long time passed, Judah's wife died and after he was somewhat consoled, he decided to go and observe his sheepshearers, so he and Hirah, his Adullamite friend went to Timnah.

Someone had told Tamar that, "behold, your father-in-law is going up to Timnah to shear his sheep." Tamar decided to take action, she took off her widow's garb, covered her head with a veil that covered her face, so that Judah would not recognize her, and she sat down at the crossroads on the way to Timnah. She could not help but notice that Shelah had grown up, and she was not given to him for a wife. This made her determined to make herself available to Judah, for she longed to bear sons from him. When Judah passed by and saw her, he thought she was a harlot, because she had her face covered and that she was sitting at the crossroads.

Judah approached her and said to her, "get ready now, I will come to you," he for sure did not suspect that she was his daughter in law, and she replied, "what will you give me that you should come to me?" Judah promised that he will send a kid from his herd," and she said, "only if you give me a pledge until you send it." Tamar was smart, Judah then said, "what is the pledge that I should give you?" and she said, "your signet, your cloak, and the staff that is in your hand." He gave them to her, and after he came to her, she conceived his likeness, mighty and righteous men like him. After she was back in her widow's garb, Judah went to look for the "harlot," to take back his pledge from the woman's hand, but he could not find her.

Judah did not want to make a big deal of the whole episode; he was afraid of being a laughingstock and he did not want people to find out about it. He did not know what else he could do to keep his word to the woman, three months later he found out that his daughter in law Tamar was

300

pregnant and accused of being a harlot. People told him, "Your daughter in law Tamar has played the harlot, and behold, she is pregnant from harlotry." So, Judah had no choice and said, "bring her out, and let her be burned." She was taken out from her father's house to be burnt, and she sent a message to her father-in-law, saying, "from the man to whom these belong I am pregnant," and she said, "please recognize whose signet ring, cloak, and staff are these?" she was hoping that he would confess by himself, and if not, let them burn me, but she refused to embarrass him. Tamar was begging in her heart that Judah would recognize his creator and not destroy three souls, because she knew she was pregnant with twins. Judah came through and recognized them, he told them, "She is right, it is from me, because I did not give her to my son Shelah," and Judah married Tamar and they really lived happily ever after.

It was always the tradition to bring the first fruits to Jerusalem as an offering to God, God also takes this opportunity to mention the prohibition of cooking meat with milk. He strongly forbids this by prohibiting the cooking of a kid in its own mothers' milk and this prohibition is written in three places in the Torah, one for the prohibition of eating meat with milk, one for the prohibition of deriving any benefit from meat with milk, and one for the prohibition of cooking meat with milk.

Niaouli

Latin Name, Melaleuca Quinquenervia
Aroma, Warm camphor scent

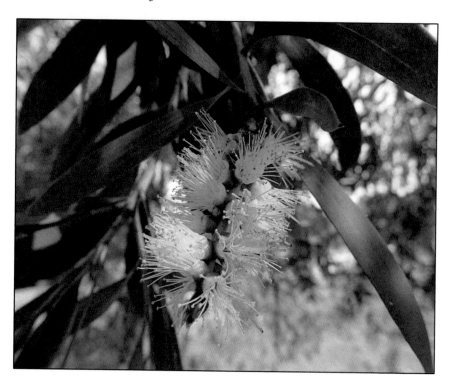

PHYSICAL

Niaouli is from the Tea Tree and Cajaput family and grows in New Caledonia, Papua New Guinea and coastal eastern Australia and are resistant to fire. Niaouli is called paper bark, because the bark looks like strips of paper, which peel from the entire height of the trunk. Aborigines used this paper bark, because of its softness for bedding and as swaddling for their babies. Its anti-fungal and antiseptic abilities make it a unique oil, it can treat all sorts of skin conditions, directly on the skin. It heals scars and skin infections and manages to destroy very difficult skin problems. This oil is a must when making moisturizer for oil and acne skin, psoriasis, and ciboria. Niaouli heals skin cancer and skin funguses, and it kills wart viruses. It is an antihistamine and helps all types of inflammations both inside and outside the body. It relieves rheumatic pains and stimulates the lymphatic system and enhances blood circulation. It has been used to treat fever successfully and respiratory problems very effectively.

Put a couple of drops in an infuser for cold, flu, bronchitis, whooping cough, sinusitis, catarrh, pneumonia, asthma, laryngitis, sore throat, tuberculosis, and coughs. Niaouli kills intestinal worms, like tape worms and round worms, you can get rid of them by simply inhaling or putting a few drops in your bath. The best thing is that it kills insects like ants, bugs, and cockroaches.

Warning, this oil is not to be administered on pregnant women or children under 5.

EMOTIONAL

Niaouli clears the clutter from the mind and this action activates very high concentration levels. It clears away all that emotional stress that have been dragging around during one's life and teaches to live with a new self. This oil is uplifting and inspiring and the tree has flowers that looks like bottle brushes, and it does exactly that. Niaouli efficiently sweeps out all negative energies that are blocking physical and mental capabilities. Its invigorating scent stimulates the body to cleanse and heal itself.

Niaouli is energetically strong and dissipates radiation, it does this by absorbing the radiation and purifying the room. Place a bottle of water with a few drops of Niaouli behind the computer, don't have to have it opened, leave it closed. Let it stay there for about a week and then obviously throw the bottle away. This oil powerfully lifts vibrations and brings one upwards to a much higher self-expectation of life values and goals and see the bigger picture of life. Use Niaouli to meditate with and to access the angel within for a very focused and possibly even an out of body experience.

BIBLICAL

A cluster of henna-flowers is my beloved to me, in the vineyards of Ein-Gedi." (Song of Songs 1:14)

"Your arid fields are as a pomegranate orchard with sweet fruit, henna and spikenard." (Song of Songs 4:13)

Spikenard and saffron, calamus and cinnamon, with all frankincense trees, myrrh and aloes, with all the chief spices." (Song of Songs 4:14)

"Your head upon you is like Carmel, and the braided locks of your head are like purple; the king is bound in the tresses." (Song of Songs 7:6)

The distinct fragrance of the henna flower was not only used as a dye but also as a perfume, henna flowers are also known because of their association with other sweet-smelling plants mentioned in the passages of the love songs of David and Solomon. A person's hair is their youth, and the braided hair of Nazirites are as beautiful as youth, they are braided as commanded by God intertwined with purple ropes, because he is bound in the locks. The purple dye probably was henna, and the paste was most likely mixed with cajaput, Ravensara or tea tree. God tells Moses to speak to the Israelites, to see if a man or woman amongst the people would set himself or herself apart, by becoming a Nazirite and making a vow to abstain from drinking wine for the sake of God. They shall abstain from new wine as well as aged wine and should he or she decide this, they may not even drink vinegar made from any wine. Neither should they drink anything immersed in grapes or even eat grapes either fresh or dried ones, not even on the Sabbath. For the entire duration of their abstinence, they shall not eat any product of grape vine, from the seeds to the skins.

For all the days of their vow of abstinence, no razor shall pass over their head until the completion of their term that they had chosen to abstain for the sake of God, they must keep it sacred and allow the growth of the hair of their heads to grow wild. During this time, they may not encounter the dead, not even for his mother and father or any of his siblings, because at this time the crown of his God is upon his head, and it may not be defiled. For the entire duration they are considered holy. If an unavoidable occurrence happened and someone died in their presence unexpectedly or suddenly, this causes the nazirite head to become defiled, they must then shave off the hair of their head on the day of their purification, as well on the seventh day and then on the eighth day commence a series of purification rituals with the high priest.

A nazirite who makes a vow has very strict laws that are uncompromising, their offering to the Lord for their naziriteship is in addition to what is within their means, whatever they commit to vow that they will do, so shall he do, in addition to the law of his naziriteship. They may vow, "I am hereby a nazirite on the condition that I shall shave my hair with one hundred burnt offerings and with one hundred peace offerings." These vows are very individual, and every Nazirite's vow vary completely, and they should not vow to do what they cannot afford or beyond their capabilities.

The Israelites love and devotion to God by use of the Tefillin for their daily prayers, these are phylacteries placed on the top of the forehead. They are worn in prayer every morning, so all the peoples of the world will see that the name of God upon them, and they will be in awe of God too. The secret of their strength and their fears are like the rock of the mount Carmel which is the most prominent of mountains. The braided hair of the Nazirites is as beautiful with their entwined purple ropes lifted onto the highest part of the head, with the name of God is bound into the locks. The winding tresses, the fringes of the sashes, with which they tie the girdles bound with love to the swiftness with which they run before God.

The Niaouli is found growing all over Israel and has basically the same qualities as Tea Tree and Cajaput, however Niaouli is a more excellent turpentine to mix with henna paste and has a milder scent than cajaput, Ravensara or tea tree.

Nutmeg

Latin Name, Myristica Fragrans
Aroma, Spicy, light, and fresh

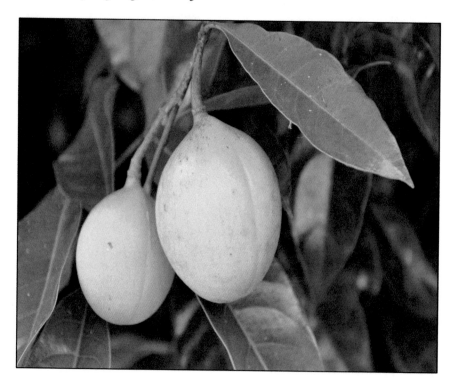

PHYSICAL

Nutmeg is the seed of the Myristica Fragrans tree which is an evergreen that is indigenous to Indonesia. Its flowers are bell-shaped, pale yellow, waxy and fleshy and nutmeg spice is made by grinding the seeds of the fragrant fruit. Nutmeg is very spicy and its hot personality heats and relaxes the digestive system, it eases that bloated stomach sensation. Nutmeg is also an anesthetic, an antiseptic, and an anti-inflammatory, with such powerful qualities it can act as a stable pain reliever. Nutmeg can tackle deep skin issues such as warts, cysts, and fungus on your toenails.

This oil can enhance the appetite and may cause the sensation of feeling hungry and in search of food all the time. It is useful for mothers of children who have problems with eating disorders. Using excessive amounts of nutmeg can result in myristicin poisoning because nutmeg has phenylpropene which is a chemical compound and too much can be poisonous.

Warning do not administer in large dosages to pregnant women and children under age 3, and do not administer to people suffering from epilepsy.

EMOTIONAL

This oil is calming and comforting, giving confidence in one's abilities. Use Nutmeg to encourage and motivate to achieve dreams, showing that dreams are possible and achievable with personal efforts. Nutmeg has Alpha and Beta Pinene and is a hallucinogen, it is an ester oil and is a sedative that has the ability to affect the emotional being giving lots of positive energy. This oil reduces aggression and fears because of its calming effects and inspires a beautiful stillness.

BIBLICAL

"And Jacob took himself moist rods of trembling poplar and hazelnut, and chestnut, and he peeled white streaks upon them, baring the white that was on the rods." (Genesis 30:37)

"You shall make an altar for bringing incense up in smoke; you shall make it out of acacia wood." (Exodus 30:1)

"And you shall bind them for a sign upon your hand, and they shall be for ornaments between your eyes." (Deuteronomy 6:8)

"Is it not so? When he smooths its surface, he scatters the black cumin and casts the cumin, and he places the prominent wheat, and the barley for a sign, and the spelt on its border." (Isaiah 28:25)

"The spirit of the Lord God was upon me, since the Lord anointed me to bring tidings to the humble, He sent me to bind up the broken-hearted, to declare freedom for the captives, and for the prisoners to free from captivity." (Isaiah 61:1)

"For, like the earth, which gives forth its plants, and like a garden that causes its seeds to grow, so shall the Lord God

cause righteousness and praise to grow opposite all the nations." (Isaiah 61:11)

"Come and let us return to the Lord, for He has torn, and He shall heal us; He smites, and He will bind us up." (Hosea 6:1)

Nutmeg was one of the spices blended with other spices and gums which were offered to God in the unique biblical blend of the Ketoret. The mystical tradition associates Ketoret with the Aramaic word, meaning "binding" or a "knot." The incense was used to reflect a harmony and connectivity within the whole universe, with the anointing oil used as an expression of nobility and greatness. It unites one's core and the essence of all forces of life, bringing tidings of redemption freeing the captive and releasing their spirit according with this recipe prescribed exactly in the bible, giving glory instead of ashes, joy instead of mourning.

God gave the Israelites commandments and statutes to perform them in the land they were about to receive, a land flowing with milk and honey. This is to teach them that they should always be in awe of God and keep his commandments forever. They should teach them to their sons and their son's sons and as a trade God will always be good to them. They should perform his commandments out of love because a person who acts out of love cannot be compared to a person who acts out of fear. A person acting out of fear will eventually resent the burden and will abandon his loyalties, whereas a person who acts out of love, and with all their heart, he will do so eagerly even if the burden is great.

As a constant reminder they will bind tefillin, known as "totafoth," meaning two, on the head between the eyes, and on the arm. Because they were never to forget that God brought them out of bondage from Egypt, should they possess all the attributes of fearing God's name, serving him with loyalty, forsaking all other gods, diligently keeping all his commandments and being cautious with their oaths to his name. Houses will become full of all good things that only God can fill, with hewn cisterns that God cleaved, vineyards and olive trees that God planted, and people will eat and be satisfied. These seeds have a warm aromatic flavor and are carminative in their properties, assisting digestion. They, like all such plants which readily yield their seed, are still beaten out with rods.

Oak

Latin Name, Quercus Calliprinos
Aroma, Light, woody, and earthy

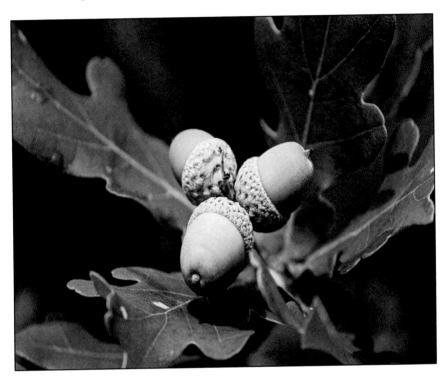

PHYSICAL

The Oak tree is a large evergreen shrub that grows in Southern Eastern Asia and in Israel's natural groves and forests. Oaks live for many years and grow very tall with a wide girth bark. It is a flowering plant and produces acorns and a single oak tree produces both male and female flowers in the spring making it possible for its own self reproduction. Oak contains tannins making it resistant to fungus and insect infestation, its leaves are toxic to lambs, sheep, cattle, goats, and horses. Oak trees are famous for their hard wood and their strength and are an excellent wood to make furniture.

The bark of the oak is used for remedies that helps hyperacid gastritis, gastro-duodenal ulcers, diarrhea, enteritis, melena, and hemorrhoids.

The leaves are a very effective antioxidant and fights free radicals this makes it capable of preventing cancer cells from forming. They also contain flavonoids which is known to support cardio functions by reducing your risk of heart disease. Flavonoids also accelerates wound healing both for external wounds and for internal stomach and peptic ulcers.

EMOTIONAL

Oak tree oil is made to cleanse homes of bad and negative energies, and in Bach Flower Therapy it is the remedy for strong, steady people who never give up under adversity. They plough on with determination, and never consider resting until they are past the point of exhaustion.

"For those who are struggling and fighting strongly to get well, or in connection with the affairs of their daily life. They will go on trying one thing after another, though their case may seem hopeless. They will fight on. They are discontented with themselves if illness interferes with their duties or helping others. They are brave people, fighting against great difficulties, without loss of hope or effort."

(Dr. Edward Bach)

BIBLICAL

"Now the Lord appeared to him in the plains of Mamre, and he was sitting at the entrance of the tent when the day was hot."
(Genesis 18:1)

"And they gave Jacob all the deities of the nations that were in their possession and the earrings that were in their ears, and Jacob hid them under the terebinth that was near Shechem."
(Genesis 35:4)

"And Saul and the men of Israel assembled, and they encamped in the Valley of the Terebinth, and they set the battle in array against the Philistines." (I Samuel 17:2)

"And Saul and they, and all the men of Israel in the Valley of the Terebinth, were at war with the Philistines." (I Samuel 17:19)

"And Absalom chanced to come before the servants of David. And Absalom was riding upon his mule, and the mule came under the thick boughs of the great terebinth, and his head caught hold in the terebinth, and he was placed between the heaven and the earth; and the mule that was beneath him passed on."
(II Samuel 18:9)

"And a man saw it and told Joab. And he said, "Behold I saw Absalom hanging in a terebinth." (II Samuel 18:10)

"And Joab said, "I shall no longer request of you." And he took three darts in his hand and thrust them into Absalom's heart while he was yet alive in the heart of the terebinth."
(II Samuel 18:14)

"And over all the cedars of the Lebanon, high and exalted, and over all the oaks of the Bashan;" (Isaiah 2:13)

"And when there is yet a tenth of it, it will again be purged, like the terebinth and like the oak, which in the fall have but a trunk, the holy seed is its trunk." (Isaiah 6:13)

"To place for the mourners of Zion, to give them glory instead of ashes, oil of joy instead of mourning, a mantle of praise instead of a feeble spirit, and they shall be called the elms of righteousness, the planting of the Lord, with which to glory."
(Isaiah 61:3)

"And you will know that I am the Lord when their slain ones will be among their idols, around their altars, upon every hill of height, on all mountaintops and under every leafy tree and under every branchy terebinth, a place where they offered up a satisfying savor to all their idols." (Ezekiel 6:13)

"Oaks from Bashan they made your oars; your rudder they made of ivory inlaid in cypresses from the isles of Kittim."
(Ezekiel 27:6)

The Hebrew name for oak is Alon and is also known as the terebinth tree. There are many oak trees in Israel, the most famous, and the oldest of them is known as "the oak of Abraham" in the hilltops of Hebron, rumored to be since the beginning of existence and still there today, it was under this oak tree that Abraham recovered from his circumcision, it was where he received visitors such as angels who had promised him a son who would be the father of great nations. It was also where he met Ephron the king of the Hittites and purchased the Machpelah cave, and it was on the third day from his circumcision, God himself came to visit him and inquired about his welfare and Abraham tried to stand in respect. God then said to him, "Sit and I will stand, and you will be a sign for your children that I am destined to stand in the congregation of the judges, and they will sit."

The cedars of the Lebanon symbolize heroes and kings of Israel and the oak from Bashan symbolizes Israel's governors. In the bible oaks are always inferior to the cedars because they do not produce fruit because of their involvement of facilitating the Israelites participating in idolatry and tree worshiping. There was a well-known oak tree near Shechem in which the bible mentions in connection with Jacob, "and Jacob hid them the idols and their ornaments under the oak." Thus, the Oak tree is mentioned in Hosea as producing acorns because when the Israelites intermarried their children were not Jewish. At the time of their expulsion when they cast off their leaves during the fall, year after year until nothing is left except for their trunk, this is where the holy seed is found right in its midst. When the tree adheres to its holiness, God will not destroy them because they were planted by him at the Gate in Jerusalem, "and there, terebinths and oaks were planted."

The oak tree redeemed its reputation when later it caught Absalom the third son of King David's hair in its branches, making it possible for Joab to kill him in battle in the "Woods of Efraim." This was a military conflict between the rebel forces of the formerly exiled Israelite Prince Absalom against the royal forces of his father king David. King David's strategy was to divide his army into three units, one was to be led by Joab, the second one by Abishai and the third by Itai, a trusted friend and commander from Gath. It was a long and bloody battle made was more difficult by the heavy forestry, which was the downfall of Absalom, where after some time of fierce battle, he was ambushed by David's army and tried to flee.

It was said about Absalom that there was not a man in all of Israel as beautiful, he was totally praiseworthy for his beauty, from the sole of his feet to the crown of his head, there was not a single blemish on him. He shaved his head at the end of every year because his hair was so thick and heavy, which the bible says weighed two hundred shekels. It was his beautiful thick hair that trapped him in the branches of a large oak tree, while he was riding his mule his hair got caught and he was unable to free himself, and the mule escaped from under him. One of the soldiers saw him trapped in the tree and told Joab that he saw Absalom hanging in a terebinth. He told Joab that he was unwilling to weigh his palms with a thousand pieces of silver against the king's son, besides it was the king's order that Avishai and Itai were not to kill Absalom, "take care whoever it may be of the youth, of Absalom." So, Joab took it upon himself against David's command and kill Absalom, killing him with three darts through the heart. After killing him they took Absalom's body and cast him in the forest into a huge pit and covered it with a very large heap of stones, then all of Israel fled to their individual tents. King David mourned for Absalom bitterly, and prayed for his son's soul, David's deep sorrow turned their "victory" into a tragedy. This enraged Joab, enflaming his resentment for Absalom whom he had viewed as an ungrateful child, and David was never able to forgive Joab for his cruel part he had taken in Absalom's death.

During Absalom's lifetime he had established for himself a monument which is in the king's valley because he said, "I have no son in order to cause people to remember my name," and he called the monument after himself, "Yad Absalom" which is still standing today. However, Absalom was survived by three sons and one daughter, Tamar who was a beautiful woman. But what Absalom had meant was that he did not have a son worthy for royalty. The Gemara says that anyone who burns the produce of another does not merit a son to inherit from him, Absalom had burned the Joab's produce. He told his servant, "Joab's field is near mine, and he has barley there; go and set it on fire, and Absalom's servants set the field on fire"

Orange

Latin name, Citrus Sinesis
Aroma, Fresh, fruity, tangy, and sweet

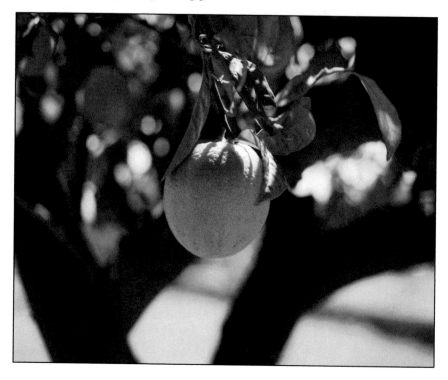

PHYSICAL

This oil is very phototoxic, it is used for scrubs and creams containing orange oil but cannot go into the sun immediately after use. The oil is taken from the fruit of the plant and contains coumarins. Its orange aroma derives from volatile organic compounds, including alcohols, aldehydes, ketones, terpenes, and esters. Like all citruses it affects the nervous system, two drops of orange oil mixed with water on lips it causes thirst and orange oil also activates the vulva during childbirth, causing them to expand and allowing the baby to be born. It also helps digest fatty foods because it doesn't allow food to be left in the digestive tract. Some studies suggest that using orange essential oil may aid in improving cognitive function, especially in Alzheimer's disease patients.

EMOTIONAL

Orange oil raises the endorphins and brings out laughter and joy. It fights stress, in fact it attacks stress. It makes one raise their head, straighten up the shoulders and put a smile on face. Remember that wonderful sensation one gets when peeling an orange when a spray of orange zest is released into the air, giving the room a burst of refreshing fragrance clearing the atmosphere instantly. Its fragrance reaches miles away giving a lighthearted positive energy just like a ray of sunlight or a beautiful shining star.

Orange oil gives spiritual guidance when listened to. It harmonizes the body, mind, and spirit. It has a very strong attraction to bring love, good fortune, balance, healing, harmony, peace, money, and riches into life. Psychologically, Orange Oil refreshes the heart and soul, it opens and lightens the heart and helps to genuinely laugh and find a sense of humor. This uplifting oil has also the ability to free up stagnant life energy. Orange is frequently thought of as and oil of abundance when allowing oneself to accept all the simple gifts of life and appreciate what one already has.

BIBLICAL

"It shall blossom and rejoice, even to rejoice and to sing; the glory of the Lebanon has been given to her, the beauty of the Carmel and the Sharon; they shall see the glory of the Lord, the beauty of our God." (Isaiah 35:2)

"I will give your rains in their time, the Land will yield its produce, and the tree of the field will give forth its fruit." (Leviticus 26:4) "

"A garden fountain, a well of living waters and flowing streams from Lebanon." (Songs of Songs 4:15)

"Awake, O north wind, and come, O south wind; blow upon my garden, that the spices thereof may flow out; let my beloved come to his garden and eat his sweet fruit." (Songs of Songs 4:16)

"And they sow fields and plant vineyards, which produce fruits and grain." (Psalms 107:37)

Th first blessing is said to God in appreciation for something we don't see often, or if we have seen it for the first time in the year. The second blessing is said before eating some fruit grown from a tree.

"Blessed are You, Lord our God, King of the universe. Who has made nothing lacking in His world and created in its goodly creatures and goodly trees to give mankind pleasure?"

Orange trees are beautiful aromatic and produce one of the most delicious fruits known to man and we say a blessing before eating it in appreciation. God mentions a garden fountain and referring it to, "arid fields" where he praises them and compares them to a fountain that waters these beautiful gardens. This is really a figure of speech where God symbolizes the immersions of purity which the daughters of Israel immerse themselves in flowing streams from Lebanon meaning a place of cleanliness, without the murkiness of mud.

God says, "since your fragrance and the beauty of your dwellings is pleasing to me, I command the north and south winds to blow on your garden so that your good fragrance should spread afar." Here God symbolizes the yielding of the diaspora and all other nations who will bring their products as an offering to Jerusalem. Then in the days of the rebuilding of the Temple where the Israelites will gather there once again for the festivals and for their pilgrimages, and Israel will say, "let my beloved come to God's gardens and if he is there, we are all there."

When the Israelites thank God for his kindness, and wonders, and when they exalt him in a communal prayer praising him, giving thanks in the presence of ten men with at least two of them being rabbinical scholars. We will see that he can make a desert into luxurious pools of water and develop wastelands into springs of water. Ruined settlements God can turn into a city of buildings and restore them into their original state. He settles the hungry there, and they will establish it into an inhabited city, where they will sow fields and plant vineyards, which produce fruits and grain.

"Blessed are You, Lord our God, King of the universe, who creates the fruit of the tree" this is the blessing we say to Godin appreciation of fruits from a tree."

Oregano

Latin name, Origanum Majorana
Aroma, Strong herbaceous

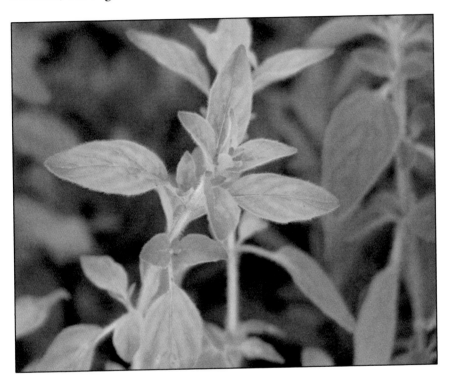

PHYSICAL

There are over twenty types of Oregano bushes and they all come from the Zaatar family known as sweet marjoram. This plant is rich in calcium, magnesium, zinc, and many other minerals. It is a very strong anti-inflammatory and antioxidant; it constricts the blood circulation and melts skin burns. Oregano boosts the immune system with support and kills pathogens which are foreign body substances which may be dormant in the body, such as candida. It completely kills these pathogens with as little as one drop on the tip of the tongue. It is also rumored that oregano oil also has a powerful effect against unwanted body fat. This oil kills ninety percent of bacterias such as, fungus, candida, and streptococcus. It is very efficient in healing flu symptoms and may even prevent being contaminated by the flu. Oregano oil is also good to cure helicobacter virus, intestinal worms, and parasite.

Oregano oil heals spasms, and though it stimulates the blood, it does not raise the blood pressure. Even though this oil is non-toxic it is still very strong and must be administered with a base oil.

Warning do not use this oil if you are pregnant, it may stimulate birth and cause a miscarriage.

EMOTIONAL

Oregano is also known as the mountain of joy. Marjoram is known for its calming effects; it completely relaxes the mind and balances the emotions. It eliminates mental fatigue and is ideal for boosting clarity of thought. Oregano oil has a long history of use in rituals and potions to guard against negative energies or influences. It builds up and balances the mood bringing positive influences on the nervous system and inhibit emotional abnormalities.

BIBLICAL

"And the Lord said to Moses, "Come up to Me to the mountain and remain there, and I will give you the stone tablets, the Law, and the commandments, which I have written to instruct them." (Exodus 24:12)

"A ritually clean person shall take the hyssop and dip it into the water and sprinkle it on the tent, on all the vessels, and on the people, who were in it, and on anyone who touched the bone, the slain person, the corpse, or the grave." (Numbers 19:18)

"When I ascended the mountain to receive the stone tablets, the tablets of the covenant which the Lord made with you, I remained on the mountain forty days and forty nights; I neither ate bread nor drank water;" (Deuteronomy 9:9)

"And the Lord gave me two stone tablets, inscribed by the finger of God, and on them was [inscribed] according to all the words that the Lord spoke with you on the mountain from the midst of the fire on the day of the assembly." (Deuteronomy 9:10)

"And it came to pass at the end of forty days and forty nights, that the Lord gave me two stone tablets, the tablets of the covenant." (Deuteronomy 9:11)

Moses came and told the people that on a certain day, the words of God will give them their new commandments and started the separation of men and women. He set boundaries around the mountain so that the people would not cross over. Moses warned them about the severity of these commandments, since at that time there were only the seven laws of Noah that they were commanded to observe. The Israelites had in addition the Sabbath, honoring one's father and mother, the laws of the red cow, and laws of mandate, which were given to them in Marah. Moses arose early the next morning and built an altar and twelve monuments for the twelve tribes of Israel at the foot of the mountain. At his orders the youths of Israel offered up burnt offerings of slaughtered bulls to God. Moses then divided up the blood into two basins of the exact same size, one half of the blood allocated for burnt offerings and the second one for the peace offerings. This blood was sprinkled over the people by Moses and the people of Israel all said in unison, "all that the Lord spoke we will do, and we will hear." Then Moses and Aaron, Nadab and Abihu, and seventy of the elders of Israel all ascended the mountain.

Unfortunately, Nadab, Abihu and the seventy elders made a fatal mistake and observed the God of Israel by peering and gazing directly at him and were thus doomed to die. However, God waited to kill them in order to not disturb the rejoicing of this special moment of the giving of the Torah, he waited until the day of the dedication of the Mishkan. Even though they all went up the mountain, only Moses alone actually approached God, Aaron, Nadab and Abihu, and seventy of the elders of Israel, all prostrated to God from afar, it was Moses who told the people about the words and laws of God. After forty days with God, Moses came down carrying the two identical stone tablets with the Law and the commandments written on them, to instruct them of all the six-hundred and thirteen mitzvoth, which included the ten Commandments. Oregano appears in the Bible as one of the most efficient healing and purification plants given to humans by God. When Moses brought down the Torah for the Jews on Mount Sinai, the Israelites purified themselves with Oregano to accept the Bible immediately.

"Arise, descend quickly from here, for your people whom you have brought out of Egypt have become corrupt; they have

quickly deviated from the way which I commanded them; they have made for themselves a molten image."

Wild oregano grows naturally in the Sinai Mountain region, ironically exactly where Moses brought down the Torah, "Tablets of Stone" with the Ten Commandments from God.

PalmaRosa

Latin Name, Cymbopogon Martini
Aroma, Sweet, rose like, with a floral lemon

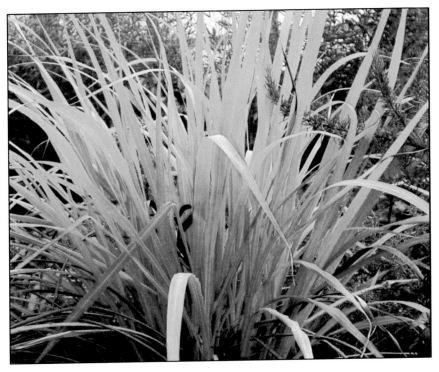

PHYSICAL

PalmaRosa comes from the Geranium, Lemongrass and Melissa family. A great oil for skin inflammations and long-term wounds. This oil reinforces the immune system and protects from bacterias and diseases. It supports the gastrointestinal system and the hormonal system, stabilizing estrogen, which stabilizes acne and post partem depression. It attacks Candida Albican, which is a single cell fungus, it is a white albino yeast causing severe itchiness and vaginal secretion. Most women know this as thrush, candidiasis, or candida. This oil attacks the candida and stops it growing and spreading in the body. Many forms of carbohydrates feed this candida and as a result takes PalmaRosa two months to kill the pathogens.

EMOTIONAL

PalmaRosa affects the adrenal hormone responsible for stress and anxiety. It controls erratic and obsessive behavior, jealousy, and self-hate, it encourages kindness and gentleness towards oneself and to tone down on the harsh and critical self-judgement. It teaches one to be loyal to the inner spirit, teaching to self-grow and development and learning to be enthusiastic, positive, emotional, and spiritual.

BIBLICAL

"Joseph fell on his father's face, and he wept over him and kissed him." (Genesis 50:1)

"And Joseph commanded his servants, the physicians, to embalm his father, and the physicians embalmed Israel." (Genesis 50:2)

"And forty days were completed for him for so are the days of embalming completed and the Egyptians wept over him for seventy days." (Genesis 50:3)

"And you, take for yourself spices of the finest sort, of pure myrrh five hundred-shekel weights; of fragrant cinnamon half of it two hundred- and fifty-shekel weights; of fragrant cane two hundred- and fifty-shekel weights," (Exodus 30:23)

"Why do I need the frankincense that comes from Sheba, and the good cane from a distant country? Your burnt offerings are not acceptable, and your sacrifices are not pleasant to Me." (Jeremiah 6:20)

Joseph embalms his father Jacob using aromatic spices such as PalmaRosa, which is part of the biblical Ketoret blend and known as the Kaneh Bosem. It is one of the fragrant canes the bible refers to, because PalmaRosa is made up of thin canes. They resemble red straws and originate from the Indian islands; it has a very pleasant fragrance. Jacob died in Egypt and there he was embalmed for forty days; blessings had come to the Egyptians while Jacob was there and when he first arrived there the famine ended, and the waters of the Nile increased. Now that Jacob was dead the Egyptians mourned him because they knew that the famine would return to their land. Joseph spoke to Pharaoh's household knowing he had an advantage here, he told Pharaoh, "My father beseeched me before he died, to bury him in his grave which he had dug for himself in the land of Canaan, there he wished to be buried, so now, please let me go up and bury my father and I will return." Pharaoh gave Joseph permission to go and bury his father, allowing him to go only because it was an oath and was fearful to transgress this oath. So, Joseph went up with all the elders of his house, as well as his brothers, his father's household and all the children to bury Jacob, also taking with them their flocks and cattle. It was a large procession of their numerous camps with their horsemen and chariots.

They arrived at the other side of the Jordan river with Jacob's coffin, there was a large threshing floor of thornbushes, and there they conducted a very great and impressive eulogy, and he made for his father a mourning of seven days. The Midrash says this was a location where all the people of Canaan and the princes of Ishmael came to fight a war, and when they saw Joseph's crown hanging on Jacob's coffin, they all stood up and hung their own crowns on it and surrounded it with crowns, resembling a threshing floor surrounded by a fence of thorns and they named the place, "Abel Mizraim" meaning Egypt mourns. Jacob's sons did as he had requested of them, they carried him to into the land of Canaan, and they buried him in the cave of Machpelah, which Abraham had bought for a burial property from Ephron the Hittite before Mamre. After burying his father, Joseph returned to Egypt, together with his brothers, and all who had gone up with him.

Patchouli

Latin Name, Pogostemon Cablin
Aroma, Earthy, woody, warm and sweet

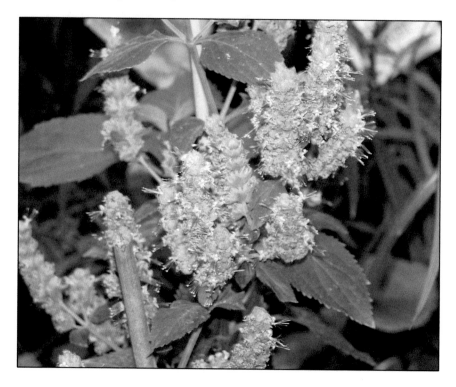

PHYSICAL

Patchouli is an herbaceous bushy plant from the mint, deadnettle family, it is indigenous of Asia and the Caribbean it has been used as perfume for hundreds of years because of its strong musky fragrance. Patchouli oil a sesquiterpene alcohol and is a thick brown almost like mold solution, its fragrance is very earthy because it grows so close to the ground. Patchouli's scent develops in three stages, earthy in the morning which develops into a lighter Earthy Smell in the late morning, and by the afternoon the fragrance is very flowery. Patchouli is an anti-inflammatory and is good for the skin, treatment for itchiness on skin, or fugus and it helps cells recover and in cell regeneration.

EMOTIONAL

Patchouli works with the base chakra; this involves the basal self and identity. It helps to understand the meaning of one's existence in the world, partnerships, duality, relationships and earning power. Patchouli helps to cross over the fence and take that leap in making a change. It gives that ability to see things not ever seen before and will view the world differently. Patchouli makes one break your boundaries, causing the self-motivation to jump and leap. This oil was used after the second world war in England to help people survive, recover, get out of their "fearful" mode, and move forward.

This oil is very dominant, even in synergies it will always be easy to identity the unique patchouli scent. This is a great oil for people who are emotionally stressed, feel frozen in time, and cannot seem to move forward. This oil is like an expensive wine, the older it gets the more powerful it becomes and does not get damaged. Use to meditate to empower and make serious changes in life. Dispel childhood issues that prevents functioning in the best possible way. Patchouli is one of the highest frequency oils and is fired with a powerful intention to achieve peace, abundance, and joy. It stimulates the conscious mind to balance with the subconscious mind for natural growth.

Patchouli cleanses energies and neutralizes raucous frequencies, making it a great purifier and space cleanser for meditation. It heals feelings of separation and isolation from loved ones and relaxes fears and anxiety by helping one feel peaceful love. Patchouli makes one feel very lucky, uplifted, with sentiments of abundance and appreciation.

BIBLICAL

"You shall make this into an oil of holy anointment, a perfumed compound according to the art of a perfumer; it shall be an oil of holy anointment." (Exodus 30:25)

"And you shall make it into incense, a compound according to the art of the perfumer, well blended, pure, holy." (Exodus 30:35)

"Instead of the briar, a cypress shall rise, and instead of the nettle, a myrtle shall rise, and it shall be for the Lord as a name, as an everlasting sign, which shall not be discontinued." (Isaiah 55:13)

"Among the shrubs they bray; under the nettles they gather."
(Job 30:7)

Patchouli is an oil that the Israelites obviously knew about because it was most likely imported via spice traders into Israel. Patchouli is a very fragrant balm and would have been valuable to them. God explains distinctly how he wants to mix the substances together, he says, "until one becomes permeated into each other with either scent or taste." The commentaries use the term "pharmaceutic" to make the mixture of spices. Each spice was measured according to its unique quantity, and it was not permitted to use the same quantities to create anything else besides this holy incense. It was also not permitted to make this same blend of ingredients for any other use besides the holy incense. If the one formulating the incense blend, decreases or increases any of the ingredients according to the measure of a hin of oil, this is permitted. The oils are made exactly according to the set formula of the incense oil, the person who anoints himself is not accountable if it is imperfect, however the one who mixes it must be responsible to make it exactly right.

The anointing incense oil sanctifies people, so they are permitted to enter the holy of holies, during that time whatever touches them also becomes holy, just as whatever service vessel the incense is placed in also becomes intrinsically holy, thus making it unfit to be used as an offering. If the oil encounters a person who has immersed himself in an uncleansed state on that day, then this oil may not be redeemed and becomes unsanctified. Only Aaron and his sons would be kohanim chosen by God and therefore, no outsider, who is not of the seed of Aaron, shall come near to the holy of holies. When Nadab and Abihu, Aaron's sons died it was because they looked into the face of God on mount Sinai with levity, while they were eating and drinking, meaning that they were drunk. They also entered the holy of holies drunk and each took a pan, put fire in them, and placed incense upon it, then they brought it before God presenting him with foreign fire, which he had not commanded of them.

The Israelites were angry at their deaths and began slandering and vilifying the incense, saying that it was a deadly poison, through which Nadab and Abihu died and because of that incident two hundred and fifty people were burnt. God said, "it is their sin that caused their deaths." When Nadab and Abihu were burned, their tunics had not been burnt, only their souls. The Commentaries say that two thread-like sparks of fire entered their nostrils and thereby destroying their souls along with all their internal organs but leaving their external body structures intact.

Peppermint

Latin Name, Mentha Piperita
Aroma, Cool, Minty

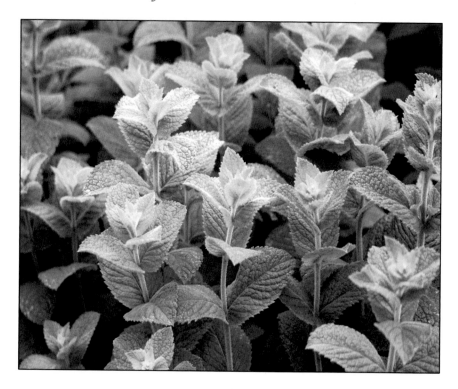

PHYSICAL

Peppermint is a menthol, mostly recognized from chewing gums and its very strong minty flavor. This oil needs to evaporate to give that cool feeling, then it gets hot like tiger balm, the oil is taken from the leaves and the flowers and is one of the first aid oils must haves at home. It freezes the recognition of pain, giving immediate relief. It is great for painful chronic problems such as a frozen shoulder or severe back pain and it helps soothe muscle spasms and headaches.

Peppermint is also used to help digestive spasms too, such as acid reflux and it is great to use for nausea. Peppermint is an anti-inflammatory, anti-flatulence, it reduces fever and relieves mucus coughs. It revives people who have fainted and calms nervousness, when inhaled. Do not use directly on the skin and do not administer to pregnant women. If there are mice and rats in the home, drop peppermint oil around your house and watch them leave. The peppermint scent is so strong for their nasal passages, it overpowers them, and it forces them to run away.

EMOTIONAL

Peppermint awakens and makes one alert and alive, it completely uplifts and rejuvenates the heart and mind. It assists relaxation and rises above nervousness, stresses, pain, and sadness. For those experiencing grief, sadness, or hopelessness this oil encourages regeneration and self-acceptance. It helps concentration, use this oil during examinations, it helps one focus and provide a view of clear pathways. If feeling bored emotionally or overwhelmed, Peppermint's vital and vibrant properties will bring fresh energy and joy for Life.

Using this oil at night may prevent sleep, due to its stimulating and invigorating properties. Peppermint is charged with intent to refresh, cleanse, and purify the mind, body, and soul, bringing spiritual protection and stimulates spiritual growth, allowing one to understand and appreciate unfolding life mysteries. It enhances the quality of dreams and increases sensitivity and perceptional awareness, it will make one more alert to signs, signals, and wisdoms from other worlds.

BIBLICAL

"And God said, "Behold, I have given you every seed-bearing herb, which is upon the surface of the entire earth, and every tree that has seed bearing fruit; it will be yours for food."
(Genesis 1:29)

"Now no tree of the field was yet on the earth, neither did any herb of the field yet grow, because the Lord God had not brought rain upon the earth, and there was no man to work the soil." (Genesis 2:5)

"And a mist ascended from the earth and watered the entire surface of the ground." (Genesis 2:6)

"For so has the Lord said to me, "I will rest, and I will look down upon My dwelling-place, like a clear heat upon herbs, like a cloud of dew in the heat of harvest." (Isaiah 18:4)

Peppermint is a common plant growing in most gardens in Israel today. Wild mints started to grow in Egypt and in biblical times, Israelites brought it with them to Israel. God says, "you will not yet fear" because the seeds were already sprouting in the ground, before man ever stepped on the earth. When the creation of the world was completed on the sixth day, before man was created, only after man worked the soil and watered the earth, did the herbs emerge from the ground. All the works of creation had been suspended specifically until the "sixth day," referring to the sixth day of Sivan, which was humanity's preparation for the giving of the bible, that was the exact date the Torah was to be given in the future. So, all the seeds of all plants and vegetations stood at the entrance of the ground until the sixth day when man was created and began to work the soil, recognizing the benefit of rain, he learned to understand that they were essential to the cycle of nature in the world.

Man comprehends that God is the Ruler and Judge over the entire world and is this defined everywhere, right under their noses, when seeing all the obvious miracles of the earth. God completed on the seventh day the creation of a human being of flesh and blood, who cannot exactly know his times and his moments, and he transforms from the profane to the holy, where he must learn about the Sabbath. God who knows his times and his moments exactly, conceived the Sabbath it seemed within a hairbreadth, therefore making it appear as if God completed his work on that day when the bible says, God rested. In fact, the Sabbath became the day of rest only when the work was completely finished.

God brought up the waters of the deep and watered the clouds to soak the earth completely, and then man was created, much like a baker, who puts water into the flour and afterwards kneads the dough. Here too, first God watered and then afterwards, God created man, he formed man of dust from the ground, by breathing into his nostrils the soul of life, and man became a living soul. God is the rock of eternity this current world was created with the Hebrew letter "hey" which is open at the bottom, so is this world open for the repentant. The World to Come was created with the Hebrew letter "yud," which is shortest and smallest of all the letters, indicating that the righteous at that future time of the world to come, will be few. This intimates that the wicked will descend below to see the netherworld, like the letter "hey," which is closed on all sides and open at the bottom, for them the wicked to descend through there.

Pine

Latin Name, Pinus Halepensis
Aroma, Crisp, clean, and fresh

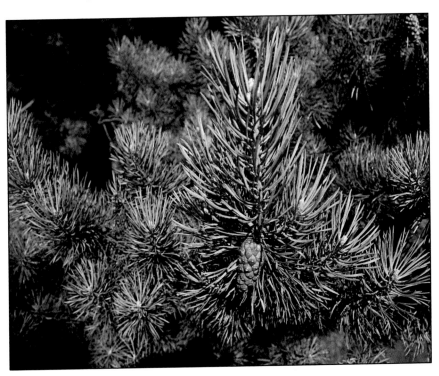

PHYSICAL

Pine is a coniferous evergreen resinous tree that grows up to eighty meters in height. Pines can live up to a thousand years, some even more. A Great Basin bristlecone pine has been recorded for living for over five thousand years. Pines mainly grow in the Northern Hemisphere, the Pinus Halepensis species are indigenous to the Middle East. Pine is great for the respiratory system because of its stimulant properties it stimulates the blood which then supplies the brain with more oxygen. When the brain has more oxygen, it automatically becomes more alert and able to learn and absorb information. One may find themselves thinking out of the box, with refreshing new ideas. Pine is an antihistamine and can help with allergies and sneezing. It is also a painkiller, useful for back or joint pain.

Plus, this oil is an antibiotic, and has been known to help with vaginal infections. If one suffers from gout or eat too much meat or animal products this oil will help because of its cleansing properties. Another great quality of this amazing tree is its needles, use it to poke and burst boils and cysts.

EMOTIONAL

Pine is a stimulant and very flammable, this oil is not suitable for people suffering from cardiovascular problems. However, it is great for those who are stuck in a rut and cannot see beyond their situation. It encourages humility and simplicity, because of its height it conveys assurance, trust, and confidence. Pine chooses its direction and goes; it trusts its choices. It displays strong characteristics of perseverance, mindfulness, and chutzpah.

Pine trees live a long time and have seen many humanities go by; we must learn to live amongst them. We inhale their fragrance and learn about life from them, this gives us a taste of their inner perception.

BIBLICAL

"I will give in the desert cedars, acacia trees, myrtles, and pines; I will place in the wilderness boxtrees, firs, and cypresses together." (Isaiah 41:19)

"To hew for himself cedars, and he took an ilex and an oak, and he reinforced it with forest trees; he planted a sapling, and rain makes it grow." (Isaiah 44:14)

"The glory of the Lebanon shall come to you, box trees, pines, and cypresses together, to glorify the place of My sanctuary, and the place of My feet I will honor." (Isaiah 60:13)

"The smallest shall become a thousand and the least a mighty nation; I am the Lord; in its time I will hasten it." (Isaiah 60:22)

"And that they should announce and proclaim in all their cities and in Jerusalem, saying, "Go out to the mountain and bring olive leaves and leaves of oil trees, myrtle leaves, date palm leaves, and leaves of plaited trees, to make booths, as it is written." (Nehemiah 8:15)

"Those who dwelt in its shade shall return; they shall revive like corn and blossom like the vine; its fragrance shall be like the wine of Lebanon." (Hosea 14:8)

"The beams of our houses are cedars; our corridors are cypresses." (Song of Songs 1:17)

"The shields of his mighty men are dyed red; the men of the army are in crimson; the chariots are in the fire of torches on the day of his preparation, and the cypresses are enwrapped." (Nahum 2:4)

The Midrash, Kohelet Rabbah says, when God created the first man, he took him on a tour and showed him all the trees of the Garden of Eden and said to him, "See my works, how beautiful and praiseworthy they are, everything that I created, I created it for you. Be careful not to spoil or destroy my world, for if you do, there will be nobody after you to repair it." Out of all his creations, God chooses the trees to symbolize the natural world, pines being the pinnacle of the plant world. Trees forms forests which as a result revolutionizes the earth from a desolate lifeless mass into a vibrant habitat bolstering all other life forms including animals and humans. A man is compared man to a tree of the field, as man is dependent on trees for his very existence and God made a special blessing for trees, *"nothing is lacking from His world, and He created good creations and good trees for the benefit of man."*

The Hebrew name for Pine is Oren, pine trees were always common in Israel during ancient times, and they are mentioned in the bible also as cedars and cypresses and always in praise for its beauty, its fragrance and good wood. Pine would have been the first-choice wood for construction and furniture, today they can be found growing in the Judean Hills able to be seen from very far away because of their tall trunks. Those who once dwelt in the shade of the Lebanon trees which they associate with God, Israel, and the Temple, and are now exiled from there, shall always yearn to return. In the Bible the pine tree is called Etz Hashemen, the "Oil Tree" because of its thick and sticky resin and high turpentine content. Pine trees have needle leaves that contain strong fibers called "forest wool." Isaiah mentions this tree among those that will fertilize in the wilderness and be redeemed. In the time of Nehemiah its branches were used for covering the "Sukkah," the temporary dwelling huts during the Jewish festival of Sukkot. In the Mishnah and other rabbinic literature, the oil tree is mentioned as a tree that was used for kindling the beacons that were lighted to announce a new month.

Ravensara

Latin Name, Ravensara Aromatica
Aroma, Camphor, herbaceous scent

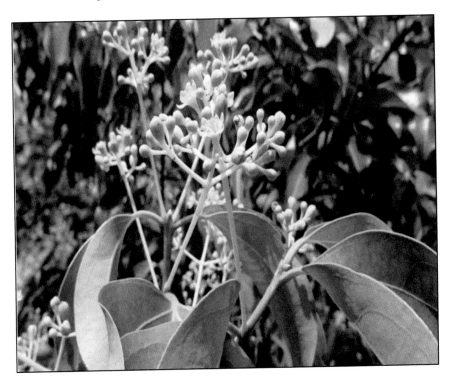

PHYSICAL

Ravensara is in a category of trees, deriving from evergreens, shrubs also the Laurel family that originated in Madagascar. Ravensara essential oil is created by distilling the leaves and twigs of the tree and mainly used for making medicine. Ravensara plants are vigorous and woody and are natives to Islands. This plant is a synergy all on its own, it helps not only in the beginning of the illness but also as the virus develops Ravensara adapt itself to into the healing mode of each stage of the illness. However, if one starts taking Ravensara when already sick, then Ravensara does not have the ability to combat the sickness. It is a very gentle oil and is suitable also for kids, its anti-fungal, anti-viral and anti-bacterial properties combats respiratory symptoms like a barking cough. Since this oil does not need to be used with a base oil, it may be applied directly onto the skin.

EMOTIONAL

Ravensara has a beautiful bright aroma and puts one in a great mood. This oil is suitable for treating multiple states of depression, anguish, mental fatigue, and lethargy. Ravensara inspires feelings of joy and hope, and even works as an aphrodisiac. It is protective and cleansing and is useful to help focus the mind to create magical ambitions that most people often dream of. It banishes anxiety and in contrast promotes courage.

Ravensara is actively protective and cleansing and should be used for healing treatments or massage. Use this oil in a diffuser to get spiritually disinfected. It analyzes the mind and memories and releases unnecessary negative emotions and responses cluttering soul. Ravensara does this gently and reassuringly every step of the way that one is doing all right and will soon be doing even better.

BIBLICAL

A cluster of henna-flowers is my beloved to me, in the vineyards of Ein-Gedi." (Song of Songs 1:14)

"Your arid fields are as a pomegranate orchard with sweet fruit, henna and spikenard." (Song of Songs 4:13)

"Behold on My hands have I engraved you; your walls are before Me always." (Isaiah 49:16)

Ravensara is one of the most useful and least harmful terpenes is terpineol, found in high concentrations in Tea Tree, Cajeput and Ravensara essential oils. Ravensara's pure terpineol darkens the henna stains because of its high levels of monoterpene alcohols, being one of the crucial ingredients used to blend into Henna Powder to improve its ability to stain the skin and facilitate its popular characteristics. We know from the bible that Henna grew in clusters of fragrant flowers was also blended with Spikenard, saffron, calamus, cinnamon, frankincense, myrrh, aloes, and other chief spices to create many aromatic incenses. Henna is a natural dye extracted from the leaves of the plant being used for centuries as a temporary tattoo in South Asia, North Africa, and the Middle East. The

Israelites used dried and powdered henna and made it into a paste which they used for dyeing their toenails, fingernails, the soles of their feet, and palms of their hands. Men were also known to have colored their beards with Henna, and even groomed their horses' tails with it. This was a cosmetic dye used a lot in Egypt at the time of Moses, this is how the Israelites learned the practice of dyeing, mainly from the Egyptian women. The bible speaks of henna flowers as a symbol of forgiveness and absolution, indicating that God forgave those who questioned him in the desert.

In Yemen, the henna dye was believed to symbolize fertility; the deeper the color of the dye, the better it was for the woman. Henna ceremonies were popular in the Yemenite society, where both Jews and Muslims shared this common custom until the Yemenite Jews were brought to Israel. Unfortunately, after this Henna ceremonies became smaller and less popular amongst their Yemenite communities. Conventionally the henna is first painted onto the palms of the bride and groom with intricate designs as a ceremonial blessing, then by the time-honored tradition the bride applies the henna paste to the palms of her guests, and once dried and removed, the henna paste leaves an orange tint, exhibiting that they have been at the celebration. In modern day Israel, Middle Eastern families have taken up the henna party celebrations prior to their weddings. Usually in a more intimate celebration for closer friends and family. The bride and groom and most of the guests dress up into traditional costumes, the henna is brought in by the grandmother.

Red Thyme

Latin name, Chemotype Linalol
Aroma, Sharp, woody, and herbaceous

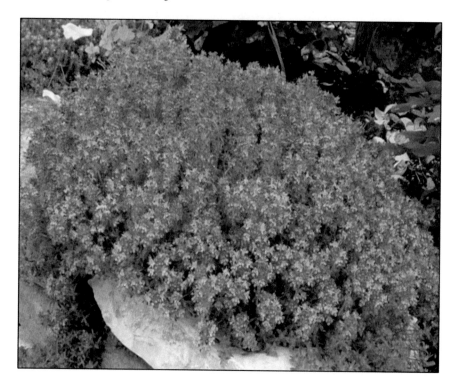

PHYSICAL

Also known at Carvacrol, it is an oil very similar to Oregano. It is an anti-inflammatory that really helps joint pains and unravel inflammation. Red thyme is also an anti-allergen and helps cope with hay fever. This oil kills streptococci and parasites and it is very effective with upper respiratory infections. Great for sinusitis, inhale it directly from the bottle or rub on the forehead or over the eyebrows. This is a very strong oil and assists the body to completely recover from illnesses, a base oil must be used with this oil, even though it does burn the skin too seriously.

The thyme family plants resemble the Zaatar plant. Thyme is connected to the throat chakra and affects the vocal cords. People that speak a lot, like teachers sometimes develop warts and swollen vocal cords. A drop on the tongue will help the vocal cords. Also good for kids with a cold or a flu, it does this by killing bacteria, Thyme oil really knows how to attack these bacteria. Children who suffer from ADHD or dyslexia, need this for their brain function. Thyme helps these kids find a different route to cope with their comprehension, almost like a bypass.

EMOTIONAL

Red Thyme blocks nightmares from accessing thoughts and emotions, it uplifts the mood and is a natural stress reliever. This oil empowers emotionally and prevents feelings that cause you to give up take control. Red Thyme is supportive and gives the backbone to cope with whatever comes by continually boosting the courage. It is a powerful cleanser of clogged up emotions like anger and resentment, it balances the emotions and mental clarity to move forward.

Red Thyme is a memory booster and helps increase concentration and brain power, this improves the quality and efficiency of work and capabilities. it energizes and revitalizers you're the allowing for release, forgiveness and let go. Other times it could be diagnosed as a blockage in the throat chakra. A drop of Thyme on the tongue helps gain courage to start to speak up for oneself. Thyme gives very thick skin and if someone is insulting, it helps to not take things to heart. The Greeks used this oil before a war to give them courage. It blends well with bitter orange and cedarwood.

BIBLICAL

"And now go, lead the people to the place of which I have spoken to you. Behold My angel will go before you. But on the day, I make an accounting of sins upon them, I will bring their sin to account against them." (Exodus 32:34)

"The kohen shall take a piece of cedar wood, hyssop, and crimson wool, and cast them into the burning of the cow." (Numbers 19:6)

"How fair is your love, my sister, my bride; how much better is your love than wine, and the fragrance of your oils than all spices!" (Song of Songs 4:10)

"Awake, O north wind, and come, O south wind; blow upon my garden, that the spices thereof may flow out; let my beloved come to his garden and eat his sweet fruit." (Song of Songs 4:16)

Aaron was ordered by God to use Thyme for his burnt offerings, Ezov, is described as a small plant found on or near walls, with an aromatic odor. Maimonides, Saadia Gaon and earlier Jewish commentators identified the connection of Ezov with Za'atar and various local herbs of that time, also including marjoram and oregano. They all have a very similar aroma as well as cleansing properties, all growing naturally wild in Israel and many times are easily bunched together and used for sprinkling. Red Thyme is of the Hyssop family plant, it is called "a species of herb that has thin stalks." The Israelites recognized them for their antibacterial, antifungal, and antimicrobial properties and were used as a part of ritual oils for cleansing lepers and purifying those who have come in contact with the dead.

The Israelite's transgression with the golden calf is perpetuated in the memory throughout the universe and future generations as a retribution, for there is no reckoning which does not include an appraisal for the calf. The commentaries say, "on the day I make an accounting of sins upon them, I will bring their sin to account." God said, "Now I have listened to you not to destroy them all at once, but always, always, when I take an accounting of their sins, I will also account a little of this sin with the other sins". This means that no punishment befalls Israel in which there is not part of the punishment for the sin of the golden calf. All Israelites since then is part of the blame for the sin and must assume responsibility also, had we been there at that time what would we have done?

When Moses went up Mount Sinai to get the Torah from God and the people saw that Moses was late in coming down from the mountain, the people gathered up against Aaron, and they said to him, *"come on! Make us gods that will go before us, because this man Moses, who brought us up from the land of Egypt we don't know what has become of him."* When Moses had gone up the mountain, he told the Israelites that he was due to return at the end of forty days, six hours from sunrise of the fortieth day. They assumed that the day Moses left was included in the calculation of the forty days, but in fact he had said to them, "forty complete days," meaning including the night. But on the day of his ascent Moses ascended in the morning and this night before was not included. So, the fortieth day of Moses' absence was the seventeenth of Tammuz and it was on the sixteenth of Tammuz that the Satan came and brought confusion into the world and displayed pitch darkness, indicating that Moses had died and therefore, Satan told them, "It is obvious that Moses has died, because it has been six additional hours and he has not returned."

Aaron was trying to delay the Israelites, in the hope that Moses would arrive before they would rebel, he told them, "Remove the golden earrings that are on the ears of your wives, your sons, and your daughters and bring them those earrings to me." The people stripped themselves of their golden earrings that were on their ears and brought them to Aaron. Aaron said to himself, *"the women and children are fond of their jewelry, perhaps their matter will be postponed, and in the meantime Moses will arrive."* But however, they did not wait for their wives and children to give them their earrings, and the men took off their own earrings. Aaron took the gold from their hands and threw it into the fire and a calf began to emerge and he shaped it an engraving tool, and made it into a molten calf, upon which the people said, "these are your gods, O Israel, who have brought you up from the land of Egypt!"

The Midrash says that as soon as the threw the gold into the fire of the crucible, sorcerers of who had left with them from Egypt, arrived at the scene and formed the calf into an ox using their sorcery. These were the mixed multitude who had accompanied the Jews from Egypt, they were the ones who gathered against Aaron, and they were the ones who made the molten gold into the calf and caused the Israelites to stray after it. Other Midrashim say that Micah was there, he had emerged from the layer of the building where he had been crushed in Egypt, and in his hand was a plate upon which Moses had inscribed "Ascend, O ox; ascend, O ox," to miraculously exhume Joseph's coffin from the Nile, the people then cast the plate into the cauldron.

When Aaron saw that it was alive, as it is said, "for the likeness of an ox eating grass," he saw that Satan's work had succeeded, and he had no words to stall them completely and keep the Israelites from worshipping the calf, so then he built an alter for God and said, "tomorrow shall be a festival to the Lord and not today," he was silently hoping that Moses would come back before they would worship the ox. During this time Aaron saw many disturbing things, he saw his sister's son Hur, who had reproved the Israelites, be assassinated, and slaughtered in front of him. The more he saw what was going on he said to himself, it is better that I should be blamed and not them. He also realized that he should be the one to build the alter and neglect his priestly work, until Moses will arrive.

The next day Satan aroused them early so that they would sin, the people offered up burnt offerings, and brought peace offerings, then the people sat down to eat and to drink, then they got up to make merry with a connotation of sexual immorality, and bloodshed, where Hur was slain. God sees what is happening to his people and says to Moses,

"Go, descend, for your people that you have brought up from the land of Egypt have acted corruptly. Now leave Me alone, and My anger will be kindled against them so that I will annihilate them, and I will make you into a great nation."

Moses pleaded to God, and said, *"Why, O Lord, should Your anger be kindled against Your people whom You have brought up from the land of Egypt with great power and with a strong hand? Why should the Egyptians say, their God brought them out of Egypt only with evil intent to kill them in the mountains and to annihilate them from upon the face of the earth. Retreat from the heat of Your anger and reconsider the evil intended for Your people."* Moses implored to God, *"Remember Abraham, Isaac, and Israel, your servants, to whom You swore by Your very Self, and to whom You said, 'I will multiply your seed like the stars of the heavens, and all this land which I said that I would give to your seed, they shall keep it as their possession forever."* God then listened to Moses and reconsidered his decision and Moses went down the mountain bearing the two tablets of the testimony in his hand, tablets inscribed from both their sides.

Joshua who was waiting for Moses on the mountain top, had no idea what was going on down below, he heard shouting, rejoicing, and laughing. The Israelites were so loud that they could be heard even from such a distance, and said he said to Moses, *"there is a voice of battle in the camp!"* Moses answered him, *"It is neither a voice shouting victory, nor a voice shouting defeat, it is the voices of blasphemy that I hear."* When they drew closer to the camp and Moses saw the calf and the dances, his anger was kindled beyond control, and he flung the tablets from his hands, shattering them at the foot of the mountain. Moses burned the ox in the fire and ground the ashes to a fine powder, he scattered this powder on the surface of their water and gave it to the Israelites to drink. There were three different death penalties meted out then. First there were the witnesses of the worship and as a warning, had been promulgated to the sinners. They were punished by the sword, according to the law, this applied to the people of a city that has been led astray and here many people had been led astray. The second penalty were those who practiced idolatry with witnesses but without warning died from a plague that God had struck them with. The third penalty were those who practiced idolatry both without witnesses and without warning died from dropsy, for the water tested them and their stomachs swelled up and they died.

Moses stood in the gate of the camp and asked, "Whoever is for the Lord, let him come to me!" And all the sons of Levi gathered around him. Moses ordered them according to words of the God of Israel, *"Let every man place his sword upon his thigh and pass back and forth from one gate to the other in the camp, and let every man kill his brother, every man his friend, every man his kinsman."* The sons of Levi did according to Moses' word; on that day some three thousand men fell from among the people.

Rose

Latin Name, Rosa Damascena
Aroma, Deep soft, hypnotic spicy rose

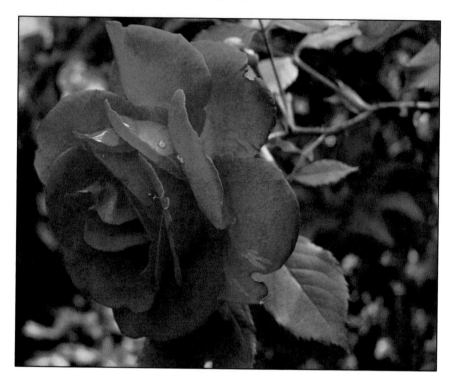

PHYSICAL

Rose is a woody flowering plant that bears flowers that vary in shape, size, color, and fragrance. They are indigenous of Africa, North America, and Asia, and are usually ornamental plants and grown for their flowers. They have an intoxicating fragrance and are used to make perfumes and flower bouquets. The oil is taken from Rosa Damascena which makes essential oil for absolute Rose oil. Rosa Damascena grows in cold countries like Romania, Bulgaria, Russia, France, and Morocco. To harvest the oil Rose petals are collected and placed into a copper pot, one hundred and seventy roses will produce one drop of rose essential oil. Roses have a short flowering season, which is only in the summer. The colors of roses are purple, pink and have a very strong scent which almost everybody loves. Rose is used for reproduction because it stimulates ovaries and sperm and helps in the ability to get pregnant. It also relieves period and PMS stress and is wonderful for shadow under the eyes and wrinkles. Rose affects the nervous system and takes care of the heart, heartrate, lowers high blood pressure as well as raising low blood pressure. Helps digestion, nausea, and skin allergies.

EMOTIONAL

For women who are having problems getting pregnant, spread rose oil onto the womb area and relax, maybe have a guided meditation session so to allow her body to conceive and to dispel fears of pregnancy. Rose is a shy quiet oil, that gives maternal confidence and hugs. This oil gives the confidence to apologize and admit mistakes. It encourages self-motivation and inner vitality; this oil is passionate and confident with a refreshing sense of freedom. Rose oil is love and devotion, with complete contentment and acceptance of love, sensuality, and purity. Rose oil will show inner awareness and freedom that will lead to completeness.

BIBLICAL

"Desert and wasteland shall rejoice over them, and the plain shall rejoice and shall blossom like a rose." (Isiah 35:1)

"It shall blossom and rejoice, even to rejoice and to sing; the glory of the Lebanon has been given to her, the beauty of the Carmel and the Sharon; they shall see the glory of the Lord, the beauty of our God." (Isiah 35:2)

"Lift up your eyes on high and see who created these" (Isaiah 40:10)

"I will be like dew to Israel, they shall blossom like a rose, and it shall strike its roots like Lebanon." (Hosea 14:6)

"His jaws are like a bed of spice, growths of aromatic plants; his lips are like roses, dripping with flowing myrrh." (Song of Songs 5:13)

"Your navel is like a round basin, where no mixed wine is lacking; your belly is like a stack of wheat, fenced in with roses."

Jerusalem was called a wasteland and Zion was called a desert, in the end they shall rejoice over the downfall of the mighty of the heathens and Persia. Strengthen weak hands, all the prophets who brought tidings of salvation consoled Israel and strengthened their weak hands. *"Be strong, you whose hands are weak,"* and to the hasty of heart who hurries to the redemption and are troubled by its delay, we say, *"with vengence God shall come and save you."* The Zohar describes the people of Israel comparing them to a single rose, with collective souls all looking up into a spiritual world. The rose is described to have thirteen petals set amongst thorns, sitting on a bed of five strong protective green leaves encasing it. Israel is the beautiful rose among the thorns whose beauty is not diminished even when she is outnumbered and surrounded by thousands of prickly neighbors. The complete rose represents the whole community of Israel, the Assemblage of Israel are the thirteen petals that make up the rose flower and the Measures of Compassion are the five protective green leaves, and the thorns are their protector.

The Kabbalah brings an interesting perception, that all physical creations in this world are expressions of spiritual forces and divine realms. It is of great significance that right at the start the Zohar commentaries of the Torah, should begin by quoting from the Song of Songs of King Solomon. There is an intense level of intimacy expressed in the Song of Songs, a love-song pouring out the intimacies of the heart and of love. This intense storyline correlates to the ethereal relationship God has with his people, and the Zohar deliberately choses to convey his observation revolving around a relatable masculine-feminine relationship. The space in between the Cherubim in the Holy of Holies in the Temple is the place of the closest, most intimate relationship between God and His People.

In the song, "your navel is like a round basin of clear water with which they wash, and the basin is made of marble," which in Arabic is called "sahar." The navel is compared to a round basin because it is shaped like a round hole. This praise does not refer to a woman's beauty as her beloved praises her, but here, her companion praises her about her deeds, saying, you are worthy to be around. No beverage will ever cease to be found, this is understood to mean that no words of instruction will cease or end from there, like the constant flow of wineries. Your belly is like a stack of wheat which everyone needs, it is hedged around with roses where a light fence suffices her, and no one will ever dream of breaching it to enter. For example, a bridegroom enters the nuptial canopy, his heart longing for the nuptials and for the love of his marriage. When he comes to cohabit with her, she says to him, *"I have perceived a drop of blood like the size of a mustard seed,"* and he turns his face the other way, no snake bit him, nor did a scorpion sting him, this is the meaning of *"she is fenced in with roses."*

Rosemary

Latin Name, Rosmarinus Officinalis
Aroma, Camphor, woody and herby

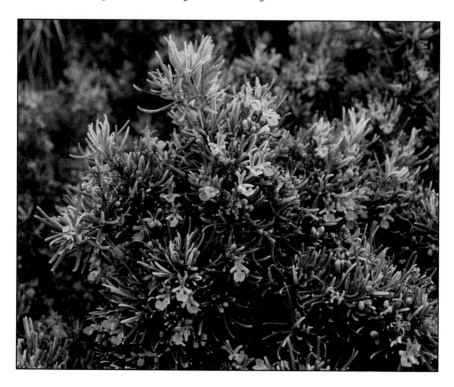

PHYSICAL

Rosemary is a woody, evergreen fragrant herb with needle leaves and purple, pink, blue or white flowers. It is native to the Mediterranean and Asia and handles being in colder climates too. It is also called Sea Dew because it can thrive by the sea. Rosemary essential oil is a very strong oil that can burn the skin. It is an anti-bacterial and effectively gets rid of mucus, dissolves phlegm. This wonder oil activates the liver by raising adrenaline levels and is used for kidney and liver cleansings and helps the gallbladder to get rid of bile and cleanse the blood stream. This oil boosts hair growth it may prevent baldness, alopecia and slows down graying and is used to treat dandruff and dry scalp and it is used in shampoo. It improves moods and clears the mind, and it prevents Alzheimer's.

Rosemary warms cold hands and fingertips helping people suffering from bad blood circulation. It balances estrogen levels in the body and helps prostate health. It contains large amounts of antioxidants, anti-inflammatories and anticancer properties that kill cancer cells. To prepare this oil at home, place rosemary in a container and then pour olive oil into it. Leave on your counter for three weeks in direct sunlight. Use the dried Rosemary to burn as incense or into teas and infusions.

Warning must not be used while pregnant, nursing, or if you suffer from high blood pressure or epilepsy.

EMOTIONAL

Rosemary dynamizes survival confidence and motivation, it stimulates movement by raising energy levels. This oil is very uplifting and high energy with lots of confidence and concentration. It brings clarity and awareness and awakens the soul, Rosemary is connected to the third eye chakra, it clears away unwanted thoughts and negative feelings. As an essential oil or in potpourris and sachets, the fragrance lifts the emotional spirit, grants a youthful outlook, and pleasant memories. Rosemary releases pressure surrounding spiritual paths, making it a great spiritual herb to keep on hand.

Rosemary is known as the symbol of faith and love, and it has grown wild all over Israel since biblical days. It is a spiritual plant that leads to a wonderful journey and is one of the major spiritually purifying herbs and can be used in herbal baths, inside cheesecloth or a coffee filter, tied with string and placed under the running bath water. Rosemary is also considered a protective herb. Place rosemary in a pillow or pillowcase to ward off bad dreams. Rosemary has an affinity for the head area. It clears away unwanted thoughts, lifts negative thinking in favor of a positive attitude, and assists with concentration.

BIBLICAL

"And he shall sit refining and purifying silver, and he shall purify the children of Levi. And he shall purge them as gold and as silver, and they shall be offering up an offering to the Lord with righteousness." (Malachi 3:3)

"The Lord is my shepherd; I shall not want."

"He causes me to lie down in green pastures; He leads me beside still waters."

"He causes me to lie down in green pastures; He leads me beside still waters."

"You set a table before me in the presence of my adversaries; You anointed my head with oil; my cup overflows."

"May only goodness and kindness pursue me all the days of my life, and I will dwell in the house of the Lord for length of days." (Psalms 23:1-6)

"Purify me with a hyssop, and I will become pure; wash me, and I will become whiter than snow." (Psalms 51:9)

Woe to the land shaded by wings, which is on the other side of the rivers of Cush to which they come in ships from a distant land, and their sails are spread out like an eagle that flies with its wings. They live in the east, and the land is hot, birds assemble there, and it is shaded by the birds' wings. This is the prophecy of the armies of Gog and Magog, as it is stated from Persia till Africa. They start by sending emissaries by sea in boats made of bulrushes floating on the surface of the water,

"Go, swift messengers, to a nation, pulled and torn, to an awesome nation from their beginning onward, a nation punished in kind and trampled, whose land the rivers have plundered."

The messengers want to see whether it is true that the Israelites have returned to their home, a nation which was pulled and torn transformed into a people that is awesome from its inception, because right from that day they were chosen as a people of God. A nation punished for their kind and given to being trampled, loathsome and rejected. All inhabitants of the world and dwellers of the earth, you need not send messengers, from the tops of the mountains shall see the gathering of the exiles, and when the shofar is sounded you shall also hear. As God said, *"I will rest, and I will look down upon My dwelling-place, like a clear heat upon herbs, like a cloud of dew in the heat of harvest."* Meaning that God will rest from paying Esau his just deserts; he will turn away from all his affairs and will look down upon his dwelling place to do good to it.

The clear heat upon herbs such as Rosemary will illuminate the desert and cause it to shine like a cloud of dew, the type for which reapers long, to refresh themselves during the heat of the harvest when the blossom is past, and the buds turn into ripening grapes. So will be the ripening of the harvest of Amalek and of Gog, when he has not yet filled his desire and his hope, that he plans to destroy his brothers, when its blossom is past and the grain is close to becoming ripe in its ears and before the buds of his vine become ripening grapes, ripened to the extent of becoming as big as a white bean. They shall be cut off from their tendrils and their branches and boughs. God shall slay all the officers and the rulers of Esau and of Gog and his armies and his allies. They shall be left to rot together for the birds of the mountains and the beasts of the earth. The birds shall spend the entire summer upon them, and the beasts of the earth shall spend the entire winter upon their corpses. The deduction of God's judgment of Gog in the future shall be twelve months, during that time, there shall be brought a gift to the Lord of Hosts, to the place of the name of the Lord of Hosts, Mount Zion.

Rosemary purifies the "mezora" the leper, the one who became unclean through contact with a corpse, or ritual impurity. Rosemary cleanses the skin from the disease tza'arat, known as leprosy. It is an eruptive plague, attacking the male genital discharges, and in women their menstruation discharge. The king Pharaoh was stricken with the plague of "Ra'athan" when he stole Sarah from Abraham and tried to have relations with her. This type of leprosy attacks the skin with painful boils, this disease makes intercourse not only very agonizing, but also harmful, this type of leprosy is debilitating and worsened by sexual intercourse.

Rosewood

Latin Name, Aniba Rosaeodora.
Aroma, Sweet, mild, spicy, and floral

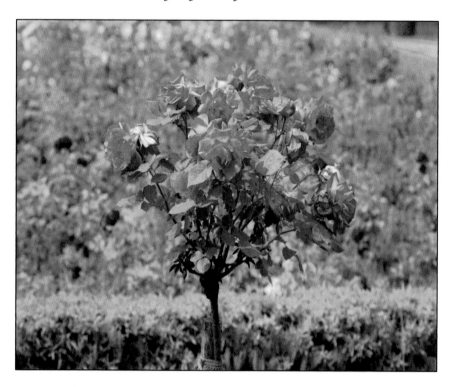

PHYSICAL

Rosewood is also known as bois-de-rose. It is an evergreen tree that grows up to forty meters. The oil is extracted from the trunk of the rosewood tree. We have all heard of rosewood furniture, which is very expensive because it is made from the bark of this tree. Rosewood oil is made from Geranium and Rose, this blend is great for the skin because it doesn't burn when applied directly on to the skin. Rosewood attacks viruses and bacterias, this is a good oil to use in moisturizer because of its anti-aging properties as well as combats acne. It strengthens skin fibers and improves blood flow; this unique blend of Rose and Geranium is also a deodorant.

It is a strong painkiller and relieves toothaches and headaches, or other oral problems like bleeding gums. It's also an antiseptic and treat insect bites, abrasions, and minor cuts. Rosewood kills cancer cells; it has components that control some cancerous cells. It is also active with the immune system, nervous system, and an anti-inflammatory.

EMOTIONAL

It soothes the mind and fine tunes the emotions and feelings and it connects with the inner self and teaches how to understand emotions. This oil gives emotional support, it is a pickup if when feeling depressed or tired. When feeling pressured, Rosewood prevents fears to attack, inhaling whenever anxiety strikes, or stress levels rise. Rosewood helps sufferers of chronic or recurring problems, such as stress, pressure, lack of sleep. It is a relaxant and due to its power can even cause hallucination.

Rosewood creates a powerful energy enrichment and works with the Third Eye. When meditating with this oil, it will stimulate the intuition to soar upwards, "Fly me to the Moon." Rosewood is connected to the heart chakra and is excellent for meditation to encourage and deep joy to come into life. This oil brings everything desired, just ask for it.

BIBLICAL

"For the conductor on shoshannim, of the sons of Korah, a maskil a song of loves."

"My heart is a stir with a good theme; I say, "My works are for a king; my tongue is a pen of an expert scribe."

"You are more handsome than other men; charm is poured into your lips. Therefore, God blessed you forever."

"Gird a sword on your thigh, O mighty one, your majesty and your glory."

"And your glory is that you will pass and ride for the sake of truth and righteous humility, and it shall instruct you so that your right hand shall perform awesome things."

"Your arrows are sharpened, nations shall fall under you, in the heart of the king's enemies."

"Your throne, O judge, will exist forever and ever; the scepter of equity is the scepter of your kingdom."

"You loved righteousness and you hated wickedness; therefore God, your God, anointed you with oil of joy from among your peers."

"Myrrh and aloes and cassia are all your garments; more than ivory palaces, those that are Mine will cause you to rejoice."

"The daughters of kings will visit you; the queen will stand at your right bedecked with golden jewelry from Ophir."

"Hearken, daughter, and see, and incline your ear, and forget your people and your father's house."

"And the King shall desire your beauty, for He is your Lord, and prostrate yourself to Him."

"And the daughter of Tyre shall seek your presence with tribute, those who are the richest of the people."

"All honor awaits the King's daughter who is within; her raiment is superior to settings of gold."

"With embroidered garments, she will be brought to the King; and virgins in her train who are her companions will be brought to You."

"They shall be brought with joy and exultation; they shall come forth into the King's palace."

"Instead of your forefathers will be your sons; you shall appoint them as princes throughout the land."

"I will mention Your name in every generation; therefore, peoples shall thank You forever and ever."

(Psalms 45:1-18)

"For the conductor, to the roses, a testimony, of Asaph a song."
(Psalms 80:1)

"O Shepherd of Israel, hearken, He Who leads Joseph like flocks, He Who dwells between the cherubim, appear." (Psalms 80:2)

Korah's band of singers called the Shoshannim, and they are playing instruments called Metzudot which were designed in the shape of a rose or lily, it is a six stringed instrument carved out of Rosewood. Korah and his sons sing a song of love, a song of praise for the Torah scholars, so making the Torah scholars endear the Torah to the people.

The Shoshannim, meaning "The Roses," was the name of the melody to which this psalm was sung which was in honor of the Torah scholars, who are described as "tender as roses and as beautiful as roses and perform good deeds as fresh as roses." Korah says "This song, which I have founded and composed, I say to one who is fit to be a king, as it is stated "King's reign with me." my tongue is, as poetic as the pen of an expert scribe".

We've all heard the expression, "Stop and smell the roses." In other words, take time out to appreciate the beauty of God's creations, particularly in the realm of smell. The Sages understood the importance of this and ordained a special set of blessings that give us the opportunity to praise God's having "perfumed the world." This song is about acknowledgment and appreciation of what is around us and that it was created for us to respect, love and care for.

Sandalwood

Latin name, Santalum Album
Aroma, Warm, balsamic, rich, and woody

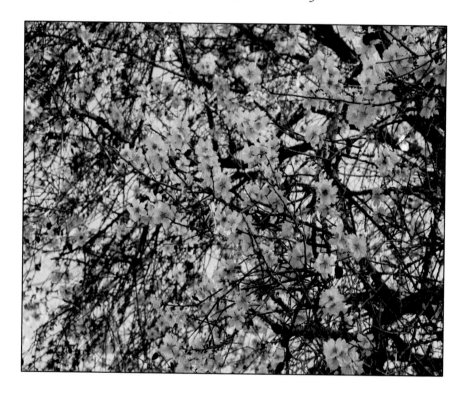

PHYSICAL

Sandalwood oil has a distinctive soft, warm, smooth, creamy, and milky precious wood scent. It gives a long-lasting, woody base to perfumes from the oriental, woody, floral and citrus fragrances. The oil is extracted from deep inside the wood from the center of the tree. The oil lasts for decades and doesn't get spoiled or damaged by bacteria. The weather doesn't affect it, it is very strong and powerful. Sandalwood is active in the immune system. People suffering with a panic attack should place a little on their wrists to calm down.

Sandalwood can be blended with oils for many problems such as, herpes simplex, acnes, ciboria, and eczema. It knows how to kill viruses on the skin, heal acne vulgaris, it can also be applied together with moisturizer. It assists the respiratory system, and kills viruses, heals bronchitis and whooping cough.

EMOTIONAL

Sandalwood is Courage! This tree exposes the hero within, it is definitely a meditation oil, it promotes ability, assertiveness because it has a strong base chakra. Sandalwood helps emotionally and encourages one to be more stable and brings out assertiveness. Sandalwood helps to understand oneself, providing the tools to identify personal issues and teaches how to deal with them. When judgement and proportions are displaced, this oil helps land back down on earth.

This is a three-step growth and awareness process; and must experience each of the three stages to reach enlightenment and realization.

> **First Stage**, is unknown Fear, Identify secret shadows
> **Second Stage**, is identified Fear, Kill these shadows
> **Third Stage**, is courage, Finding the hero within

Warning do not administer to people who had an organ transplant, this oil will cause them to reject their new organ.

BIBLICAL

"They extend like streams, like gardens by the river, like aloes which the Lord planted, like cedars by the water."
(Numbers 24:6)

"Also, Hiram's ships that delivered gold from Ophir, brought from Ophir a huge quantity of almog-wood and precious stones."
(I Kings 10:11)

"And the king made of the almog-wood a path to the House of the Lord and to the king's palace, harps and psalteries to accompany the vocalists, there had come no such almog-wood nor has there been seen to this day." (I Kings 10:12)

"Spikenard and saffron, calamus and cinnamon, with all frankincense trees, myrrh and aloes, with all the chief spices."
(Song of Songs 4:14)

"Myrrh and aloes and cassia are all your garments; more than ivory palaces, those that are Mine will cause you to rejoice."
(Psalms 45:9)

Sandalwood known as aloes and almog wood in the Bible, it produces a sweet balsamic scent and used as a fragrant perfume. It was imported via the Ophir region from India by King Solomon and used to build musical instruments for the Holy Temple of Jerusalem. This imported wood is hard, heavy, close-grained, and of a fine red color instead of the white fragrant sandalwood found in Israel. It was a rare wood whose tree does not grow with the firs and cedars in Lebanon. Hiram was the Phoenician king of Tyre, was originally his father David's friend, and maintained his alliance with the family and became Solomons loyal friend also. He supplied Solomon with much of the Algom wood to build the holy temple of Jerusalem. It was his servants and Solomon's servants, who transported the gold from Ophir, imported the algom wood and precious stones. The Algom wood melted and bent easily because of its unique softness, Solomon used this wood to make a path to the House of God and to the king's palace. He also designed harps and psalteries for the singers, nothing like they had ever seen before in the land of Judah. He created them for the Levites who like to sing with musical instruments, these were secular songs that he composed for them to sing to him.

During the year following the Queen of Sheba's visit, King Solomon accumulated huge wealth, in one year alone he earned six hundred sixty-six talents of gold. Guides and the merchants were afraid to pass from province to province or from kingdom to kingdom without a hiring a guide from the king. They would give Solomon a fee to rent these guides, by word of mouth this brought all the kings of Arabia and their regents of the land, thus bringing with them gold and silver for Solomon, these merchants would bring him gold on a pretext to witness his wisdom. King Solomon made two hundred shields of malleable gold and it took six hundred malleable gold pieces to go into one shield. Then Solomon took three hundred shields of malleable gold, using three hundred gold pieces into one shield, and Solomon placed them in the house of the forest of Lebanon. Solomon built a huge house in Jerusalem which he built from an abundance of the large trees of Lebanon, and it was there that he deposited those shields, Next Solomon made an immense ivory throne using the ivory of elephants and overlaid it with pure gold. He made six steps up to ascend the throne as well as a ramp of gold attached to the throne. Solomon added armrests on either side with two lions also made of gold standing beside them. There were twelve lions in total, two on each step at either end nothing like anything ever made for any kingdom.

All King Solomon's drinking vessels were gold, particularly all the vessels of his house in the forest of Lebanon were made of a more superior gold, and silver was not even considered by Solomon. The king's ships would go to Tarshish with Huram's servants once in three years, and these ships from Tarshish would return bearing and abundance of gold, silver, ivory, apes, meerkats, long-tailed monkeys, and peacocks. Now Solomon transcended all the kings of the earth in affluence as well as in wisdom, and in turn all the kings of the earth sought Solomon's presence to hear the wisdom with which God had endowed him. Obviously each one would bring him a gift of vessels of silver, gold, garments, weapons, spices, horses, mules plus tribute their due for the year. God came to Solomon in a dream and said to him, "if you walk in My ways, to keep My statutes and My commandments, as your father David did walk, then I will lengthen your days." When Solomon awoke from his dream, he realized when he heard a bird chirp and a dog bark, he understood their language. Solomon then came to Jerusalem and stood before the ark of the covenant of God, and offered up burnt offerings, peace offerings and made a feast for all his servants.

"I have also given you that which you have not asked, both riches and honor, so that there shall not be any among the kings like you all your days." (I Kings 3:13)

Solomon accumulated four thousand stables of horses and chariots and twelve thousand horsemen, and he placed them in the chariot cities and with the king in Jerusalem, but he transgressed God's commandment of, "Only he shall not multiply horses to himself." Solomon ruled over all the kings, from the river until the land of the Philistines and right to the border of Egypt. He succeeded in making silver as common in Jerusalem as stones, and he made cedar trees as common as the sycamores that are in abundance in the lowlands of Israel. Solomon received many horses as gifts from Egypt and other lands. All in all, Solomon reigned in Jerusalem and over all Israel for forty years, unlike his father David, who reigned seven years in Hebron and thirty-three years in Jerusalem. Solomon's final resting place is with his fathers, he is buried in the City of David alongside his father, and Rehoboam his son reigned in his place.

Spikenard

Latin Name, Nardostachys Jatamansi
Aroma, Warm, heavy, and musty

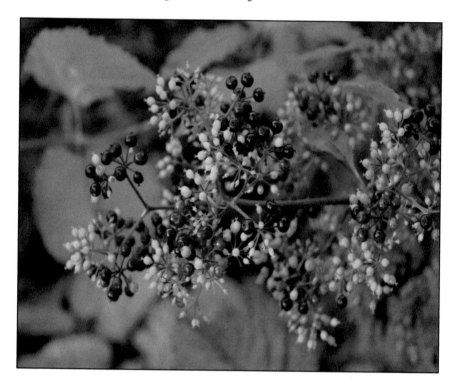

PHYSICAL

Nardostachys Jatamansi is a flowering plant that grows and originates from the Himalayas. It is the main source of a unique type of intensely aromatic, amber-colored essential oil. Since ancient times Spikenard has been used as a perfume, medicine and for religious services. This oil is used as an herbal medicine and it does so naturally, it treats insomnia, stress, digestive problems, infections, stimulates the immune system and nervous system. When taken orally it cleanses the uterus, helps with infertility, and treats menstrual disorders.

Spikenard helps treat sleeping problems depression, stress, anxiety, and chronic fatigue syndrome. It stops the growth of bacteria from inside the body and out. Spikenard treats bacterial infections in the kidneys, urinary bladder, and urethra. It's also known to treat toenail fungus, athlete's foot, tetanus, cholera, and food poisoning. Relieves inflammations and fights diseases, allergic diseases like asthma, arthritis, and Crohn's disease, as well as Alzheimer's disease, cancer, cardiovascular disease, diabetes, high blood pressure, high cholesterol levels and Parkinson's disease.

EMOTIONAL

Spikenard is a relaxing and soothing oil for the skin and mind; it's used as a sedative and calming agent. It's also a natural coolant, so it rids the mind of anger and aggression. The anti-depressive qualities of spikenard sedate feelings of depression and restlessness and can serve as a natural way to get rid of stress. It encourages forgiveness, fearlessness and brings on a grounded sense of balance.

BIBLICAL

"While the king was still at his table, my spikenard gave forth its fragrance." (Song of Songs 1:12)

"Your arid fields are as a pomegranate orchard with sweet fruit, henna and spikenard." (Song of Songs 4:13)

"Spikenard and saffron, calamus and cinnamon, with all frankincense trees, myrrh and aloes, with all the chief spices." (Song of Songs 4:14)

"And they said to him, "Say now 'Shibboleth,' " and he said "Shibboleth," and he was not prepared to pronounce it properly, and they grabbed him and slaughtered him at the fords of the Jordan; and there fell at that time of Ephraim, forty-two thousand." (Judges 12:6)

Spikenard was one of the crucial eleven ingredients of the incense to serve at the altar of the Holy Temple of Jerusalem. The Ketoret was a specific and inherent incense made of a careful pharmaceutical formula of spices, the recipe was given by God to enable prayer service and offerings at the Holy Temple in Jerusalem. The commentaries explain the passage above "my spikenard gave forth its fragrance", God said this instead of saying "gave forth its stench." Which is what He really wanted to say. God promised Solomon if he continued to walk in his ways he will rewarded with a long life, riches, and honor, all this for unconditional belief in God's law. God promised to grant the king all the above whether he deserved it or not, however, only for the longevity and a hereditary monarchy God imposed conditions in his law, that Solomon must never turn aside from the commandments. Likewise, for the continuation of the monarchy for his descendants after him God said the same thing.

Solomon's wisdom reached two women, who came to see to the king, they had an argument about which of them was the real mother of a baby. One woman said, "Oh, my lord, I and this woman dwell in one house; and I gave birth to a child with her in the house, and on the third day after I had given birth, this woman also gave birth; and we were both together and alone in the house." She continued, "this woman's son died at night; because she had lain on him, so she arose in the middle of the night and took my son from beside me, while the handmaid slept, and laid him in her bosom, and laid her dead son in my bosom. When I woke up in the morning to nurse my son, I saw that he was dead, but as I looked more closely at him, I saw that it was not my son whom I had given birth to."

The other woman said, "That is not so, the living baby is my son, and the dead baby is your son," the first woman disagreed " That is not so, the living baby is my son, and the dead baby is your son." And so, they argued in front of the king. Suddenly the king said, "Fetch me a sword," when the sword was brought to the king, he said "divide the living child into two, and give half to one, and the second half to the other." The woman whose son was the live one, said to the king, with great compassion and fear naturally aroused for her son, "O my lord, give her the living child, and by no means slay him." Contrarily the other woman said, "let it be neither mine nor yours, lets divide it." Then the wise king answered and said, "Give her the living child, and by no means slay him, for she is his real mother." When all of Israel heard of this judgment of their king, they feared him because they saw that the wisdom of God was within him.

When God was still at Sinai and the Jews sinned with the Golden Calf and the Scripture says it was with an expression of love that God said, "gave forth its fragrance," and did not write, "stank," or "became putrid," because the Scriptures are always polite. The Hebrew word for Spikenard is

"Shibboleth" which means acceptance, because of God's unconditional love for His people.

Sweet Marjoram

Latin name, Origanum Majorana
Aroma, Warm, spicy, and herbaceous

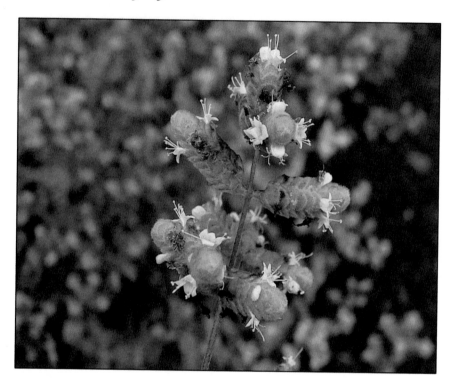

PHYSICAL

Sweet Marjoram is a terpene oil that is very similar to Oregano and originates in Mediterranean regions. It evaporates and constricts; it activates the nervous system and is used as a relaxant and a painkiller. It is an antioxidant and strengthens the immune system, and heart and blood cells. It lowers blood pressure, relaxes your brain, soothes PMS and other stomach cramps such as constipation, by allowing stool to be released.

Sweet Marjoram improves digestion and improves appetite and releases good digestive enzymes into the system. It is also an anti-inflammatory and helps with muscle aches and pains. Marjoram treats epilepsy, convulsions, poisons, headaches, asthma, and fevers.

EMOTIONAL

Sweet Marjoram reduces craving and obsessing about food and depression, nervousness, and hyperactivity. Great for relaxation and blackouts, with a few drops in a diffuser. This oil encourages and calms the senses; however, this calming voice ignites the soul, it heats up and flares an inner spark. Sweet Marjoram give a sense of balance and integrity, a certain pride in oneself for perseverance and of principles to maintain one's own personal high standards of sincerity.

BIBLICAL

"Purify me with hyssop, and I shall be clean" (Psalms 51:9)

"From the cedar tree that is in Lebanon even unto the hyssop that springeth out of the wall" (1 Kings 5:13)

"And you shall take a bunch of hyssops and immerse it in the blood that is in the basin, and you shall extend to the lintel and to the two doorposts the blood that is in the basin, and you shall not go out, any man from the entrance of his house until morning." (Exodus 12:22)

"There were men who were ritually unclean because of contact with a dead person, and therefore could not make the Passover sacrifice on that day. So, they approached Moses and Aaron on that day." (Numbers 9:6)

Sweet Marjoram was another form of Hyssop which is mentioned in the bible many times as use to purify the Alter in the Temple of Jerusalem and to purify lepers and it was their solution for use as a disinfectant. Our forefathers were familiar with this herb and used it as food, as a ritual plant and as a medicinal plant. David wrote a song sharing his guilt about his affair with Bathsheba, who at the time was married to Uriah the Hittite, who was also one of David's mighty men. David approached the prophet Nathan about Bathsheba begging him to be gracious to him, "O God, according to Your kindness; according to Your great mercies, erase my transgressions." David never recovered from his guilt and was always looking for forgiveness from God and to be washed thoroughly of his sin and be purified from it. "For I know my transgressions, and my sin is always before me." His sin always stood in his face, and it was a constant cause of worry because of it.

"Against You alone have I sinned, and I have done what is evil in Your sight, in order that You be justified in Your conduct, and right in Your judgment."

He told God only your power can forgive me, even though my sin was against Uriah, I still sinned against you. David never took heed of God's warning in this matter, in this case, "the servant overpowered his master." David always said to God, "Test me, O Lord, and try me," and God really did test him, and he realized that he was not perfect, and God taught him wisdom. David is now begging to hear joy and gladness once again and hopefully forgiveness for his sin. He asks God to create for him a pure heart, and a renewed steadfast spirit within him. David never wanted to stumble again and have the holy spirit taken away from him. He was fearful that he would die by the sword as a punishment for Uriah, whom he had killed by the sword. He begs God not to despise his broken and crushed heart and with God's will to be good to Zion and build the walls of Jerusalem to build God's temple in its midst in the days of his son, Solomon.

Tea Tree

Latin name, Melaleuca Alternifolia.
Aroma, Camphoraceous

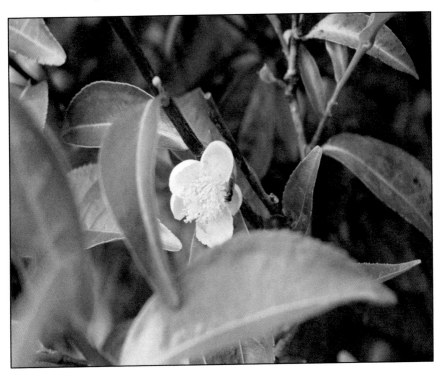

PHYSICAL

Raised in Australia under very harsh conditions where survival of plants is very hard, this oil is from the Cajaput and Niaouli family. Tea Tree oil is made from the leaves of the tree, this tree likes to grow in wet places and can absorb water and dry. The oil is made up of short molecules that evaporate very quickly, it is a protection oil, like Eucalyptus and Pine. It is a very multi-talented oil and protects against viruses, bacterias, infections and funguses, and can be used in a diffuser.

This oil is not able to work alone, it is not strong enough to combat these problems without help even though it has antibiotic properties and attacks bacterias very aggressively. Tea Tree cannot be used directly on the skin and must be used with a base oil or part of a synergy. Tea Tree oil was a hero during the 2nd world war, where it was used on soldiers' wounds, and it killed all their infections. This is another first aid oil and a must always have in all homes. Tea tree oil is an efficient insect deterrent and killer. It repels parasites and other bugs like mosquitoes, fleas, lice, and flies. No insect will come near someone who has applied this oil.

Do not administer to children under the age of five, Pregnant Women or people suffering from high blood pressure. Also, do not use every day, Tea Tree oil can kill good cells along with the bad, so give your body the time to regenerate.

EMOTIONAL

Tea Tree oil gives an overall sense of all well-being, it assists to establish complete positive health both physically and emotionally. This oil eases mental stress and purifies the body and soul of emotional wounds. It assists in calming down, it is self-sufficient and teaches how to start coping alone. Tea Tree helps break negative behavior patterns created over the years and trust one's own abilities. It builds up healthy boundaries and helps disconnect from unhealthy toxic relationships, codependences and any other relationships that are unstable, draining and preventing growth. Tea Tree treats those unpredictable mood swings, it calms panic attacks, soothes manic episodes, calms anxieties and depression.

The spiritual roots are often associated with distrust of self or others, guilt, and shame. This can be released with the assistance of Tea Tree. In the center of the body, are the seven chakras that the inner-body energy that flows through. The oil will expand all the chakras and then align them with the Crown Chakra. The Crown Chakra is the highest and symbolizes the ability to be connected spiritually. This chakra represents inner and outer beauty. The location is magically on top of the head. The corresponding chakra colors are yellow and blue. Yellow represents the Solar Plexus Chakra, and the location in the upper abdomen area. This affects self-worth, confidence, and self-esteem. Blue is the Throat Chakra which symbolizes communications skills and self-expression. Signifying trust and the ability of keeping secrets.

BIBLICAL

"All the days of his vow of abstinence, no razor shall pass over his head; until the completion of the term that he abstains for the sake of the Lord, it shall be sacred, and he shall allow the growth of the hair of his head to grow wild." (Numbers 6:5)

"O maidens of Zion, go forth and gaze upon King Solomon wearing the crown that his mother gave him on his wedding day, on the day of the gladness of his heart" (Song of Songs 3:11)

"Your arid fields are as a pomegranate orchard with sweet fruit, henna and spikenard." (Song of Songs 4:13)

"Spikenard and saffron, calamus and cinnamon, with all frankincense trees, myrrh and aloes, with all the chief spices." (Song of Songs 4:14)

"Grace is deceitful, and beauty is vain, but a woman that fears the Lord, she shall be praised" (Proverbs 31:30)

Since terpineol is found in high concentrations in Tea Tree, Cajeput and Ravensara, it the same compound the Israelites would use to blend with Henna flowers to darken and strengthen the potency of the paste. Henna flowers have an extraordinary fragrance and is used in many perfume blends and is associated with other sweet-smelling plants mentioned in the bible. Henna was used in the bible as a hair coloring by both men and women, hair in the biblical days was recognized as a characteristic of divine beauty and both men and women are encouraged to care for their appearance and to make the effort to always look presentable. In fact, married Jewish women traditionally cover their hair to protect their marriage and create privacy from outsiders, modesty is not supposed to detract from beauty but rather to maintain it within the marriage.

One of the happiest days in the Jewish calendar is the fifteenth of Av, this was the day the daughters of Jerusalem would go out in borrowed white garments and dance in the vineyards for the boys. They would say to them, "young man, lift up your eyes and see what you choose for yourself. Do not set your eyes on beauty but set your eyes on the family." The daughter of the king borrowed white garments from the daughter of the High Priest; the daughter of the High Priest borrowed from the daughter of the deputy High Priest; the daughter of the deputy High Priest borrowed from the daughter of the priest anointed for war, who read verses of Torah and addressed the army as they prepared for battle. The daughter of the priest anointed for war, borrowed from the daughter of a common priest; and all the Jewish people would borrow from each other. The reasoning was that no one would be embarrassed if she did not own her own garments, and all the garments would be immersed before they were worn so that they would be pure. This was the only day people from different tribes were allowed to intermarry. So instead of the girls having to chase the boys, the girls would go out to the field and let the boys come and chase them, allowing the boys to choose their brides for themselves.

"Give her of the fruit of her hands; and let her works praise her in the gates"

All hair, whether for a man or a woman, besides the obvious physical qualities and their own personal psychological significance, has very distinct spiritual qualities too. These elements affect men and women differently, in intensity but not in type, a man is allowed to grow his hair in a moderate way if he desires, as long as there is no impediment to his putting on phylacteries. A Nazerite's hair is forgiven a harsh judgment for that of a merciful one due to his austere spiritual commitment to God. Hair is the part of the human being that is viewed as a reflection of the divine consciousness and attributes, known as Mochin. There are ten characteristics that make up the "Mochin" which are, crown, knowledge, comprehension, measure, kindness, strength, glory, everlasting, splendor, foundation and majestic. These are the attributes depicted by the kabbalah as the analogy of human like form, hair is said to originate as an excess of the Mochin's processing and receptivity of the divine light from the infinite realm. The fifteenth of Av was also the day of the Giving of the Torah, and the day of the building of the holy Temple of Jerusalem, so the fifteenth of Av became a day of double celebration, the Mishnah says that this was also the date when most families would have made their wood donations.

Vanilla

Latin Name, Achillea Orchid
Aroma, Sweet, woody, and musty

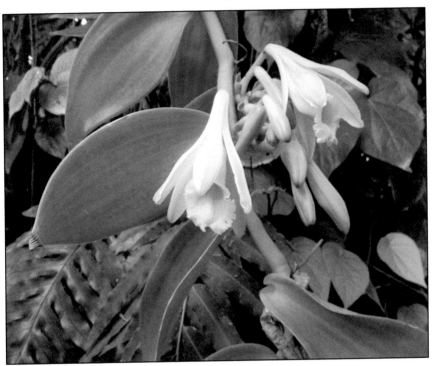

PHYSICAL

Vanilla Bean Orchid is a plant known as an orchid fruit, Vanilla is native to the Americas and responsible for natural vanilla flavor. It has oval shaped, bright green leaves and may grow up to twenty-four inches, its bell-shaped flowers blooms in white, yellow, or pink. The vanilla extract comes from the seed pods, known as vanilla beans giving that familiar exotic flavor. Vanilla is attributed to curb the appetite and control food urges. It has a numbing characteristic that anesthetizes and relaxes the body and even the soul. Vanilla is often used flavoring food, drinks, and cosmetics, it is also a popular flavor choice for ice cream flavor. It is a popular ingredient in western sweet baked goods, such as cookies and cakes.

Vanilla fights skin infections and wounds with its anti-bacterial qualities. This oil contains antioxidants and combats free radicals, it also has many anti-cancer possibilities because of its robust antioxidant contents. It is a natural aphrodisiac; it stimulates the secretion of hormones like testosterone and estrogen treating many sexual problems. Vanilla is an anti-depressant and a sedative; it has a very relaxing tranquilizing effect on your brain. It's amazing aroma is so soothing that it also lowers blood pressure and decreases your risk for heart attacks and diabetes.

Since there really is no way to make a Vanilla essential oil, you can make your own extract, this also may be done in oil with and organic oil of choice.

⇒ TAKE 6 VANILLA STICKS THAT YOU PURCHASED FROM A REPUTABLE AND RELIABLE SOURCE.
⇒ CUT OPEN THE STICKS LENGTHWAYS, THOUGH DON'T SPLIT IT.
⇒ IMMERSE IN A JAR OF 150MLS OF VODKA OR OIL
⇒ LEAVE IN A DARK AND COOL PLACE FOR 3 WEEKS WHEN YOU WILL SEE THE LIQUID TURN VERY DARK BROWN.
⇒ USE FOR BAKING, ADDING TO YOUR COFFEE OR WHATEVER ELSE YOU LOVE VANILLA FOR.

Warning do not administer to Pregnant women or Nursing Mothers.

EMOTIONAL

Vanilla helps solve difficult problems and enables dealing with them well. Helps when feeling lonely and knows how to help one to feel brave when blended with sandalwood. It helps to recover from deep sorrow and pain, or a lack of coping and the feeling of impotence.

BIBLICAL

"And the Lord said to Moses, "Take for yourself aromatics, balsam sap, onycha and galbanum, aromatics and pure frankincense; they shall be of equal weight." (Exodus 30:34)

"And you shall make it into incense, a compound according to the art of the perfumer, well blended, pure, holy." (Exodus 30:35)

"And you shall crush some of it very finely, and you shall set some of it before the testimony in the Tent of Meeting, where I will arrange meetings with you; it shall be to you a holy of holies." (Exodus 30:36)

"The kings came and fought; then fought the kings of Canaan in Taanach by the waters of Megiddo; they took no gain of money.' (Judges 5:19)

"And this is the matter of the tax levy which king Solomon raised; to build the Temple of the Lord, and his own house and the Milo, and the wall of Jerusalem and Hazor and Megiddo and Gezer." (I Kings 9:15)

"In his days, Pharaoh-Neco went up against the king of Assyria by the Euphrates River, and King Josiah went toward him, and he killed him in Megiddo when he saw him." (II Kings 23:29)

"And his servants transported him dead from Megiddo, and they brought him to Jerusalem and buried him in his grave. And the people of the land took Jehoahaz the son of Josiah and anointed him and made him king instead of his father." (II Kings 23:30)

"The king of Ta'nach, one; the king of Megiddo, one." (Joshua 12:21)

"Manasseh had in Issachar and in Asher: Beth-shean and her towns, and Ibleam and her towns, and the inhabitants of Dor and her towns, and the inhabitants of 'En-dor and her towns, and the inhabitants of Taanach and her towns, and the inhabitants of Megiddo and her towns, the three regions." (Joshua 17:11)

An analysis of burial offerings at a Canaanite tomb in Megiddo, northern Israel, found Vanilla residue in a three-thousand-six-hundred-year-old tomb, giving evidence of the use of vanilla in biblical days. Either the vanilla orchids or their beans reached Megiddo via trade routes that first passed through Mesopotamian society in southwest Asia. Vanilla extracted oils were used as additives for foods and medicines, as well as for ritual incense sacrifices. Even in those days, vanilla was an expensive imported spice, there were small jugs of vanilla extract placed in the tomb of a man, woman and child who were wearing ornate gold, silver, and bronze jewelry for their burial. Megiddo was the site of quite a few battles, it is in the land of the tribe of Menashe, and it guarded the western branch of a narrow pass and trade route connecting Ancient Egypt and Assyria. Also known as "Hill of the Ruler" and after the Israelites captured it, it became one of the most important cities of biblical times until it was destroyed by Aramaean raiders. It overlooks the Jezreel Valley, which is a great strategic location, Megiddo is a mound created by many generations of people living and rebuilding on the same spot and the hill of Megiddo is named in the bible as the site of the future "Battle of the End of Days."

Vanilla has been discovered to have been a well-known and popular spice in biblical times and like with most plants and spices were infused in olive oil by the Israelites. This was the most convenient method they had to extract the essence of the plants, spices and gums used to prepare the ketoret and anointing oils for the Kohen's offerings in the holy temple for God or even used it as a perfume, medication or to enhance their food.

Verbena

Latin Name, Verbena Bonariensis
Aroma, Bitter

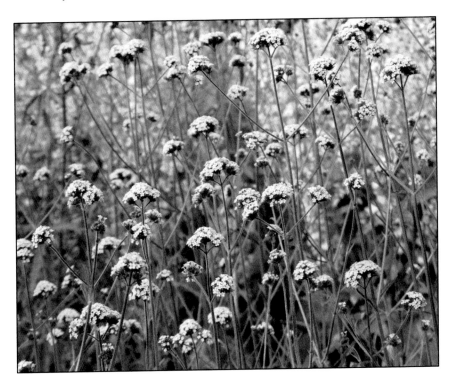

PHYSICAL

Verbenas are native of America and Asia and are herbaceous woody plants with very small blue, white, or pink flowers. They have mainly been used as ornamental plants; the Egyptians called it the tears of Isis. This plant has long bitter leaves which affects the nervous system via the heart. It grows above ground and makes a great medicine that protects the heart by relaxing the central nervous system and spasms and it helps symptoms of depression, hysteria, and seizures.

Verbena treats sore throats and respiratory diseases, such as asthma and bronchitis. It is also used to help digestive disorders and other diseases connected to the kidneys and liver. Verbena has a relaxing effect while giving birth, because it calms the contractions, it is hormonal and so also balances menstruation and lactation for nursing mothers.

Verbena balances liver functions because of its bitter taste it excretes poisons. It heals sun fungus, tinea versicolor which is a skin eruption that appears on human skin. It also helps dermatophytosis also known as ringworm which is very contagious.

Warning, this is a very strong oil and must never be used without a base.

EMOTIONAL

Verbena is the Vervain plant used in Bach Flower Therapy.

"The patient may be too stern, too rigid in principle, too narrow-minded in outlook, endeavoring to mold the world too much to his own ideals. Of highest principle, yet into "A great wish to convert" (Dr. Edward Bach, 1936)

Dr. Bach's description
"Those with fixed principles and ideas, which they are confident are right, and which they very rarely change. They have a great wish to convert all around them to their own views of life. They are strong of will and have much courage when they are convinced of those things that they wish to teach. In illness they struggle on long after many would have given up their duties".

Verbena releases anger and balances the emotions. This Uplifting oil relaxes over enthusiastic and overbearing tendencies, it soothes strong will that causes stress to the point of being inflexible. This oil is great for people who are too much of a perfectionist and demand unreasonable justice. Are blessed with extreme mental energy, willing to deliver one hundred percent into causes believed to make the world a better place. Verbena balances the maintenance of amazing personalities and drive while at the same time relaxing and de-stressing.

BIBLICAL

"And the Lord shall plague Egypt, plaguing and healing, and they shall return to the Lord, and He shall accept their prayer and heal them." (Isaiah 19:22)

"From heaven, you let judgment be heard; the earth feared and became calm." (Isaiah 38:9)

"I made myself gardens and orchards, and I planted in them all sorts of fruit trees." (Ecclesiastes 2:5)

"I made myself pools of water, to water from them a forest sprouting with trees." (Ecclesiastes 2:6)

Verbena is a wild flora and similar to the flowers that grow wild all over the mountains of Israel. It used to grow in Jerusalem at the time of the bible, known in Israel today as Louisa. For every plague and disease, God promised to create a cure for them which must be reconciled by prayer. "There will be a highway built with a paved road by which they will always travel through from Egypt to Assyria. This is how the Assyrians will discover the Egyptians, and the Egyptians will discover the Assyrians, and the Assyrians will wage a war with the Egyptians." God's harsh prophesy that the Egyptians will have no power to save their people from the messengers of the king of Assyria, their idols shall quake from before God and the hearts of the Egyptians shall melt in their midst. As a continued punishment for enslaving the Israelites, God said he will stir up Egyptians against Egyptians, and they shall war each man against his own brother, then each man against his friend. It will continue from city against city and province against province. They shall turn in vain to their idols, their sorcerers, their necromancers and to those who prophesize by the divine jidoa bone.

Verbena is known as a very spiritual plant that assists in attuning to the higher spiritual self, in attempting to complete the harmonization between mind and spirit. Isaiah prophesied the episode concerning the retribution of the mighty king Sennacherib of Assyria, where kings and princes in the neighboring lands feared him greatly. Sennacherib gathered his entire army and prepared for an invasion of Judah and King Hezekiah. First, he sent forty-five thousand princes riding in golden and silver chariots to lead the way, then he sent eighty thousand knights in armor and sixty thousand swordsmen. He finally sent two and a half million cavalrymen which made up his army. Sennacherib advanced his army towards Judah and easily captured all the fortified cities of Judah, until he came to the high walls of the city of Jerusalem. His men at his command piled up their pillows to the same height as the walls and when they climbed to the top of the pile and looked down into the city, he was disappointed and scorned, "Why did I have to bring my entire army to take this poor little village, only a few of my legions could had razed it down to the ground!"

Sennacherib told his eager men, "No hurry; we shall spend the night by the walls of this city and refresh ourselves after the weary journey, and in the morning let every warrior bring me but one brick from the walls of the city." Rabshakeh, the leading general of Sennacherib's army, called out to the defenders of the city of Jerusalem, "let not your king Hezekiah deceive you that your God will save you. Has any god of other nations delivered his land from the hand of the king of Assyria? Has Hezekiah put his faith in that broken rod, the king of Egypt, to save your land? Or might it be that Hezekiah relies upon his warriors to defend his capital? Now, then, let him make a wager with my master, the king of Assyria, and I will give him two thousand horses, if he is able to set riders on them." Rabshakeh managed to convince the defenders of Jerusalem to revolt against Hezekiah and surrender the city to Sennacherib. When Hezekiah heard this, he rent his clothes in grief and despair and prayed to God, only one of the king's ministers remained loyal to him.

Eliakim, Shebna and Joah said to Rabshakeh, "Please speak to your servants in Aramaic for we understand it; do not speak with us in Judean within the hearing of the people who are on the wall." Shebna the scribe a strong leader by nature, explained to him that the Judeans people are frightened by your words, at first, they thought that he did not come to scare the people since Rabshakeh was an apostate Jew. They assumed that even though his master's orders were incumbent upon him to observe, they thought that maybe his heart was attracted to his family, and he would take pity upon them. But instead, Rabshakeh was loyal to Sennacherib, and he said, "Did my master send me to speak these words to your master and to you? Is it not to the men who sit on the wall to eat their dung and drink their urine with you?" God took note of the words of Rabshakeh whose king of Assyria, his master, sent him to blaspheme against God, believing that he is stronger than the God of Israel himself. Isaiah told king Hezekiah's men, to give him a message from God, "have no fear of the words you have heard, that the servants of the king of Assyria have blasphemed Me. Behold I will imbue him with a desire, and he will hear a rumor and return to his land, and I will cause him to fall by the sword in his land."

Rabshakeh returned to his army unit and found out the king of Assyria was waging war against Libnah, and he heard that Sennacherib had left

Lachish. Then he heard that Tirhakah the king of Cush, was saying that he was going to wage war against the king of Assyria. He also heard that the king of Cush sent emissaries to Hezekiah, and even though these were rumors, Rabshakeh accepted all these reports from his messengers as facts. It appealed to him to withdraw from Jerusalem to fight first against Cush. Isaiah sent a message to Hezekiah, the king of Judah, "let your God, in whom you trust, not delude you, Jerusalem shall not be given into the hands of the king of Assyria. He shall not enter this city, neither shall he shoot there an arrow, nor shall he advance upon it with a shield, nor shall he pile up a siege mound against it. By the way he comes he shall return, and this city he shall not enter." Then an angel of God advanced and slew one hundred eighty-five thousand of the camp of Assyria and when the Israelites arose the next morning, they were all dead corpses.

This was the second time Sennacherib came to siege Jerusalem, after he went and battled with Cush, he returned and came to Jerusalem, and it was at this time that the angel killed them. This was in retaliation for Sennacherib sweeping Shebna the scribe and his men, leading them in chains, all the way to Cush. When he came back to Jerusalem, to fulfill what he had started, they did not come back with Rabshakeh he only brought kings with crowns tied to their heads, and the lowest ranking of them was an officer with over two thousand men, and all these armies fell. Sennacherib, the king of Assyria, left and went away the way he came, and he returned and dwelt in Nineveh. When this prophecy was fulfilled, the people finally became calm. Anger of the wicked results in their downfall which results in the creatures of the earth thanking God, and when people show their anger against his people, God punishes them, and they will see that their anger is powerless against the Israelites. A great example is of Nebuchadnezzar, when he threw Hananiah, Mishael, and Azariah into the fiery furnace, and they said,

"Blessed be the God of Shadrach, Meshach, and Abed-nego, who sent His angel and rescued His servants, who trusted Him, deviated from the command of the king, and risked their lives in order not to worship or prostrate themselves to any god except to their God." (Daniel 3:28)

God will prevent and stop the residue of wrath of wicked men who mean harm to Israel, he will restrain them from being able to show their pride via their wrath. In the expression "residue" when describing their wrath should be of no account, because the only one who is able to gird all wrath to man is God alone.

Vetiver

Latin Name, Chrysopogon Zizanioides
Aroma, Green, Soft, earthy, and musty

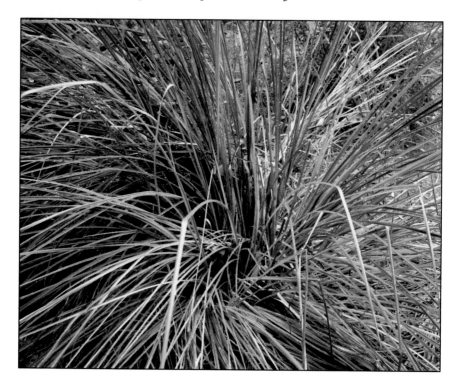

PHYSICAL

This tree has very long leaves, reaching up to one and a half meters as well as roots also reaching one and a half meters. In Indonesia it is used on roofs. It is mainly cultivated because of its fragrance; it is used widely around the world as a fixative in perfumes. It is a fragrant grass that is like Lemongrass, and it is grown to stabilize the soil and protects it against pests and weeds. Vetiver's odor is described as deep, sweet, woody, smoky, earthy, amber and balsam very much resembling Patchouli and Sandalwood. This plant was around in Biblical times, and it would have been the fragrance that Israelites used for incense, perfumes, and medications.

It's essential oil produces a thick amber fluid that smells thick, woody and earthy the perfect consistency for creams and soaps. It is used for its antiseptic properties to treat acne and sores. It affects the nervous system and because of its deep roots it is able to excrete toxins from the body. It balances stress and is very calming, vetiver reduces swellings, helps with constipation and asthma. Another great asset is its ability to rid the body and pets of lice, fleas, and prevents parasites. This oil also kills termites.

EMOTIONAL

Vetiver has a calming grounding effect on emotions and moods and generates happiness. It helps to collect up feelings and heal any state of consciousness and brightens feelings of blah. Its ability to affect emotions is water based, bringing out tears to release pent up anger or frustrations. Vetiver encourages emotional growth and wisdom; it strengthens the integrity giving the inner strength to honor peers.

Vetiver protects from negative thoughts and land sliding into bad places. It raises self-esteem and grounds to slow the fast-paced freak out from taking over and even stops the success of built-up agitation in the mind to flourish.

BIBLICAL

"The woman conceived and bore a son, and when she saw him that he was good, she hid him for three months." (Exodus 2:2)

"When she could no longer hide him, she took for him a reed basket, smeared it with clay and pitch, placed the child into it, and put it into the marsh at the Nile's edge." (Exodus 2:3)

"His sister stood from afar, to know what would be done to him." (Exodus 2:4)

"Pharaoh's daughter went down to bathe, to the Nile, and her maidens were walking along the Nile, and she saw the basket in the midst of the marsh, and she sent her maidservant, and she took it." (Exodus 2:5)

"Can papyrus shoot up without a marsh? Can the reed-grass grow without water?" (Job 8:11)

"When it is still in its greenness, it will not be plucked, but before any other grass, it will dry up." (Job 8:12)

"Who sends emissaries in the sea and in boats of bulrushes on the surface of the water, "Go, swift messengers, to a nation, pulled and torn, to an awesome nation from their beginning onward, a nation punished in kind and trampled, whose land the rivers have plundered."
(Isaiah 18:2)

While the Jews were in slavery in Egypt, Pharaoh issued yet another evil decree, this time he ordered that all Jewish male babies were to be killed as soon as they were born. Because of this decree Moses' parents Yocheved and Amran decided to sperate so they would not get pregnant and have their baby only to be killed by Pharaoh. Miriam their daughter begged them to remarry pointing out that their separation will be seen as a weakness, both by the Israelites who may emulate them and separate also, and by the Egyptians. They took Miriam's words to heart and remarried, then Yocheved conceived and was pregnant with Moses. She miraculously gave birth safely to Moses at six months and one day of her gestation, and since Pharaoh calculated her due date from the day, she came back to her husband Amram, they came searching for her after nine months to capture the baby. However, since she had already secretly given birth, she managed to hide Moses for three months. The Midrash says that when Moses was born, the entire house was filled with light.

After three months Yocheved saw that she could no longer hide her baby, and she designed a special basket made of reed. She coated the outside of the basket with a thick water-resistant resin made from plants and on the inside, she lined it with clay. Yocheved placed the basket with Moses inside into the area of the river with the most thickly dense marshes and reeds. There were many canes and reeds surrounding these wetlands mentioned in the bible, they were the reeds that supported Moses' basket keeping him sturdy and safe, thus preventing him from drowning. The commentaries say that these varieties of Nile grasses were of a pliable substance that could withstand both soft and hard pressure like water currents running down rivers. Vetiver grows in culms and slows water flows by building a barrier in the form of a mat, keeping Moses safe in his basket. Pharaoh's own daughter saw him floating in the river and decided to adopt him knowing that he was an Israelite baby and she prophesized that he would be a great man, understanding that he would lead the Israelites and not the Egyptians.

She raised him like her own son and was the one who had named him, Moses meaning drawing out, "for I drew him from the water." Moses grew up both in height and in greatness, and Pharaoh appointed him to manage his house where he became exposed to the distress and the burdens of his own people. One day he was on his daily rounds when he saw an Egyptian whose responsibility it was to be a taskmaster over the Israelites team leaders, waking them up at the crack of dawn with the roosters. The Egyptian was striking and lashing at an Israelite, Moses saw this and making sure there was no one around so he killed the Egyptian and hid his body in the sand. The Midrash says the Israelite man was the husband of Shulamit the daughter of Dibri, and the taskmaster had seen her and liked what he saw. He woke the Israelite man in the middle of the night and kicked him out of his own house, then the taskmaster entered the house and was intimate with his wife. His wife mistakenly thought that the taskmaster was her husband, when the man returned home and realized what the Egyptian had done to him under his own roof. The Egyptian saw that the Israelite knew of his actions, so he beat him up and drove him hard all day, so Moses slew the Egyptian and thought that he was not seen.

After this incident Moses saw two Israelites fighting, he asked the aggressive one, *"why are you going to strike your friend?"* The man retorted back,

> *"Who made you a man, a prince, and a judge over us? Do you plan to slay me as you have slain the Egyptian?"* Moses became frightened and said, "Indeed, the matter has become known!"*
> (Exodus 2:13)

The man scolded Moses because he was still young and inexperienced in life, he challenged Moses to slay him. The Midrash says that Moses slew the Egyptian using an ethereal name that caused him to die. Once Moses realized that he was seen he became afraid that Pharaoh would kill him, now that it was known that he had slain the Egyptian. Pharaoh indeed had heard of this incident from the Israelite informant, and he sought to kill Moses who had already fled. When Pharaoh did catch up with Moses, he delivered him to his executioner to execute him, but the sword had no power over him, and they could not kill him. and Moses said, "God saved me from Pharaoh's sword."

Moses stayed in hiding in the land of Midian, where he lived by a well and there, just like Jacob, who met his wife at a well, Moses was hoping to meet his wife too by the well and he camped there for a short while. As it happened the chief of Midian who had seven daughters, who came regularly to draw water to fill the troughs to water their father's flocks. Recently the chief who was the most prominent Midianite among them had decided to abandon idolatry, so the people banned him from living with them. Midianite shepherds came and drove the girls away and Moses arose and rescued them by driving the shepherds away and watering their flocks. When they arrived back home their father Jethro was surprised to see them back home so quick, when he asked them what happened, they told him "An Egyptian man rescued us from the hands of the shepherds, and he also drew water for us and watered the flocks." So, he says to his daughters, "where is he? Why have you left the man? Invite him and let him eat bread."

The Midrash says that Jethro recognized Moses as being of the seed of Jacob, for the water rose towards him, hinting to his daughters, perhaps he will marry one of you. At this offer, Moses agreed to stay with them, and Moses swore to Jethro that he would not move from Midian without his consent and gave him Zipporah to marry. They soon had a son and Moses named him Gershom, meaning, "I was a stranger in a foreign land." After some time, while Moses was still in Midian, Pharaoh died and Israel required salvation, and who Moses was pasturing his livestock, realized that the salvation must come through him. The people of Israel were tired of their hard labor and cried out to God,

> "God heard their cry, and God remembered His covenant with Abraham, with Isaac, and with Jacob." (Exodus 2:24)

Gid focused his attention on his people and felt much love for them, God did not conceal his eyes from them and sent an angel to appear to Moses in a flame of fire from within the thorn bush, it was burning with fire, but was not being consumed by the fire. Moses was surprised at this and stared at the bush, God saw that he caught Moses' attention and God called him from within the thorn bush, and he said, "Moses, Moses!" And Moses said, "Here I am!" God said,

> "I am the God of your father, the God of Abraham, the God of Isaac, and the God of Jacob. I have surely seen the affliction of My people who are in Egypt, and I have heard their cry because

of their slave drivers, for I know their pains. I have descended to rescue them from the hands of the Egyptians and to bring them up from that land to a good and spacious land, to a land flowing with milk and honey, to the place of the Canaanites, the Hittites, the Amorites, the Perizzites, the Hivites, and the Jebusites. And now, behold, the cry of the children of Israel has come to Me, and I have also seen the oppression that the Egyptians are oppressing them. So now come, and I will send you to Pharaoh, and take My people, the children of Israel, out of Egypt." (Exodus 3:6-10)

Wormwood

Latin Name, Artemisia Absinthium, Sheba
Aroma, Bitter, gentle

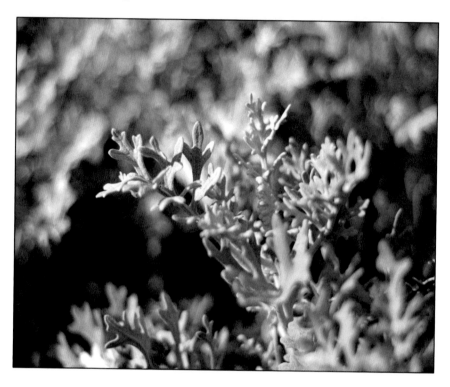

PHYSICAL

This oil is very often used in medication, it has very powerful qualities and effective in many areas. It was once forbidden to grow in private gardens because of its hallucinating properties and is now grown in almost every garden in Israel. Artemisia is very bitter and can be drunk as a tea, it cleanses the liver and kills intestinal parasites and is safe for all ages. Wormwood relaxes muscles and spasms and chronic joint pains. It reduces fever by cooling down the body temperature.

Artemisia has a strong tradition in ancient herbal medicine and folklore. Its oil is extracted from the leaves and flowering tops, and it has antiseptic and antifungal properties, and is also said to relieve itching, burning and stinging sensations when freshly crushed leaves are applied to the skin.

Warning do not administer to Pregnant Women and Nursing Mothers; this oil may cause an allergic reaction for people who in general suffer from allergies. The chemicals in the plant indicate that it is slightly toxic and is not for long term use.

EMOTIONAL

Artists in the old days used to take them to change their mood and relax. According to Chinese Medicine, bitterness signals the body to start healing itself and it then proceeds to destroy toxins. Smoking dried Artemisia leaves is said to produce a mild and pleasant stimulation that can increase to euphoria that some compare to cannabis intoxication. Its soothing and relaxing effects of this oil on the brain and the nervous system calms down any epileptic and hysteric attacks when they occur

Consumed internally as a tea or extract, Artemisia is said to cause mild clear relaxation. Smoking or consuming a tincture of Artemisia is said to increase the intensity of dreams, as well as lucidity in the dreams and an increase in recall. Artemisia maintains proper health of the uterus and kills intestinal parasites. It is also used to improve concentration and memory.

BIBLICAL

"Perhaps there is among you a man, woman, family, or tribe, whose heart strays this day from the Lord, our God, to go and worship the deities of those nations. Perhaps there is among you a root that produces hemlock and wormwood."
(Deuteronomy 29:17)

"He has filled me with bitterness; He has sated me with wormwood." (Lamentations 3:15)

"Remember my affliction and my misery, wormwood and gall."
(Lamentations 3:19)

"Therefore, so thus said the Lord of Hosts, the God of Israel; Behold, I will feed them this people with wormwood and will give them poisonous water to drink." (Jeremiah 9:14)

"Therefore, so said the Lord of Hosts concerning the prophets, Behold I will feed them wormwood and give them poisonous

water to drink, for from the prophets of Jerusalem has falseness emanated to the whole land." (Jeremiah 23:15)

"Those who turn justice to wormwood, and who leave righteousness on the ground." (Amos 5:7)

"Will horses run on the rock, or will one plow with cattle, for you have perverted justice to hemlock and the fruit of righteousness to wormwood?" (Amos 6:12)

"But her end is as bitter as wormwood, as sharp as a two-edged sword." (Proverbs 5:4)

Wormwood is mentioned several times in the bible usually in the context of something evil, and when translated from Hebrew "La'anah," which means bitterness, humbled or when more harshly translated, a curse. Wormwood is described in the bible to be very bitter and is referred to as the number one punishment for evil deeds or to be humbled. When Moses and Aaron came to Pharaoh and said to him, "So said the Lord, the God of the Hebrews, how long will you refuse to humble yourself before Me? Let My people go, and they will worship Me." They were telling Pharaoh you have refused to be humble and meek before God.

Wormwood was used like a lie detector, it was drunk with poisonous water, possibly containing snake venom and hemlock. if a person was caught and arrested for a criminal act, he would be forced to drink this mixture. The true verdict was whether he died or not, this tincture caused a very painful death and violent stomach pains and vomiting. It was relied upon as a judge and juror, if the person lived, he was set free, however if he died it was considered equitable and got his just punishment. In the Bible it is implied that if a person commits a bad deed, this means the person had the bad thoughts that caused him to do the criminal act already thriving and developing within him for a while.

Joseph lived in Egypt with his brothers and children until the age of one hundred and ten and witnessed the birth of his great grandchildren, the grandchildren of Ephraim and Manasseh. This means that Ephraim's children were all born and living in Egypt and not in Israel. So going by this assumption, both Ephraim and Manasseh and their children died in Egypt, like their father Joseph. It was Ephraim's descendants who entered the land of Israel with Joshua, son of Nun who led the conquest, and not Ephraim himself. The descendants of Ephraim who waged war with the Philistines, they made an error in their calculations and left some thirty years before the prophesized date to be the end of their slavery. They fled Egypt on their own initiative and unfortunately fell into the raid in Gath, they trusted in their might and in their arrows, but ultimately, they were forced to retreat and fled on that day of battle. When Pharaoh finally let the Israelites go, God did not lead them on the road through the Philistine country even though it would have been closer because he didn't want the people to face war and possibly causing them to change their minds and return to Egypt.

"For though he flourishes among the marshes, an east wind shall come, a wind of the Lord, ascending from the desert, and his spring shall dry up, and his fountain shall be parched; he shall plunder the treasure of all coveted vessels." (Hosea 13:15)

The sons of Ephraim; were all killed by the men of Gath, who were then natives of the land, this was in retaliation to the sons of Ephraim who came down to raid their cattle. Their father Ephraim mourned for them for many days, and his brothers came to comfort him. Ephraim then came to his wife, and she conceived and had another son who he named Beriah, in memory of the disaster had befallen his house. As a comfort the tribes of Judah and Ephraim, both will finally play an important role in the leadership of Israel in the last days, being the ultimate fulfilment of the part of the blessing of Jacob, of Joseph and his sons.

Yarrow

Latin Name, Achillea Nobilis
Aroma, Herbal, and slightly camphorous

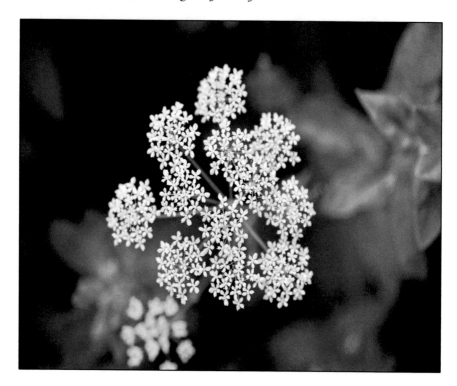

PHYSICAL

Yarrow essential oil is blue in color and a strong antibiotic; its flowers are pale yellow and is used very efficiently for scars and applied immediately after an operation. This oil improves circulatory disorders such as varicose veins and bleeding hemorrhoids. Their fresh leaves were used to stop bleeding wounds and lessen menstrual bleeding and helps regulate them. Yarrow also eases menopausal problems, cystitis, and infection, it was use in wound healing particularly in the military during the second world war, when it was also called bloodwort.

Yarrow combats bacteria because it is an antiseptic, decongestant, and an astringent. Use for chest infections where there is a lot of phlegm. It is also good for weeping eczema when the skin is very itchy.

Warning do not administer to Pregnant Women and Nursing Mothers, and this plant in oil form or herb form should not be used long term because it may cause photosensitivity to the sun.

EMOTIONAL

It is a great oil for skin wounds such as acne, skin problems are associated with stress. Yarrow is a relaxant especially for teenagers, whereas Ylang Ylang awakens too many emotions for them. Yarrow encourages harmony, equilibrium, and intuition. It centers and helps to reach for dreams, visions, and aspirations. It helps to clarify boundaries especially for overbearing people.

BIBLICAL

"Now no tree of the field was yet on the earth, neither did any herb of the field yet grow, because the Lord God had not brought rain upon the earth, and there was no man to work the soil." (Genesis 2:5)

"And it will cause thorns and thistles to grow for you, and you shall eat the herbs of the field." (Genesis 3:18)

"And on this night, they shall eat the flesh, roasted over the fire, and unleavened cakes; with bitter herbs they shall eat it." (Exodus 12:8)

"Better a repast of herbs where there is love, then a fattened ox where there is hatred." (Proverbs 15:17)

"Instead of wheat, thistles shall emerge, and instead of barley, noisome weeds. Job's words are ended." (Job 31:40)

"Truth will sprout from the earth, and righteousness will look down from heaven." (Psalms 85:12)

"Behold I am making a new thing, now it will sprout, now you shall know it; yea I will make a road in the desert, rivers in the wasteland." (Isaiah 43:19)

Yarrow is an herbaceous plant which grows naturally all-over central Israel and are always seen as capable of growing in abundance; however, it must be worked for. It is important to plant each herb separately and not to mix their seeds, Achillea Nobilis, or Yarrow may be both a blessing and a curse in the home garden, is often also called yarrow weed. Normally weeds in Israel grow freely in fields of grain, the most conspicuous being the tares weed which grows among grain, particularly wheat, because its grains are very similar to wheat. Other species of weeds are mustard, scolymus thistle and noisome weeds, which thistles may emerge instead of wheat, the bible says, "in a field beset with thistles it is advisable to sow wheat, and in a field beset with weeds, it is advisable to sow barley." When Israel will speak truth, the charity that they perform on earth will look down from heaven. God too will give good, He will open His treasury, the heavens, to give rain, in order that His land yield its produce.

"Cause the heavens above to drip, and let the skies pour down righteousness; let the earth open, and let salvation and righteousness be fruitful; let it cause them to sprout together; I, the Lord, have created it." (Isiah 45:8)

Ylang Ylang

Latin name, Cananga Odorata
Aroma, Sweet, exotic and balsamic

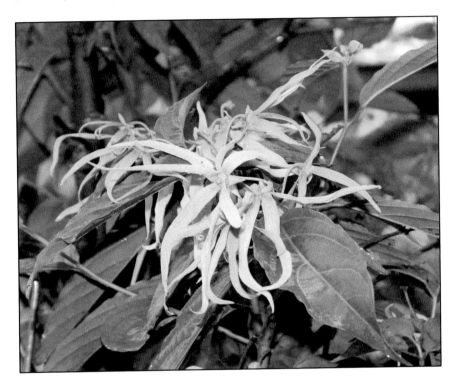

PHYSICAL

Much of this amazing oil qualities are based on its pleasant flowery scent. This is a tropical plant that originates in Indonesia, it is known as poor man's Jasmine. It was first used in China for its unique healing abilities. Ylang Ylang lowers blood pressure and sugar levels as well as help epilepsy. It balances oily and dry skin and promotes hair growth. The flower is obtained through steam distillation of the flowers and is widely used in the perfume industry because of its unique combination of floral, fruit and wood aroma.

EMOTIONAL

It relaxes fears and anger and helps people who were sexually abused in childhood. It is also an anti-inflammatory, though it is mainly used for emotional issues. This oil is so powerful emotionally, it is best not to administer alone to teenagers, but it is ok in a synergy. It may be too overpowering and intense for them to handle, it exposes old situations, problems, and depressions.

Ylang Ylang is rebellious and has a euphoric and sedative effect on the nervous system and a formidable aphrodisiac quality is useful for impotence and frigidity. It is an anti-stress and helps anxiety, tension, shock, fear, and panic. it is great for meditation and connecting with the subconscious mind. It is also a time giver and teaches patience.

BIBLICAL

"And she gave the king one hundred and twenty talents of gold and very many spices and precious stones; there had never arrived such an abundance of spices as those which the Queen of Sheba gave to king (Solomon." 1 Kings 10:10)

"Judea and the land of Israel they are your peddlers; with wheat of Minnith, balsam trees, honey, oil, and balm, they gave your necessities." (Ezekiel 27:17)

"Go up to Gilead and take balm, O virgin daughter of Egypt; in vain have you increased medicines, you have no cure." (Jeremiah 46:11)

"Suddenly, Babylon has fallen and has been broken; wail over her, take balm for her pain, perhaps she may be healed." (Jeremiah 51:8)

"And Hezekiah rejoiced over them, and he showed them his entire treasure- house, the silver, the gold, the spices, and the good oil, and the entire house in which he kept his vessels, and everything that was found in his treasures; there was nothing that Hezekiah did not show them in his palace and in his kingdom." (Isaiah 39:2)

In the Bible one of the names referring to balm is Bosem which means perfume, which young women used as a cologne to seduce young men.

Ylang Ylang is an aphrodisiac balsam and was imported into Israel by spice traders from Indonesia. The wheat of Minnith is the name of a place that produced wheat of the highest quality, it was said, "until you come to Minnith." The Midrash explains that it was excellent with thick wheat kernels, which are sold by number, an expression used in those days as gathering of many numbers, bundles, or bunches. The same type of expression was, "just as the myrtle is crowded with leaves, so was Leah crowded with sons." Minnith is also a definition of prepared portions of food as in multitude. Balsam trees also called pannag mainly found in Jericho, and because of their fragrant scent, and Jericho is called Jericho because of its balsamic fragrance. The Queen of Sheba came to visit King Solomon and she also brought with her many gifts, one of which was sweet balsamic woody and florally aromatic spices and oils.

Tyre was a city situated on the seaport where traffickers of peoples of many isles, and God says that Tyre is the perfection of beauty. Until now everyone said that about Jerusalem now Tyre the ultimate extreme of beauty is incorporated together. With a multitude of wealth merchants were confident to find merchandise fit for them. Javan, Tubal, and Meshech were peddlers of living people for slavery, filling copper vessels of both male and female slaves. There was merchandise from Tyre to be bought as gifts, such as ivory, horns of ibexes, bones of elephants, birds, and peacocks. Many spices, balms, oils, gold, and precious stones were bought in by traders and merchants which the Israelites bought to make up all their creams and incenses. It was the custom of trafficking that merchants arriving from the south were not allowed to conduct commerce with one another. Rather, the inhabitants of the city would purchase from this one and sell to that one.

Ships come up to the wall and the gates, and in Israel many large cities are situated by the sea, but not all of them are a good place for a port, and the ships cannot approach them. From the heart of the seas, borders are seen from the ship buildings of perfected beauty by architects, just like the ships designed from junipers from Senir. They fashion the mast from planks of cedars from Lebanon where they were prevalent, and since it was built on the sea, it was destroyed by the sea, like any superior ship whose cargo in its hold was too heavy for it, can sink by the east wind. They made the oars from oaks from Bashan and the rudder from ivory inlaid in cypresses from the isles of Kittim. The Sail was made of linen with embroidery from Egypt designed with pictures and embroideries, of blue and purple colors, and from the isles of Elishah there was a tent with a roof covered over the entire surface of the ship. Citizens from Sidon and Arvad were the oarsmen, wise men from Tyre, were the mariners who repaired cracks on all the ships of the sea with a guarantee.

Formulas

Acne

Essential Oils
3 Drops Lemon
3 Drops Cypress
3 Drops Eucalyptus
3 Drops Lavender
Base
10mls Shea Butter
Or
30mls Natural Gel
Warning do not administer on pregnant women or people suffering from high blood pressure, or hay fever sufferers during hay fever season.

Acne - Inflamed Skin

Essential Oils
4 Drops Cypress
4 Drops Lemon
4 Drops Clove
4 Drops Sandalwood
Base
10mls Almond Oil
Spread on clean face.

After Birth

Essential Oils
30 Drops Lavender
30 Drops Lemon
Base
30mls Almond Oil
A few drops on Sanitary Towel/ Pad.

Angina

Essential Oil – NO BASE (Synergy)
4 Drops Amni Visnaga
3 Drops Rosemary
3 Drops Ravensara
Rub directly on chest.

Anti-Allergan

Essential Oil – NO BASE (Synergy)
5 Drops Pine
5 Drops Chamomile Roman
5 Drops Lavender
Blend and put 4-6 drops in diffuser.

Aphrodisiac

Essential Oils
4 Drops Ylang Ylang
4 Drops Geranium
4 Drops Sandalwood
4 Drops Bergamot
Base
20mls Almond Oil

Asthma in Adults

Essential Oils
6 Drops of Amni Visnaga
6 Drops of Ravensara
Base
10ml Almond Oil
Rub on Chest.

Asthma in Diffuser

Essential Oil – NO BASE (Synergy)
5 Drops Amni Visnaga
5 Drops Ravensara
5 Drops Nigella

5 Drops Pine
5 Drops Eucalyptus Dives
Blend and Use a few drops in diffuser, or just inhale.

Asthma in Kids

Essential Oils
2 Drops Amni Visnaga
2 Drops Ravensara
Base
10ml Almond Oil
Rub on soles of feet.

Athletes Foot

Essential Oils
3 Drops Clary Sage
3 Drops Rosemary
3 Drops Lavender
3 Drops Myrrh
Base
10mls Olive Oil

B

Baby Oil

Essential
5 Drops Rose
5 Drops Chamomile
5 Drops Lavender
Base
50mls Macadamia Oil

Bad Reaction to Essential Oils

Essential Oils
1 Drop Cardamom
Base
5mls Honey

On your tongue.

Bacteria, E-Coli, Salmonella - Pathogens

Essential Oils
2 Drops Wormwood
2 Drops Marigold
2 Drops Thyme
2 Drops Sage
2 Drops Cajaput
2 Drops Lavender
2 Drops PalmaRosa
Base
10mls Wine
Swallowed with the wine, one time.

Birth and Labor

Essential oils
2 Drops Rosemary
2 Drops Clary Sage
2 Drops Bitter Orange
2 Drops Jasmine
Base
20mls almond oil
5ml Vitamin E oil
Rub on back and stomach.

Blood Pressure - Hypertension

Essential Oils
24 Ginger
12 Black Pepper
12 Cardamom
Base
30mls Almond Oil
Rub on your back three times a day.

Blood Pressure Hypertension

Essential Oils – NO BASE (Synergy)
1 Drop Ylang Ylang

1 Drop Melissa
Drop in diffuser and relax or place a few drops on wrists three times a day.

Blood Pressure and Stress Reliever

Essential Oils – NO BASE (Synergy)
1 Drop Ylang Ylang
1 Drop Marjoram
1 Drop Lemongrass
Drop in diffuser and relax.

Bruising

Essential Oils
10 Drops Lavender
10 Drops Juniper
5 Drops Helichrysum
Base
20mls Vitamin E Oil

Burns

Essential Oils
5 Drops Lavender
5 Drops Marigold
Base
5mls Oblipicha
5mls Vitamin E
Use directly on burn.

C

Cancer Avoidance

Essential Oil
30 Drops Grapefruit
Base
5mls Cannabis Oil
Take three drops three times a day.

Cancer Killer

Essential Oils
4 Drops Lemon
Base
5mls Honey
5mls Hemp Oil
Take three drops three times a day.

Cancer Protection

Essential Oils – (Synergy)
10 Drops Lemongrass
10 Drops Melissa
10 Drops Verbena
Base
100mls Water
Blend oils in small bottle and drip 3 drops in a cup of water, take three times a day.

Candida

Essential Oil
2 Drops Oregano
Base
1 tsp Olive Oil
Use this blend divided into 3 times for the day.

Candida Albicans

Essential Oils
3 Drops PalmaRosa
Directly on tongue and three drops on pad three times a day.

Car Sickness

Essential Oil
1 Drop Ginger
Base
1tsp Honey

Cellulitis

Essential Oils
15 Drops Juniper
15 Drops Grapefruit
15 Drops Geranium
15 Drops Eucalyptus
Base
50mls Almond Oil
Scrub over area with hard sponge or stone.

Colds, Flu and Phlegm

Essential Oils
15 Drops Eucalyptus Globulus
15 Drops Peppermint
10 Drops Amni Visnaga
Base
40mls Linseed Oil

Colic

Essential Oils
1 Drop Lavender
1 Drop Chamomile
Base
10mls Almond Oil
Rub on babies' stomach as needed.

Cough - Respiratory Phlegm

Essential Oils – NO BASE (Synergy)
2 Drops Cardamom
2 Drops Cedarwood
2 Drops Myrtle
2 Drops Pine
Spread on throat – also good for kids

Cough with Phlegm

Essential Oils
1 Drop Cardamom

1 Drop Thyme
Base
½ tsp Honey
Take four times a day

Cradle Cap

Essential Oils
1 Drop Myrtle
Base
5mls Almond Oil
5mls Macedonia Oil
Apply one minute before shower, after shower comb gently.

Deodorant for Women

Essential Oils
10 Drops Cypress
10 Drops Lavender
10 Drops Geranium
10 Drops Lemon
Base
200mls Natural Gel

Deodorant for Women - Summer

Essential Oils
10 Drops Cypress
10 Drops Grapefruit
10 Drops Lemon
10 Drops Lavender
Base
200mls Natural Gel

Deodorant for Men

Essential Oils
15 Drops Lavender

15 Drops Patchouli
10 Drops Bergamot
Base
200mls Natural Gel

Dry Skin for Babies

Essential Oils
5 Drops Rose
5 Drops Chamomile Roman
5 Drops Lavender
Base
50mls Macadamia Oil

E

Eczema

Essential Oils
5 Drops Achillea Yarrow
5 Drops Chamomile
5 Drops Kimmel
5 Drops Vanilla
5 Drops Lavender
Base
10mls Olive Oil
10mls Flaxseed Oil

Eczema – Between Toes

Essential Oils
20 Drops Myrrh
20 Drops Lavender
20 Drops Chamomile Blue
Base
10mls Vitamin E
40mls Almond Oil

Eczema - Strong

Essential Oils
60 Drops Lavender and Propolis
10 Drops Myrrh
10 Drops Vanilla
10 Drops Myrtle
Base
20mls Palm Oil
20mls Shea Butter

Emotional Support Perfume - Unisex

Essential Oils
4 Drops Jasmine
4 Drops Sandalwood
4 Drops Rosewood
4 Drops Patchouli
2 Drops Clove
2 Drops Cinnamon
Base
20mls Almond Oil
Rub on wrists and behind ears as needed.

Emotional Support - Opening Up

Essential Oils – NO BASE (Synergy)
10 Drops Pine
10 Drops Eucalyptus
10 Drops Lavender
10 Drops Frankincense
Rub on wrists, inhale or use in diffuser.

Eyesight Improvement

Essential Oils
1 Drop Carrot Seed
Base
½ tsp Sesame Oil
½ tsp Honey
Mix into a cream and take orally twice a day.

F

Facial Cleanser

Essential Oils
6 Drops Litsea Cubeba
6 Drops Thyme
6 Drops Juniper
Base
10mls Alcohol
50mls Purified Water
Put ingredients into a spray bottle and cleanse your face.

Facial Scrub Acne

1 Tbsp Lemon Juice
1 Tbsp Sugar
Scrub and clean, enjoy.

Fear - Anger and Hysteria

Essential Oils
1 Drop Melissa
2 Drops Bitter Orange
Base
5mls Honey

Fear - Anger and Hysteria

Essential Oil – NO BASE (Synergy)
42 Drops Bitter Orange
10 Drops Bergamot
10 Drops Orange
Blend and Use a few drops in diffuser, or just inhale.

Fear, Empowerment, Immune System

Essential Oil
4 Drops Cedarwood
Base
1 Tbsp Almond Oil

Spread along your spine at night, our immune system works better through the night.

Fear - Existence

Essential Oil – NO BASE (Synergy)
5 Drops Frankincense
5 Drops Eucalyptus Smithii
5 Drops Cedarwood
5 Drops Pine
5 Drops Bergamot
Blend and Use a few drops in diffuser, or just inhale.

Fear - Identified

Essential Oil – NO BASE (Synergy)
3 Drops Cedarwood
3 Drops Ylang Ylang
3 Drops Mandarin
Rub along your spine.

Fear - Courage

Essential Oil
3 Drops Cedarwood
3 Drops Ylang Ylang
3 Drops Mandarin
3 Drops Sandalwood
Base
15mls Almond Oil
Rub along your spine.

Fear - Children

Essential Oil – NO BASE (Synergy)
5 Drops Cedarwood
5 Drops Lavender
5 Drops Chamomile Roman
5 Drops Mandarin
Blend and Use a few drops in diffuser, or just inhale.

Fear – Teenagers

Essential Oil – NO BASE (Synergy)

5 Drops Cedarwood
5 Drops Ylang Ylang
5 Drops Mandarin
5 Drops Sandalwood
Blend and Use a few drops in diffuser, or just inhale.

Fear – Unknown

Essential Oil – NO BASE (Synergy)

3 Drops Cedarwood
3 Drops Ylang Ylang
Rub along your spine at night.

Feeling Blah!

Essential Oil – NO BASE (Synergy)

4 Drops Vetiver
4 Drops Patchouli
Rub 2 or 3 drops on wrist.

Fever – Babies

Essential Oils - NO BASE (Synergy)

2 Drops Wormwood
2 Drops Black Pepper
Run with your fingers up baby's spine.

Fever

Essential Oils – NO BASE (Synergy)

3 Drops Marigold
3 Drops Black Pepper
3 Drops Wormwood
Rub along spinal cord or on sole of feet from toe to heel.

Fleas on Pets

Essential Oils - NO BASE (Synergy)

4 Drops Vetiver

4 Drops Lemongrass
Put a few drops on back of your pet's neck to rid them of fleas.

Fungal Infections

Essential Oils
2 Drops Thyme
2 Drops Lavender
2 Drops Marigold
2 Drops Cinnamon
2 Drops Wormwood
2 Drops Bergamot
2 Drops Eucalyptus Globulus
2 Drops Juniper
2 Drops Clove
2 Drops Lemon
2 Drops Sage
Base
20ml Olive Oil
Olive oil is a heavy oil and stops the oxygen supply to the fungus imprisoning the fungus and strangling the infection. Apply three times a day.

Fungus Athletes Foot

Essential Oils
4 Drops Lemongrass
4 Drops Marigold
4 Drops Geranium
4 Drops Cinnamon
4 Drops Tea Tree
4 Drops Eucalyptus
4 Drops Oregano
Base
30mls Shea Butter
Apply twice a day.

Fungus on Fingernails

Essential Oils
5 Drops Achillea
5 Drops Cardamom

Base
10ml Neem Oil

G

Gassy Stomach Kids

Essential Oils
3 Drops Myrtle
Base
10mls Sesame Oil
Massage on stomach as needed.

Gout - General

Essential Oils
10 Drops Cypress
10 Drops Juniper
10 Drops Sage
10 Drops Lavender
Base
50mls Almond Oil

Gout Pain

Essential Oils
10 Drops Nutmeg
10 Drops Peppermint
10 Drops Verbena
10 Drops Lavender
Base
40mls Sesame Oil

#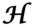

Hair Cream

Essential Oils
12 Drops Lavender

12 Drops Cypress
12 Drops Rosemary
12 Drops Eucalyptus
12 Myrtle
Base Cream
50ml Castor Oil
50ml Almond Oil
100ml Coconut Oil
20g Beeswax
Use a small amount on your fingertips and rub into scalp after washing.

Hair Mask

Essential Oils
7 Drops Geranium
7 Drops Eucalyptus
7 Drops Rosemary
Base
20mls Coconut Oil
Leave on for 30 minutes then wash off.

Hair Mask - Hair Loss from Stress

Essential Oils
10 Drops Myrtle
10 Drops Geranium
10 Drops Eucalyptus
10 Drops Rosemary
Base
10mls Oblipicha
30mls Jojoba Oil
Leave on for 30 minutes then wash off.

Hand Cold Dry Rough Skin

Essential Oils
5 Drops Lemon
5 Drops Patchouli
5 Drops Lavender
20 Drops Cassia
Base
35mls Palm Oil

5mls Wheatgerm Oil

Hand/Foot Cream

Essential Oils
15 Drops Lavender
15 Drops Lemon
15 Drops Patchouli
15 Drops Rosewood
Base
30mls Shea Butter
20mls Palm Butter
10mls Coconut Oil
40mls Almond Oil
10mls Beeswax

Headache

Essential Oils
6 Drops Lavender
6 Drops Mint
Base
15mls Almond Oil
Spread over forehead and around eyes, just be careful to not get into your eyes.

Headache from Stress

Essential Oils – NO BASE
3 Drops Cardamom
Rub with fingertips on skull

Hematomas

Essential Oils – NO BASE (Synergy)
10 Drops Lavender
10 Drops Juniper
10 Drops Sandalwood
Use as needed.

Hemorrhoids Fissura - Cream Based

Essential Oils
10 Drops Cardamom
10 Drops Geranium
10 Drops Myrtle
Base
40mls Shea Butter
40mls Palm Butter
20mls Sea Buckthorn
10mls Beeswax
Apply twice a day.

Hemorrhoids - Cream Based

Essential Oils
5 Drops Cypress
5 Drops Juniper
5 Drops Lemon
5 Drops Geranium
5 Drops Clary Sage
5 Drops Myrrh
5 Drops Myrtle
5 Drops Lavender
Base
50mls Shea Butter
10mls Oblipicha
1 tsp. Vitamin B
Apply twice a day.

Hemorrhoids Fissura - Oil Based

Essential Oils
3 Drops Cypress
3 Drops Lemon
3 Drops Juniper
3 Drops Geranium
3 Drops Sage
3 Drops Myrrh
3 Drops Myrtle
3 Drops Lavender
Base

50mls Shea Butter
This version is good if you are bleeding, the cream may be painful to administer.

Herpes

Essential Oils
3 Drops Eucalyptus
3 Drops Melissa
3 Drops Myrtle
Base
5mls Olive Oil
5mls Flaxseed Oil

Herpes Simplex

Essential Oils
4 Drops Melissa
4 Drops Lavender
4 Drops Eucalyptus
Base
10mls Olive Oil
Spread on area as needed, will go away after 4 days but keep using for 3 months to completely get rid of it.

Hyperactivity

Essential Oils – NO BASE (Synergy)
10 Drops Bergamot
10 Drops Sweet Marjoram
Use a few drops in diffuser, or just inhale.

I

Immortality - Living Healthy

Essential Oils – NO BASE (Scent)
30 Drops Melissa
30 Drops Lemon
15 Drops Clove

10 Drops Cinnamon
5 Drops Coriander
3 Drops Marjoram
3 Drops Angelica
Inhale every day for as long as you feel a need for it!

Immune System

Essential Oils
10 Drops Pine
10 Drops Cedarwood
10 Drops Lavender
10 Drops Tea Tree
Base
50mls Almond Oil

Inflammation of Joints

Essential Oils
10 Drops Nutmeg
10 Drops Thyme
10 Drops Rosemary
10 Drops Lavender
10 Drops Black Pepper
Base
40mls Sesame Oil
10mls Arnica

Inflammation of Ligaments

Essential Oils
10 Drops Nutmeg
10 Drops Clove
10 Drops Ginger
10 Drops Thyme
Base
30mls Almond Oil
Massage over painful area.

Intestinal Worms

Essential Oils NO BASE (Synergy)

2 Drops Wormwood
2 Drops Oregano
Drop on your tongue 5 times a day.

Intestinal Worms (Kids)

Essential Oils
1 Drop Myrtle
Base
1 tbsp Olive Oil
Administer for three weeks.

J

Jericho Rose Bite

Essential Oils
5 Drops Lavender
5 Drops Tea Tree
5 Drops Marigold
Base
5mls Oblipicha
5mls Vitamin E
Use directly on burn.

Jetlag

Essential Oils NO BASE (Synergy)
2 Drops Lemongrass
2 Drops Rosewood
Inhale or rub on wrists.

#

Kidney and Bladder Rehabilitation

Essential Oils
2 Drops Carrot
Base

5mls Honey
Take three times a day.

Kidney Cleanse

Essential Oils
4 Drops Geranium
Base
10mls Hemp Oil
Drink 1tsp three times for one day.

L

Lice Killer

Essential Oils
8 Drops Eucalyptus
8 Drops Lavender
8 Drops Geranium
10 Drops Rosemary
Base
30mls Almond Oil
Leave on head for a minimum of one hour.
Use fine comb dipped into 50mls water/50mls Vinegar.
Comb hair and dip into the vinegar mix.

Lip Balm

Essential Oils
1 Drop Orange
Base
5mls Palm Oil

Liver Cleanse

Essential Oils
3 Drop Carrot Seed
3 Drop Rosemary
Base
10mls Hemp Oil

Drink 1tsp 3 times a day for as long as you need.

Liver Cleanse (Fatty Liver)

Essential Oils
1 Drop Carrot Seed
1 Drop Rosemary
Base
1tsp Olive Oil
Drink 3 times a day for as long as you need.

M

Massage Blend - All Round Health

Essential Oils
3 Drops Rosemary
3 Drops Eucalyptus
3 Drops Pine
3 Drops Lavender
Base
30mls Almond Oil

Massage Blend - Anger

Essential Oils
2 Drops Bergamot
2 Drops Orange
2 Drops Grapefruit
2 Drops Mandarin
2 Drops Lemon
2 Drops Anise Star
Base
20mls Almond Oil
This blend is very phototoxic, do not go into sun for 4 hours after massage.

Massage Blend - Aphrodisiac

Essential Oils
5 Drops Nutmeg

5 Drops Ylang Ylang
5 Drops Cardamom
5 Drops Patchouli
5 Drops Sandalwood
5 Drops Rose
5 Drops Jasmine
5 Drops Black Pepper
Base
50mls Almond Oil

Massage Blend – Pain

Essential Oils
5 Drops Nutmeg
5 Drops Clove
5 Drops Lavender
5 Drops Cajaput
5 Drops Vanilla
Base
10mls Sesame
20mls Almond

Massage Blend – Sadness

Essential Oils
2 Drops Rosemary
3 Drops Mint
3 Drops Lavender
2 Drops Orange
Base
10mls Sesame Oil
Do not go out into the sun for two after putting on your skin.

Mastectomy Breast Cancer

Essential Oils
10 Drops Lavender
10 Drops Sandalwood
10 Drops Juniper
10 Drops PalmaRosa
Base
10mls Almond Oil

10mls Oblipicha

Mastectomy Wound

Essential Oils
10 Drops Helichrysum
10 Drops PalmaRosa
Base
20mls Vitamin E
Drip freely over wound, no need to rub in.

Master Blend

Essential Oils NO BASE (Synergy)
15 Drops Pine
15 Drops Eucalyptus
15 Drops Thyme
15 Drops Rosemary
15 Drops Lavender
15 Drops Lemongrass
15 Drops Coriander
15 Drops Cardamom
15 Drops Cajaput
15 Drops Mint
15 Drops Oregano
15 Drops Tea Tree
15 Drops Black Pepper
15 Drops Sage
This makes up a 10ml bottle.

Master Blend is a magic synergy of all the above oils because there are equal amounts of each of these essential oils, they lose their harm to our skin and can be used directly without a base oil.

This blend is a protection and prevention of colds, flu, respiratory infections and viruses.

Put onto your pulse and gently rub in, or you can simply smell them straight from the bottle.

Melancholy

Essential Oils
4 Drops Eucalyptus Globulus
Base
10mls Almond Oil
Have rubbed along your spinal cord downwards.

Mice & Rat Deterrent

Essential Oils
50 Drops Peppermint
Base
20mls Almond Oil
Make cotton wool balls, douse in oil mixture and place each cotton ball in corners all over your house.

Migraine

Essential Oils
1 Drop Lavender
1 Drop Mint
Base
5mls Honey
To be taken orally

Moisturizer – Day Care

Essential Oils
20 Drops Geranium
10 Drops Pine
15 Drops Rosewood
15 Drops Clary Sage
10 Drops Niaouli
Base
50mls Almond Oil
30mls Coconut Oil
10mls Oblipicha
10mls Vitamin E Oil
10mls Jojoba Oil
Water Base
1 tbsp Sodium Borate (Borax) – dissolved

50mls hot water
2 tbsp Beeswax – melted
Blend all ingredients in high-speed blender.

Moisturizer – Night Care

Essential Oils
20 Drops Geranium
15 Drops Rosehip
15 Drops Lavender
15 Drops Lemon
10 Drops Neroli
10 Drops Niaouli

Base
50mls Almond Oil
30mls Avocado Oil
10mls Oblipicha
10mls Vitamin A Oil
10mls Jojoba Oil

Water Base
1 tbsp Sodium Borate (Borax) – dissolved
50mls hot water
2 tbsp Beeswax – melted

Mosquito Bites – From Newborn

Essential Oils NO BASE (Synergy)
5 Drops Eucalyptus Limonite
5 Drops Fir
5 Drops Lavender
5 Drops Geranium
One drop on each arm and leg. You can also use in humidifier.

Mosquito Bites – Infected

Essential Oils NO BASE (Synergy)
4 Drops Eucalyptus Limonite
4 Drops Fir
4 Drops Lavender
4 Drops Geranium
½ teaspoon honey
Blend all ingredients in high-speed blender, Spread over the bite.

Mosquito and Insect Bites

Essential Oils
2 Drops Lavender
2 Drops Tea Tree
Base
5mls Honey

Mouth Ulcers - Option 1

Essential Oils
2 Drops Clove
Base
50mls Warm Water
Gargle and spit out 4 times a day.

Mouth Ulcers - Option 2

Essential Oils
2 Drops Myrrh
Base
50mls Warm Water
Gargle and spit out 4 times a day.

Mouth Ulcers - Option 3

Essential Oils
2 Drops Tea Tree
Base
50mls Warm Water
Gargle and spit out 4 times a day.

Mouth Ulcers - Option 4

Essential Oils
4 Drops Grapefruit
2 Drops Clove
Base
50mls Warm Water
Gargle and spit out 4 times a day

Muscle Cramp after Sport

Essential Oils
6 Drops Silver Fir
6 Drops Eucalyptus
6 Drops Cardamom
6 Drops Lemongrass
6 Drops Cajaput
6 Drops Ginger
Base
30mls Sesame Oil

Muscle Cramps - Lactic Acid

Essential Oils
4 Drops Wormwood
4 Drops Lemongrass
4 Drops Lavender
Base
10mls Sesame Oil

Muscle Pain

Essential Oils
8 Drops Wintergreen
8 Drops Clove
8 Drops Mint
Base
20mls Natural Gel
10mls Sesame Oil

Muscle Stress - Fatigued

Essential Oils
3 Drops Cardamom
3 Drops Lemongrass
Base
10mls Sesame Oil

N

Nausea

Essential Oils – NO BASE (Synergy)
1 Drop Cardamom
1 Drop Ginger
Directly on Tongue

O

Oral Bacteria

Essential Oils NO BASE (Synergy)
2 Drops Wormwood
2 Drops Marigold
2 Drops Thyme
2 Drops Sage
2 Drops Cajaput
2 Drops Lavender
2 Drops PalmaRosa
Take 2 drops of this blend with 1tsp of Olive Oil six times a day.

Ovarian Cysts

Essential Oils
10 Drops Nutmeg
10 Drops Clove
Base
20mls Almond Oil
Gently massage over ovarian area on your body.

P

Pain Killer - Analgesic

Essential Oils
10 Drops Mint
10 Drops Clove

10 Drops Lavender
10 Drops Nutmeg
Base
30mls Almond Oil

Pain Killer - Extreme

Essential Oils
5 Drops Coriander
5 Drops Cinnamon
Base
10mls Sesame Oil

Pain Killer - First Aid

Essential Oil
10 Drops Eucalyptus
10 Drops Peppermint
Base
20mls Sesame Oil

Pain Killer - Inflamed Pain

Essential Oils
3 Drops Nutmeg
3 Drops Clove
3 Drops Mint
3 Drops Cedarwood
3 Drops Myrrh
3 Drops Vanilla
3 Drops Frankincense
Base
20mls Sesame Oil
20mls Hemp Oil
10mls Arnica Oil
Warning do not administer on pregnant women or people suffering from epilepsy.

Pain Killer - Inflamed Frozen Shoulder

Essential Oils
3 Drops Black Pepper

3 Drops Peppermint
3 Drops Cedarwood
3 Drops Capsicum
3 Drops Red Thyme
3 Drops Marigold
3 Drops Wormwood
Base
20mls Sesame Oil
20mls Hemp Oil
10mls Arnica Oil
Warning do not administer on pregnant women or people suffering from epilepsy.

Pain Killer – Intense Pain
Essential Oils
2 drops Silver fir
2 drops Cedarwood
4 drops Helichrysum
4 drops German chamomile
2 drops Rosemary
Base
30mls (1 oz) of jojoba Oil

Pain Killer – Motoric
Essential Oils
5 drops of rosemary
5 drops of cajuput
Base
10mls Almond oil

Phlegm Excretion

Essential Oils
15 Drops Eucalyptus
15 Drops Mint
7 Drops Amni Visnaga
Base
30mls Flaxseed Oil
Rub on Throat as needed.

PMS

Essential Oils
3 Drops Grapefruit
Base
50mls Water
Drink as needed

Problem Solving for Success

Essential Oils – NO BASE (Synergy)
20 Drops Clove
20 Drops Juniper
20 Drops Patchouli
Put few drops in diffuser or inhale.

Psoriasis

Essential Oils
5 Drops Bergamot
5 Drops Eucalyptus Globulus
5 Drops Geranium
5 Drops lavender
Base
10mls Vitamin E Oil
10mls Almond Oil
This formula doesn't heal Psoriasis, but it does calm it down.

R

Reduce Size after Pregnancy

Essential Oils
6 Drops Geranium
6 Drops Ylang Ylang
Base
20mls Almond Oil
Rub on stomach, thighs, breasts to stimulate elastin and collagen.

Relaxant Emotional

Essential Oils
3 Drops Nutmeg
3 Drops Jasmine
3 Drops Sandalwood
3 Drops Rosewood
3 Drops Patchouli
3 Drops Clove
3 Drops Cinnamon
Base
20mls Almond Oil

Relaxant General

Essential Oils
6 Drops Lavender
3 Drops Bergamot
3 Drops Grapefruit
Base
10mls Almond Oil
Relaxes and helps you sleep.

Respiratory

Essential Oils – NO BASE (Synergy)
5 Drops Cajaput
5 Drops Rosemary
5 Drops lavender
5 Drops Thyme
Blend and place one drop on tongue with 1tsp of honey.

Ringworm

Essential Oil
30 Drops Verbena
Base
10mls Any Alcohol or Vodka, do not go into the sun after use.

Room Deodorizer

Essential Oils

8 drops silver fir oil
4 drops juniper oil
4 drops cypress oil
4 drops cedarwood oil
Diffused or spritzed as desired.

S

Scar Prevention - Immediately After Operation

Essential Oils
5 Drops Achillea
10 Drops Lavender
5 Drops Sandalwood
Base
20 ml Obliphica
This blend must be oily and not creamy so as not to damage sensitive stitched skin. Apply freely as needed.

Scar - Fresh Skin Scar

Essential Oils
10 Drops Lavender
10 Drops Helichrysum
10 Drops Pine
10 Drops Cedarwood
10 Drops Patchouli
10 Drops Juniper
10 Drops Eucalyptus
Base
60mls Almond Oil
10mls Avocado Oil
10mls Oblipicha
10mls Shea Butter
10mls Stellaria

Scar - Ripped Muscle Fibers

Essential Oils

4 Drops Lavender
4 Drops Ylang Ylang
4 Drops Mint
Base
10mls Almond Oil
5mls Vitamin E Oil
Spread freely on scar.

Seborrhea

Essential Oils
10 Drops Geranium
10 Drops Patchouli
Base
20mls Almond Oil

Self-Confidence

Essential Oils – NO BASE (Synergy)
5 Drops Patchouli
5 Drops Vetiver
5 Drops Cypress
5 Drops Rosemary
Blend Oils and place a few drops in diffuser or inhale.

Self-Confidence - Stuttering

Essential Oils – NO BASE (Synergy)
10 Drops Bergamot
10 Drops Cinnamon
Blend Oils and place a few drops in diffuser or inhale.

Skin Itchiness

Essential Oils
20 Drops Lavender
10 Drops Myrrh
10 Drops Myrtle
10 Drops Vanilla
Base
50mls Coconut Oil

Skin Lightening Pigmentation

Essential Oils
7 Drops Lemon
5 Drops Eucalyptus Global
5 Drops Mint
5 Drops Lavender
5 Drops Marigold
Base
15mls Flaxseed Oil
15mls Dissolved Dead Sea Salt
15mls Sweet Soap
Rub into Skin until absorbed and leave on for one minute, apply every day for 5 months – Do not go into sun after use. Best applied at night.

Skin Protection Cancer Prevention

Essential Oils
10 Drops Niaouli
Base
10ml Shea Butter

Skin Protection - Gangrene

Essential Oils
10 Drops Lavender
Base
5ml Shea Butter
5ml Cannabis Oil

Skin Rash Eczema

Essential Oils
6 Drops Lavender
6 Drops Niaouli
6 Drops Myrtle
6 Drops Propolis
Base
20mls Linseed Oil

Skin Suffering from Cold

Essential Oils
3 Drops Lemon
3 Drops Patchouli
3 Drops Lavender
20 Drops Cassia
Base
35mls Palm Oil
5mls Sesame Oil

Skin Wounds - Acne, Whiteheads, Blackheads.

Essential Oils
5 Drops Chamomile
5 Drops Plantago
5 Drops Sage
5 Drops Rutha
5 Drops Myrtle
Base
30ml Castor Oil
½ tsp Ginger root crushed
½ tsp Turmeric root crushed

Spinal Pain

Essential Oils NO BASE (Synergy)
10 Drops Ginger
10 Drops Lavender
10 Drops Cajaput
10 Drops Black Pepper
10 Drops Thyme
Run along spine especially the painful part.

Spinal Pain

Essential Oils NO BASE (Synergy)
10 Drops Lavender
10 Drops Cajaput
Run along spine especially the painful part.

Sprain with Swelling

Essential Oils
10 Drops Lavender
10 Drops Juniper
Base
20mls Vitamin E Oil

Stress – Overworked Student

Essential Oils NO BASE (Synergy)
5 Drops Lavender
5 Drops Chamomile Blue
5 Drops Mandarin
5 Drops Cedarwood
Blend and Use a few drops in diffuser, or just inhale.

Sun Burn

Essential Oils
20 Drops Lavender
20 Drops Patchouli
15 Drops Clove
Base
50mls Sesame Oil
10mls Oblipicha
10mls Vitamin E

Sunscreen 8UV Protection

No Essential Oils
Base
20mls Jojoba Oil
20mls She butter
20mls Coconut Oil

Sweating Profusely

Essential Oils
10 Drops Juniper
10 Drops Sage
Base

20mls Gel

T

Tick Killer

Essential Oils NO BASE (Synergy)
2 Drops Vetiver
2 Drops Lemongrass
2 Drops Mint
Drop onto the back of your pet's neck and on their paws.

Toothache

Essential Oils
5 Drops Clove
Rub directly onto the gum and tooth area as needed.

Triglycerides

Essential Oils
2 Drops Grapefruit
Directly on tongue 3 times a day.

V

Varicose Veins - Swollen Veins

Essential Oils
6 Drops Rosemary
6 Drops Cypress
Base
10mls Almond Oil
Rub upwards and keep legs raised using a pillow for as much as possible.

Virus Protection

Essential Oils NO BASE (Synergy)
10 Drops Eucalyptus Globulus

10 Drops Pine
10 Drops Lemon
10 Drops Cyprus
10 Drops Myrtle
10 Drops Juniper
10 Drops Rosemary
10 Drops Oregano
Blend oils and use in diffuser, rub a few drops on wrists or inhale.

Weight Loss Aid

Essential Oil
5 Drops Grapefruit
Base
50mls Water
Drink ½ an hour before meals.

Wrist Inflammation

Essential Oils
5 Drops Peppermint
5 Drops Ginger
Base
5mls Sesame
5mls Almond

Worms

Essential Oils
1 Drop Cajaput
Base
5mls Olive Oil
One-time treatment.

Worms Kids

Essential Oils
3 Drops Myrtle

Base

10mls Olive Oil

Take 1tsp three times a day for three weeks.

Wounds – Infectious

Essential Oil

3 Drops Lavender

3 Drops Geranium

3 Drops Tea Tree

Base

10mls Obliphica

Use as needed, also great after operations.

First Aid

Must Have at Home Oils

Essential Oils
Chamomile Roman
Clove
Eucalyptus
Lavender
Lemon
Oregano
Patchouli
Peppermint
Rosemary
Tea Tree

Base Oils
Avocado
Almond
Olive
Sesame

Quick Look Reference

Acne
Carrot Seed, Cedar wood, Chamomile, Cypress, Frankincense, Geranium, Lavender, Lemon, Litsea Cubeba, Myrrh, Palma Rosa, Pine, Rosemary, Sage, Tea Tree, Yarrow, Ylang Ylang.

Adrenal, Kidney Function
Amni Visnaga, Geranium.

Allergies
Chamomile, Eucalyptus Limonite, Fir, Geranium, Lavender, Myrtle, Pine, Rose.

Anti-Bacteria, Anti-biotic
Eucalyptus Global, Eucalyptus Limonite, Lavender, Lemongrass, Litsea Cubeba, Marigold, Nutmeg, Oregano, Verbena, Yarrow.

Anti-Depressants
Angelica, Artemisia, Basil, Bergamot, Bitter Orange, Cardamom, Cassia, Cinnamon, Cistus, Clove, Grapefruit, Jasmine, Kimmel, Lavender, Lemon, Lemongrass, Mandarin, Marjoram, Melissa, Myrrh, Neroli, Orange, Patchouli, Rose, Sandalwood, Vanilla, Ylang Ylang.

Anti-Inflammatory
Angelica, Artemisia, Basil, Bitter Orange, Black Pepper, Cajuput, Cardamom, Cedar wood, Chamomile, Cinnamon, Clary sage, Clove, Coriander, Cypress, Eucalyptus Dives, Eucalyptus Global, Eucalyptus Limonite, Eucalyptus Smithii, Fennel, Fir, Frankincense, Geranium, Ginger, Grapefruit, Helichrysum, Juniper, Lavender, Lemon, Lemongrass, Litsea Cubeba, Mint, Myrrh, Myrtle, Nutmeg, Orange, Oregano, Raven Sara, Red Thyme, Rose, Rosemary, Rosewood, Sage, Sandalwood, Star of Anise, Tea Tree, Thyme, Ylang Ylang.

Antioxidant
Black Pepper, Chamomile, Cinnamon, Cistus, Clove, Coriander, Ginger, Lavender, Lemon, Lemongrass, Litsea Cubeba, Mandarin, Orange, Oregano, Rose, Sage.

Anti-Viral, Colds, Flu
Cedar wood, Eucalyptus Smithii, Eucalyptus Dives, Eucalyptus Global, Fir.

Aphrodisiac
Black Pepper, Cardamom, Coriander, Jasmine, Nutmeg, Patchouli, Rose, Sandalwood, Ylang Ylang.

Appetite Enhancers
Ginger, Nutmeg.

Appetite Suppressants
Grapefruit, Sweet Marjoram, Vanilla.

Astringents
Black Pepper, Cypress, Eucalyptus Limonite, Geranium, Lavender, Lemon, Marigold, Nutmeg, Rose, Rosemary, Sage, Sandalwood, Thyme.

Babies
Artemisia, Black Pepper, Eucalyptus Dives, Eucalyptus Limonite, Eucalyptus Smithii, Fir, Lavender, Pine.

Blood Circulation
Angelica, Black Pepper, Cassia, Cinnamon, Clove, Cypress, Grapefruit, Helichrysum, Lavender, Lemon, Rose, Rosemary, Sandalwood.

Brain
Neroli, Rosemary.

Burns
Lavender, Marigold, Vitamin E.

Cancer
Basil, Black Pepper, Cannabis, Cardamom, Chamomile, Coriander, Fennel, Grapefruit, Hemp, Lemon, Lemongrass, Litsea Cubeba, Marigold, Myrtle, Oregano, Rose, Sage, Verbena.

Cardiovascular, Blood Pressure
Amni Visnaga, Angelica, Black Pepper, Cinnamon, Lavender, Litsea Cubeba, Melissa, Oregano, Patchouli, Raven Sara, Rose, Rosemary, Sage, Verbena, Ylang Ylang.

Cellulite
Eucalyptus, Grapefruit, Juniper.

Cholesterol, Triglycerides
Ginger, Grapefruit.

Confidence, Feel Good, Euphoria
Mandarin, Myrtle, Tangerine, Vetiver, Ylang Ylang.

Coughs, Phlegm, Cystic Fibrosis
Amni Visnaga, Anise Star, Bergamot, Cardamom, Carrot Seed, Coriander, Eucalyptus Global, Eucalyptus Limonite, Eucalyptus Smithii, Ginger, Marjoram, Mint, Myrrh, Myrtle, Oregano, Pine, Sage, Yarrow.

Cuts, Bites
Eucalyptus Global, Helichrysum, Lavender, Lemon, Marigold, Tea Tree.

Deodorant
Bergamot, Cypress, Geranium, Grapefruit, Lavender, Lemon, Patchouli.

Diabetes, Pancreas
Anise Star, Cinnamon, Eucalyptus Dives, Eucalyptus Global, Mint, Ylang Ylang.

Digestive System
Anise Star, Artemisia, Basil, Bitter Orange, Caraway, Cardamom, Chamomile, Cinnamon, Coriander, Fennel, Frankincense, Ginger, Grapefruit, Juniper, Kimmel, Lavender, Lemongrass, Mandarin, Marjoram, Myrtle, Nutmeg, Oregano, Palme Rosa, Rose, Sage, Thyme, Vanilla, Vetiver.

Diuretic
Coriander.

E-Coli, Salmonella
Artemisia, Cajuput, Lavender, Marigold, Palma Rosa, Sage, Thyme.

Emotional Support, Neurotransmitters
Angelica, Bergamot, Bitter Orange, Eucalyptus Dives, Eucalyptus Global, Frankincense, Geranium, Grapefruit, Helichrysum, Jasmine, Lavender, Lemon, Mandarin, Neroli, Nutmeg, Orange, Patchouli, Pine, Rose, Sandalwood, Tangerine, Violet, Ylang Ylang.

Excretes Toxins, Bad Smells
Angelica, Eucalyptus Dives, Ginger, Grapefruit, Litsea Cubeba.

Eyes
Bergamot, Cannabis, Carrot Seed.

Face Whitening, Pigmentation
Angelica, Cyprus, Eucalyptus Global, Lavender, Lemon, Marigold, Mint, Ylang Ylang.

Facial Skin
Geranium, Lavender, Neroli, Pine, Rosewood, Sage, Vitamin E.

Fatigue
Geranium.

Fear, Hysteria
Bitter Orange, Cedar wood, Cypress, Eucalyptus Global, Ylang Ylang.

Fever
Artemisia, Black Pepper, Marigold.

Fungus, Cysts, Warts
Artemisia, Basil, Bergamot, Cardamom, Chamomile, Cinnamon, Clove, Eucalyptus Global, Frankincense, Geranium, Juniper, Lavender, Lemon, Lemongrass, Marigold, Melissa, Myrrh, Nutmeg, Oregano, Rose, Rosemary, Sage, Tea Tree, Thyme, Verbena, Yarrow, Ylang Ylang.

Hair
Eucalyptus Global, Geranium, Myrtle, Rose, Rosemary.

Hallucinate
Artemisia, Cannabis, Coriander.

Headache
Black Pepper, Cardamom, Mint.

Hemorrhoids
Cardamom, Cypress, Geranium, Juniper, Lavender, Lemon, Myrrh, Myrtle, Sage, Yarrow.

Herpes
Eucalyptus Global, Melissa, Myrtle.

Immune System
Cedar wood, Eucalyptus Limonite, Fir, Geranium, Lavender, Oregano, Pine.

Insomnia
Cedar wood, Frankincense, Melissa, Vetiver.

Joint Pain, Rheumatism, Arthritis
Anise Star, Artemisia, Cajuput, Cedar wood, Clove, Coriander, Eucalyptus Smithii, Fir, Frankincense, Ginger, Mint, Myrrh, Nutmeg.

Kids
Anise Star, Bitter Orange, Cedar wood, Eucalyptus Limonite, Eucalyptus Smithii.

Lice, Fleas, Mosquitoes
Eucalyptus Global, Eucalyptus Limonite, Geranium, Lavender, Lemongrass, Rosemary, Vetiver.

Liver Function, Cleanse
Artemisia, Caraway, Carrot Seed, Eucalyptus Dives, Eucalyptus Global, Grapefruit, Mint, Rosemary, Verbena.

Lymphatic System
Grapefruit.

Mouth, Dental
Clove, Ginger, Myrrh, Sage.

Meditation
Eucalyptus Global, Frankincense, Myrtle, Sandalwood.

Mental Stress, Relaxants Sedatives
Angelica, Artemisia, Bergamot, Bitter Orange, Coriander, Geranium, Grapefruit, Lavender, Litsea Cubeba, Marjoram, Melissa, Nutmeg, Rose, Sandalwood, Vanilla, Verbena, Ylang Ylang.

Milk Production Enhancers
Caraway, Chamomile, Fennel.

Moods, Depression, Anger
Angelica, Anise Star, Basil, Cardamom, Geranium, Helichrysum, Melissa, Patchouli, Rose, Rosewood, Sandalwood, Vanilla, Verbena, Vetiver, Ylang Ylang.

Muscles Cramps, Pain
Anise Star, Artemisia, Basil, Bergamot, Black Pepper, Cajaput, Cannabis, Cardamom, Cassia, Cedarwood, Chamomile, Cistus, Cinnamon, Clary sage, Clove, Coriander, Cypress, Eucalyptus Dives, Eucalyptus Global, Eucalyptus Limonite, Eucalyptus Smithii, Fennel, Fir, Frankincense, Geranium, Ginger, Grapefruit, Hop, Jasmine, Juniper, Kimmel, Lavender, Lemon, Lemongrass, Litsea Cubeba, Mandarin, Marigold, Marjoram, Melissa, Mint, Myrtle, Neroli, Nutmeg, Orange, Oregano, Palma Rosa, Patchouli, Pine, Rose, Rosewood, Sage, Sandalwood, Tea Tree, Thyme, Vanilla, Winter Green.

Nausea
Ginger.

Nervous System
Angelica, Artemisia, Bitter Orange, Coriander, Grapefruit, Litsea Cubeba.

445

Nervous Pain
Angelica, Artemisia, Bitter Orange, Cedarwood, Eucalyptus Dives, Eucalyptus Global, Eucalyptus Limonite, Eucalyptus Smithii, Fir, Grapefruit, Nutmeg, Oregano, Yarrow, Ylang Ylang.

Neurologic System
Angelica, Cedar wood, Coriander, Eucalyptus Global, Mandarin, Ylang Ylang.

Pain, Analgesic
Black Pepper, Cajuput, Cardamom, Cedar wood, Clove, Coriander, Eucalyptus Smithii, Frankincense, Ginger, Lavender, Mint, Myrrh, Nutmeg, Rose, Vanilla, Yarrow, Ylang Ylang.

Parasites
Artemisia, Helichrysum, Myrtle, Oregano, Vetiver.

Pre-Pregnancy Strengthening
Geranium, Rose Angelica, Sage.

Psoriasis
Bergamot.

Relaxants Sleep
Artemisia, Bergamot, Bitter Orange, Cardamom, Chamomile, Clary, Sage, Hop, Jasmine, Lavender, Melissa, Neroli, Nutmeg, Patchouli, Rose, Rosewood, Vanilla, Verbena, Ylang Ylang.

Respiratory System
Amni Visnaga, Anise Star, Basil, Cajaput, Cardamom, Cassia, Cedarwood, Chamomile, Coriander, Eucalyptus Dives, Eucalyptus Global, Eucalyptus Limonite, Eucalyptus Smithii, Fennel, Fir, Ginger, Grapefruit, Kimmel, Lavender, Lemongrass, Mandarin, Myrrh, Myrtle, Neroli, Orange, Oregano, Pine, Raven Sara, Rose, Sage, Sandalwood, Tea Tree, Thyme, Yarrow.

Sub-Cutaneous Inflammation
Coriander, Cypress, Fennel, Frankincense, Geranium, Helichrysum, Lemon, Litsea Cubeba, Rosemary, Yarrow.

Skin, Scars, Wounds, Stretch Marks
Angelica, Bergamot, Cardamom, Carrot Seed, Cedar wood, Chamomile, Cistus, Clary Sage, Clove, Coriander, Cypress, Eucalyptus, Eucalyptus Dives, Frankincense, Geranium, Grapefruit, Helichrysum, Jasmine, Juniper, Kimmel, Lavender, Lemon, Marigold, Melissa, Myrrh, Myrtle, Neroli, Niaouli, Orange, Palma Rosa, Patchouli, Pine, Rose, Rosemary, Rosewood, Sage, Sandalwood, Tea Tree, Thyme, Vanilla, Verbena, Yarrow.

Stomach Pain
Anise Star, Artemisia, Bitter Orange, Coriander, Nutmeg.

Swellings, Bruises
Benzoin, Cedar wood, Coriander, Fir, Helichrysum, Oregano, Raven Sara, Sage, Sandalwood, Thyme, Vetiver.

Thyroid
Geranium.

Urinary and Sexual Organs
Caraway, Cypress, Eucalyptus Global, Ginger, Jasmine, Marjoram, PMS, Rose, Sage, Vanilla.

Vaginal Infections
Artemisia, Chamomile, Myrrh, Oregano, Sage, Tea Tree, Ylang Ylang.

Varicose Veins, Water Retention
Cypress, Juniper.

Weight Management
Cinnamon, Grapefruit, lemon.

Women, Hormonal
Anise Star, Artemisia, Basil, Carrot Seed, Clary sage, Cypress, Fennel, Geranium, Jasmine, Kimmel, Marjoram, Oregano, Rose, Sage, Tea Tree, Vanilla, Verbena, Ylang Ylang.

Worms
Artemisia, Myrtle, Oregano.

References

Websites

https,//www.chabad.org/
https,//www.neot-kedumim.org.il/
https,//www.ou.org/
https,//www.revolvy.com/main/index.php
https,//www.israel21c.org/
http,//flora.org.il/en/plants/
http,//www.wildflowers.co.il/
https,//gardenerdy.com/
https,//www.jewishvirtuallibrary.org/
https,//www.spiritualscents.com/
http,//hebrewnations.com/
http,//www.flowersinisrael.com/
http,//www.lgbotanicals.com/
http,//israelphilately.org.il/
https,//escentualweb.com/
https,//scienceblog.com/
http,//www.jojobaisrael.com/
http,//www.balashon.com/
https,//www.bible-history.com/

Disclaimer

Last updated: December 12, 2020

The information contained in this book Essential Oils and their Relevance to the Bible, or any information derived from either of my websites https://holylandoils.com or http://estherlehman.com is for general information purposes only. HolyLand Oils and Esther Lehman assumes no responsibility for errors or omissions in the contents of my books or my service.

In no event shall Essential Oils and their Relevance to the Bible be liable for any special, direct, indirect, consequential, or incidental damages or any damages whatsoever, whether in an action of contract, negligence or other tort, arising out of or in connection with the use of the service or the contents of the service.

This book, HolyLand oils and Esther Lehman reserve the right to make additions, deletions, or modification to the contents of our book and formulas at any time without prior notice. HolyLand Oils and Esther Lehman does not warrant that the website is free of viruses or other harmful components.

ABOUT THE AUTHOR

Esther Lehman lives in Israel, in Maale Adumim which is a town just outside Jerusalem, Israel. She is a personal trainer and a holistic nutritionist, and aromatherapist.

She studied exercise physiology at the Wingate Institute for physical education and sports in Israel, and studied naturopathy at the Bina Academy, Jerusalem, Israel,

Esther is a black belt 4th Dan in Krav Maga. She teaches a wide range of exercise and fitness classes such as Pilates, body sculpting, aerobics, aqua, Krav Maga, and more for over 25 years.

Esther is also a massage therapist and reiki master; she believes that the body is a mirror of its own thoughts. Thinking positively, with kindness and self-respect, gives you the best opportunity to allow positive changes to occur in your life which affects your general health and wellbeing.

The first purpose of writing this book is to connect the trees, plants and flowers living among us today to the Old Testament. Esther finds it fascinating to see how our daily lives today are parallel to those in biblical days. It is beautiful and therapeutic to have this unique connection with the Bible in our daily lives.

Another reason for writing this book is to help people achieve their goals and change their life through the eyes of the Bible. Ultimately the force of the changes must be generated from within you, but nature is surrounding us to make it is easier for us to combat the difficulties and continue the journey to success.

Contact Esther Lehman at, www.holylandoils.com/contact-us/.
Visit online at,
www.estherlehman.com
www.holylandoils.com,

Other Books by this Author
10 Best Ways to Start Losing Weight

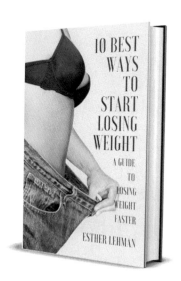

https://amzn.to/3yFxUiH

10 Best Ways to Start Losing Weight is going to give you a big PUSH into taking responsibility for your health. When you are overweight and stuck, feeling like you have no solution, it is of the utmost importance to realize that you do. In this book I have compiled ways to motivate you into starting your weight loss journey, but we both know that YOU are the only person who can actually cause this action to happen.

Once you made this decision, you will quickly see that it is a daily decision running at you constantly all through your day. Preventing declination is an art. Every microsecond of our day we make these decisions, whether when we prepare our meals or if we exercise. It is a privilege to learn to build up this inner power that takes advantage of our opportunity to control what we put into our bodies.

Once you have mastered this art, the solution will be so simple, so obvious, and you will know exactly what to always do. You have taken over the implementation of this far from simple concept and made it your own personal system. Your friends will wonder how this happened and you will be able to help them too, thus helping yourself even more.

You will always be motivated into making the right choices of the foods you eat, because you now know how poor food choices are avoidable. Life is a bundle of stresses that can cause havoc to our digestion. Learning to cope with stress together with eating healthy regularly will affect your journey to weight loss and good health forever.

Lose Fat by Reducing Stress

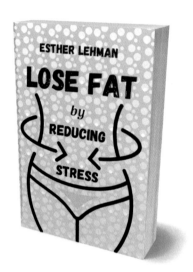

https://amzn.to/2NKU4Yo

This book is your guide to weight loss. There are systematic diet and eating methods that ensures you lose weight. Human nature is to always strive for the perfect body, even if they have a great physique. This book is a must have if you really want to lose weight. Weight loss is not only for women and men who want to lose belly fat, but also for everyone who wants to learn to lose fat, build muscle mass and change their body composition.
Most women feel their perfect body is petite, slim, and fit.

Most men feel their perfect body is a set of six-pack abs and shirt ripping biceps.

Women and men are always struggling with their body image, and with the right nutrition and exercise program, it is possible. In fact, weight loss does gives you that extra confidence in yourself, and it is your confidence that makes you more attractive to the opposite sex.

Let us not forget that the focus on being thin is to stay healthy and active, maintaining a healthy weight range is the recipe for youth.
Bodies comes in many shapes and sizes; how would you define the perfect body for you?

Maintaining your motivation to lose weight by remaining emotionally strong and focused on your goal is the underlying key to your success. In most cases, stress was probably the cause of your weight gain, to prevent further weight gain, you must identify and solve the source of your stress. Stress also prevents weight loss, regardless of your diet and exercise routines.

Stay motivated and stick to your goals, and you will get through and succeed.

Don't give up because you have not seen results quickly enough.
Give your workout sometime and don't depend on scales alone. This is a journey that you owe yourself, being as little as 10% overweight can cause serious damage to our health, both from the perspective of our physical health and our emotional health too. Doctors are not as relaxed about obesity as they once were. The obesity epidemic is one of the biggest health risks of this century, it is associated with heart disease, cancer and diabetes. Our bodies give us early warning signs way before we become sick. It constantly gives us opportunities to solve minor health issues before they become serious.

Lose weight by eating a healthy diet starting now, prevent any future diseases that may threaten to develop due to your current extra weight and lifestyle. My guide to losing weight is real, you will receive step by step help and the tools to start dropping those pounds. So, start this exciting journey now, buy this book and learn the secrets of your body and how to teach it to respond to the methods in this book so that you reach and achieve health and happiness.

This book is a guide to lose weight and keep off the extra pounds forever. Change your lifestyle because Fad Diets don't work!

Women of the Bible

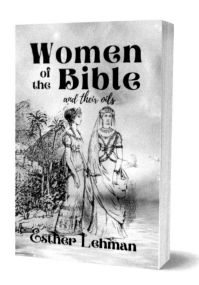

https://amzn.to/2J9YhJe

All of us live in the reflection of these fascinating Women of the Bible, and we may even ask why are they so special? Beginning at the beginning we meet Eve who was created in just one clear day by God, how would that make you feel if you were in her shoes? Suddenly you are a fully grown woman and wife given the heavy responsibility to populate the entire world. A lot was expected of her, she was created for the sole purpose to be Adam's wife, to be his companion and emotional support. She instantly became aware of her desires, and we probably think of Eve as a pious and mature woman. Since she was the template of all women, she probably felt then exactly as you and I feel right now.

All women ever own exactly the same emotions so you will identify with the women written about in this book. Their experiences in their relationships with their husbands and their trials of their lives will be exactly like ours. Even though these women were prophetesses and mothers of humanity, it is amazing to see how they have the same dramas in their lives. They have sagas with loving but tactless husbands, jealous rival wives, when men like king David married many wives and women had to deal with the emotions of being not the favorite wife, or if she was, then her desperation of maintaining her "main wife" status. Why did Sarah our barren matriarchs seek the recognition of motherhood through her surrogate handmaiden Hagar, which ended up being a solution that brought more grief than honor.

I have compiled the stories of the lives of thirty women, in this book you will get to look into the human qualities of all the women written about, we will bring them back to life and feel their joys and sorrows in real time.

"I will plant in the wilderness the acacia tree, and the myrtle and the Etz Shemen "Oil Tree" I will set in the Arava cypress, maple and box-tree together."
(Isaiah 41:19)

Made in the USA
Middletown, DE
03 September 2023